Challenging Concepts in Oral
and Maxillofacial Surgery

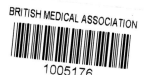

Published and forthcoming titles in the Challenging Concepts in series

Anaesthesia (Edited by Dr Phoebe Syme, Dr Robert Jackson, and Professor Tim Cook)

Cardiovascular Medicine (Edited by Dr Aung Myat, Dr Shouvik Haldar, and Professor Simon Redwood)

Emergency Medicine (Edited by Dr Sam Thenabadu, Dr Fleur Cantle, and Dr Chris Lacy)

Infectious Disease and Clinical Microbiology (Edited by Dr Amber Arnold and Professor George Griffin)

Interventional Radiology (Edited by Dr Irfan Ahmed, Dr Miltiadis Krokidis, and Dr Tarun Sabharwal)

Neurology (Edited by Dr Krishna Chinthapalli, Dr Nadia Magdalinou, and Professor Nicholas Wood)

Neurosurgery (Edited by Mr Robin Bhatia and Mr Ian Sabin)

Obstetrics and Gynaecology (Edited by Dr Natasha Hezelgrave, Dr Danielle Abbott, and Professor Andrew Shennan)

Oncology (Edited by Dr Madhumita Bhattacharyya, Dr Sarah Payne, and Professor Iain McNeish)

Oral and Maxillofacial Surgery (Edited by Mr Matthew Idle and Mr Andrew Monaghan)

Respiratory Medicine (Edited by Dr Lucy Schomberg and Dr Elizabeth Sage)

Challenging Concepts in Oral and Maxillofacial Surgery
Cases with Expert Commentary

Edited by

Mr Matthew R. Idle FRCS (OMFS)

Specialty Registrar in Oral and Maxillofacial Surgery, West Midlands Deanery and Queen Elizabeth Hospital Birmingham, University Hospitals Birmingham NHS Trust, UK

Mr Andrew M. Monaghan FRCS (OMFS)

Consultant in Oral and Maxillofacial Surgery, Birmingham Children's Hospital NHS Trust and Royal Air Force - Royal Centre for Defence Medicine, UK

Series editors

Dr Aung Myat BSc (Hons) MBBS MRCP

BHF Clinical Research Training Fellow, King's College London British Heart Foundation Centre of Research Excellence, Cardiovascular Division, St Thomas' Hospital, London, UK

Dr Shouvik Haldar MBBS MRCP

Electrophysiology Research Fellow & Cardiology SpR, Heart Rhythm Centre, NIHR Cardiovascular Biomedical Research Unit, Royal Brompton & Harefield NHS Foundation Trust, Imperial College London, London, UK

Professor Simon Redwood MD FRCP

Professor of Interventional Cardiology and Honorary Consultant Cardiologist, King's College London British Heart Foundation Centre of Research Excellence, Cardiovascular Division and Guy's and St Thomas' NHS Foundation Trust, St Thomas' Hospital, London, UK

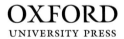

OXFORD
UNIVERSITY PRESS

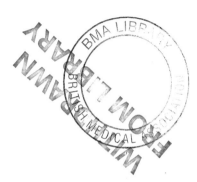

UNIVERSITY PRESS

Great Clarendon Street, Oxford, OX2 6DP,
United Kingdom

Oxford University Press is a department of the University of Oxford.
It furthers the University's objective of excellence in research, scholarship,
and education by publishing worldwide. Oxford is a registered trade mark of
Oxford University Press in the UK and in certain other countries

Impression: 1

Published in the United States of America by Oxford University Press
198 Madison Avenue, New York, NY 10016, United States of America

British Library Cataloguing in Publication Data

Data available

Library of Congress Control Number: 2015952459

ISBN 978-0-19-965355-3

Printed in Great Britain by
Ashford Colour Press Ltd, Gosport, Hampshire

FOREWORD BY
PROFESSOR FERNANDES

Frequently, books address the common aspects of an oral and maxillofacial surgery practice while neglecting problematic or challenging cases. We are all familiar with the adage that we learn best from the difficult cases or those cases where the outcome was different from what we planned; either because of errors in planning, execution, and/or postoperative care. This book tackles the challenging concepts in oral and maxillofacial surgery and uses recognized experts in our specialty to address the issues that commonly arise.

The book is well structured and covers a wide range of topics. The manuscript authors have done a good job in framing the questions addressed in their respective chapters. I would recommend this book to all trainees. As they progress through their training, this book will be more relevant to their understanding of the specialty. Equally, practicing surgeons will find the book to be of benefit when faced with infrequently managed challenging cases.

I extend my congratulations to Drs. Idle and Monaghan for putting together a well thought out and structured book, and for their hard work in bringing *Challenging Concepts in Oral and Maxillofacial Surgery* to fruition.

Rui Fernandes, DMD, MD, FACS
Associate Professor
Chief of Head Neck Surgery
University of Florida College of Medicine Jacksonville

FOREWORD BY PROFESSOR WOODWARDS

This book presents an attractive departure from the standard format of most surgical texts. The concept of case-based discussions is now well-established in the toolkit of surgical training and is well-founded in educational theory. Having a real case on which to base a learning point is always going to lead to a clearer understanding of theory as well as to retention of knowledge.

The authors, in their scenarios, take the reader through diagnosis, case planning, surgical management and the management of complications in a clear and attractive format. The highlighted boxes containing learning points, clinical tips and evidence base add considerably to the wealth of information this publication provides.

Seeking knowledge is not always easy; learning is often attempted at the end of a busy day and the way in which this book breaks learning down into single case studies lends itself ideally to the often brief opportunities for study available to busy surgical trainees.

The topics chosen cover a good spectrum of the practice base of oral and maxillofacial surgery, and the additional insight in trauma that the experience some of the authors have in battlefield trauma care brings an additional dimension to the content.

The authors are to be congratulated on producing this work, which brings together an impressive range of contemporary knowledge, expertise and evidence, making it a valuable resource for all oral and maxillofacial surgeons.

R T Woodwards MD FRCS FDSRCS
Consultant OMF/Head and Neck Surgeon
Manchester UK

PREFACE

The specialty of oral and maxillofacial surgery has advanced dramatically over the last century, notably during periods of conflict. The additional surgical demands presented by war fuel the adage that 'necessity is the mother of invention'. As we advance into the 21st century with the availability of novel surgical and non-surgical methods, including tissue engineering, the multidisciplinary team must use the available evidence to appropriately apply these techniques. Ultimately the patient's needs must be placed at the centre of this decision-making process.

We present a unique format as part of this Challenging Concepts series of 26 scenarios including all aspects of the oral and maxillofacial surgery syllabus. These are intended to provide the clinician with examples of problems that may present in day-to-day practice and provoke thought regarding management options. Highlighted boxes containing 'Learning Points', 'Clinical Tips', and the 'Evidence base' underscoring the management, accompany the main body of the text. The intention is that these will add flesh to the bones of the case and provide an aide-mémoire for the reader. The case has then been peer reviewed by a renowned expert in the field in the form of the 'Expert comments' boxes. This opportunity to mine the experience provided by opinion leaders is original to this series of textbooks.

We are also privileged in having the permission to present three complex battle-field cases from the conflict in Afghanistan. Understandably these carry their own inherent challenges that can be transferred into the management of civilian cases.

This text is aimed primarily at trainees in oral and maxillofacial surgery but we hope that some aspects may appeal to senior clinicians alike. Several chapters will be relevant to related specialties such as otolaryngology, oral surgery, orthodontics and dentistry. Allied professionals in the fields of speech therapy, dietetics and specialist nurses will hopefully find use in the text as well.

We hope that you enjoy this textbook and find it applicable to your practice.

Matthew Idle
Andrew Monaghan

ACKNOWLEDGEMENTS

We would like to thank all of the Experts and Trainees who have kindly given their time and knowledge to contribute to this book. Nicola Wilson, Caroline Smith, and Angela Butterworth at Oxford University Press have provided invaluable guidance and support that has ensured this book came to fruition and for this we would like to express our sincere gratitude.

Matthew Idle
Andrew Monaghan

Additionally, I would like to give thanks and dedicate the book to the following individuals:

To my wife, Amy, for your love, support, exhaustive proofreading, and modelling for the front cover. For the advice and understanding I will be forever grateful.

To my parents, Heather and Tony, for your unconditional love and sacrifices that enabled me to pursue a career in surgery.

To my brother, sister-in-law and nephew, Toby, Susie, and Rory for your love, support, and golfing companionship.

To my grandparents, Jeanne and Leslie.

Finally, to my mentor and co-author, Andrew, for his friendship and guidance through my training.

Matthew Idle

CONTENTS

EXPERTS

Robert Bentley
Director for Trauma
King's College Hospital
London
UK

Christopher Bridle
Consultant Oral and Maxillofacial Surgeon
Oral and Maxillofacial Surgery Centre
The Royal London Hospital
London
UK

Lachlan Carter
Consultant Oral and Maxillofacial Surgeon
Leeds Teaching Hospitals NHS Trust
UK

Andrew Currie
Consultant Oral and Maxillofacial Surgeon
Oxford University Hospitals NHS Trust
Oxford
UK

Stephen Dover
Consultant Oral and Maxillofacial/Craniofacial
Surgeon, Queen Elizabeth Hospital Birmingham
University Hospitals Birmingham NHS Trust
Birmingham
UK

Martin Evans
Consultant Oral and Maxillofacial/Craniofacial
Surgeon, Queen Elizabeth Hospital Birmingham
University Hospitals Birmingham NHS Trust and
Birmingham Children's Hospital
Birmingham
UK

Andrew Gibbons
Consultant Oral and Maxillofacial Surgeon, Royal Air
Force/ Peterborough and Stamford Hospitals NHS
Foundation Trust
UK

Jason Green
Consultant Oral and Maxillofacial Surgeon
Queen Elizabeth Hospital Birmingham
University Hospitals Birmingham NHS Trust
Birmingham
UK

Nicholas Grew
Consultant Oral and Maxillofacial/Head and Neck
Surgeon, The Royal Wolverhampton NHS Trust
UK

Simon Holmes
Consultant Oral and Maxillofacial Surgeon
Barts and the London NHS Trust
London,
UK

Graham James
Consultant Oral and Maxillofacial Surgeon
Royal Worcester Hospital NHS Trust
Worcester
UK

Tim Martin
Consultant Oral and Maxillofacial/Head and Neck
Surgeon, Queen Elizabeth Hospital Birmingham
University Hospitals Birmingham NHS Trust
Birmingham
UK

Mark McGurk
Professor of Oral and Maxillofacial Surgery
Guy's Hospital and King's College Hospital
London
UK

Ahmed Messahel
Consultant Oral and Maxillofacial Surgeon
The Shrewsbury and Telford NHS Trust
UK

Andrew Monaghan
Consultant Oral and Maxillofacial Surgeon
Birmingham Children's Hospital NHS Trust
and Royal Air Force - Royal Centre for Defence
Medicine
Birmingham
UK

Sat Parmar
Consultant Oral and Maxillofacial/Head and Neck
Surgeon, Queen Elizabeth Hospital Birmingham
University Hospitals Birmingham NHS Trust
Birmingham
UK

Khaleeq-Ur Rehman
Consultant Oral and Maxillofacial/Head and Neck
Surgeon, The Royal Wolverhampton NHS Trust
Birmingham
UK

Simon Rogers
Consultant Oral and Maxillofacial Surgeon
Aintree Hospital
Liverpool
UK

Andrew Sidebottom
Consultant Oral and Maxillofacial Surgeon
Nottingham University Hospitals NHS Trust
Nottingham
UK

Mike Simpson
Consultant Oral and Maxillofacial Surgeon
Luton and Dunstable University Hospital
UK

Ken Sneddon
Consultant Oral and Maxillofacial Surgeon
Queen Victoria Hospital
East Grinstead
UK

Dilip Srinivasan
Consultant Oral and Maxillofacial Surgeon
Nottingham University Hospitals NHS Trust
Nottingham
UK

Simon Van Eeden
Consultant Oral and Maxillofacial/Cleft Surgeon
Alder Hey Children's NHS Foundation Trust
Liverpool
UK

Rhodri Williams
Consultant Oral and Maxillofacial Surgeon
Queen Elizabeth Hospital Birmingham
University Hospitals Birmingham NHS Trust and
Birmingham Children's Hospital
Birmingham
UK

CONTRIBUTORS

Anwer Abdullakutty
Specialty Registrar, London Deanery and Queen
Victoria Hospital East Grinstead
East Grinstead
UK

Hiba Aga
Specialty Registrar, West Midlands Deanery and The
Royal Wolverhampton NHS Trust
Wolverhampton
UK

Nabeela Ahmed
Specialty Registrar, Trent Deanery and Nottingham
University Hospitals NHS Trust
Nottingham
UK

Laith Al-Qamachi
Specialty Registrar, West Midlands Deanery
The Royal Wolverhampton NHS Trust
Wolverhampton
UK

Atheer Ujam
Specialty Registrar, Barts and the London NHS Trust /
King's College Hospital NHS Trust
London
UK

Alan Attard
Consultant Oral and Maxillofacial Surgeon
University Hospital Birmingham
Edgbaston
UK

John Breeze
Specialty Registrar
Queen Elizabeth Hospital Birmingham
University Hospitals Birmingham NHS Trust
Birmingham
UK

Richard Burnham
Specialty Registrar, Barts and the London NHS Trust
Oral and Maxillofacial Surgery Centre
The Royal London Hospital
London
UK

Jacob D'Souza
Consultant Oral and Maxillofacial Surgeon, Royal
Surrey County and Nuffield Health Guildford Hospitals
UK

Christopher Fowell
Specialty Registrar, West Midlands Deanery and
Queen Elizabeth Hospital Birmingham
University Hospitals Birmingham NHS Trust
Birmingham
UK

Barbara Gerber
Specialty Registrar, Oxford Deanery and Oxford
University Hospitals NHS Trust
Oxford
UK

Lisa Greaney
Specialty Registrar, London Deanery and Queen
Victoria Hospital East Grinstead
UK

Elizabeth Gruber
Specialty Registrar, West Midlands Deanery and Royal
Worcester Hospital
Worcester
UK

Douglas Hammond
Specialty Registrar, West Midlands Deanery and
Queen Elizabeth Hospital Birmingham
University Hospitals Birmingham NHS Trust
Birmingham
UK

Jahrad Haq
Specialty Registrar, London Deanery
King's College Hospital
London
UK

Matthew Idle
Specialty Registrar, West Midlands Deanery and
Queen Elizabeth Hospital Birmingham
University Hospitals Birmingham NHS Trust
Birmingham
UK

Kevin McMillan
Craniofacial Fellow
Birmingham Children's Hospital NHS Trust
UK

Grigore Mihalache
Specialty Doctor in Oral and Maxillofacial Surgery,
The Shrewsbury and Telford Hospitals NHS Trust
UK

Neil Opie
Specialty Registrar, West Midlands Deanery and
Queen Elizabeth Hospital Birmingham
University Hospitals Birmingham NHS Trust
Birmingham
UK

Alan Parbhoo
Consultant Oral and Maxillofacial Surgeon
Luton and Dunstable University Hospital
UK

Francine Ryba
Specialty Registrar, London Deanery and King's
College Hospital
London
UK

Rabindra Singh
Consultant Oral and Maxillofacial/Head and Neck
Surgeon, University Hospital Southampton NHS
Trust
UK

Chris Sweet
Cleft Fellow
North West Deanery
UK

Suraj Thomas
Specialty Registrar, Barts and the London NHS Trust/
King's College Hospital NHS Trust
London
UK

Luke Williams
Specialty Registrar, London Deanery and King's
College Hospital
London
UK

ABBREVIATIONS

ADDWR	anterior disc displacement with reduction		MDT	multidisciplinary team
AJCC	American Joint Commission on Cancer		MIO	maximal interincisal opening
AOB	anterior open bite		MMF	maxillomandibular fixation
ATLS	Advanced Trauma Life Support		MRI	magnetic resonance imaging
BAD	British Association of Dermatologists		NICE	National Institute of Health and Care Excellence
BCC	basal cell carcinoma			
BCLP	bilateral cleft lip and palate		NMSC	non-melanoma skin cancer
BSSO	bilateral sagittal split osteotomy		NOE	nasoethmoidal
CBCT	cone-beam computed tomography		NSAID	non-steroidal anti-inflammatory drug
CNS	cleft nurse specialist		OB	open bite
C-spine	cervical spine		OKC	odontogenic keratocyst
CSA	circumflex scapular artery		OKOC	orthokeratinized odontogenic cysts
CSF	cerebrospinal fluid		OPG	orthopantomogram
CT	computed tomogram		ORIF	open reduction and internal fixation
DCIA	deep circumflex ileac artery		ORN	osteoradionecrosis
DO	distraction osteogenesis		PCR	progressive condylar resorption
ECSL	extra-corporeal shockwave lithotripsy		PEEK	polyetheretherketone
ED	emergency department		PET	positron emission tomography
EVD	external ventricular drain		PMMA	polymethymethacrylate
FGR	fibroblast growth factor receptor		PNI	penetrating neck injuyr
FMPA	Frankfort-mandibular plane angle		RCT	randomized controlled trial
GBR	guided bone regeneration		SCC	squamous cell carcinoma
GCS	Glasgow Coma Scale reported		SLNB	sentinel lymph node biopsy
GDP	general dental practitioner		SLT	speech and language therapist
GMP	general medical practioner		SMAS	superficial musculoaponeurotic system
HA	hydroxyapatite		S-N	sella–nasion
HBOT	hyperbaric oxygen therapy		SSCMDT	specialist skin cancer multidisciplinary team
IAN	inferior alveolar nerve			
ICP	intracranial pressure		SSM	superficial spreading melanoma
ICU	intensive care unit		SSO	sagittal split osteotomy
IP	inverted papilloma		TMD	temporomandibular disorder
IVC	inferior vena cava		TMD	temporomandibular dysfunction
KCOT	keratocystic odontogenic tumour		TMJ	temporomandibular joint
LAFH	lower anterior face height		TNM	tumour, node, metastasis
LASCCHN	locoregionally advanced squamous cell carcinoma of the head and neck		US	ultrasound
			UV	ultraviolet
LM	lentigo maligna		VCFS	velocardiofacial syndrome
LPFH	lower posterior face height		VF	videofluoroscopy
LRP	locking reconstructive plate		VME	vertical maxillary excess
MCA	middle cerebral artery		VPI	velopharyngeal incompetence

CURRICULUM MAP

Challenging Concepts in Oral and Maxillofacial Surgery Chapter:

1. Complex midface reconstruction following tumour ablation
2. Cutaneous malignancy
3. Management of osteoradionecrosis of the mandible
4. Frontal sinus fractures
5. Management of panfacial injuries: top down or bottom up?
6. Adult orbital wall fracture repair
7. Biomechanics of the mandible and current evidence for treatment of the fractured mandible
8. High-energy ballistic injuries to the face
9. Reconstructive challenges following blast injuries to the facial soft tissue and skeleton
10. Low-energy explosive fragmentation injuries to the neck and face
11. Cranial vault reconstruction following decompressive craniectomy
12. Distraction osteogenesis: a reconstructive option
13. Posterior calvarial osseodistraction for syndromic craniosynostoses
14. The anterior open bite
15. Severe class II skeletal deformity
16. The segmental maxillary osteotomy
17. TMJ replacement
18. Osteochondroma of the mandibular condyle / temporo-mandibular joint
19. Management of the Wilkes Grade III TMJ
20. Salivary calculi
21. Sagittal split osteotomy for the removal of a lower third molar
22. Implant restoration of the atrophic maxilla with concurrent mandibular rehabilitation
23. Keratocystic odontogenic tumours (KCOT) and orthokeratinised odontogenic cysts (OKOC)
24. Paediatric temporo-mandibular joint ankylosis
25. Cleft palate related velopharyngeal incompetence
26. Paediatric maxillofacial trauma

	1	2	3	4	5	6	7	8	9	10	11	12	13	14	15	16	17	18	19	20	21	22	23	24	25	26
1. Management of a patient with dento-alveolar pathology							X					X									X	X	X		X	
1.1 Surgical extraction of unerupted / impacted teeth and roots							X														X				X	
1.2 Apical surgery / excision of jaw cyst																							X			
2. Management of infections of the head and neck								X	X	X																
2.1 Drainage of tissue space infection								X	X	X																
3. Management of patient with compromised airway	X		X					X	X	X								X								
3.1 Surgical access to airway (tracheostomy / cricothyroidotomy)	X		X					X	X	X																
4. Management of maxillofacial trauma				X	X	X	X	X	X	X	X															X
4.1 Repair of facial lacerations					X	X		X	X	X	X															

	1	2	3	4	5	6	7	8	9	10	11	12	13	14	15	16	17	18
4.2 Reduction and fixation of fracture of mandible					X	X	X	X		X								X
4.3 Fracture of mandibular condyle – open reduction and fixation																		X
4.4 Elevation and fixation of fractured zygoma			X															
4.5 Fracture of orbital floor --- repair and graft			X	X														X
5. Management of salivary gland swellings														X				
5.1 Submandibular gland excision														X				
5.2 Parotidectomy														X				
6. Management of oro-facial pain / temporomandibular joint dysfunction												X	X	X		X		
6.1 Temporo-mandibular joint arthrocentesis													X					
7. Management of a patient with benign jaw tumour													X		X			
7.1 Resection of odontogenic tumour / fibro-osseous lesion													X		X			
7.2 Harvest of bone graft	X		X					X		X	X				X			
8. Potentially malignant and malignant epithelial tumours of the mucosa and skin	X	X																
8.1 Local skin flaps	X	X																
8.2 Excision of malignant skin tumour		X																
9. Management of patient with a neck lump / swelling	X	X																
9.1 Neck dissection(s)	X	X	X															
10. Management of a patient with developmental / acquired deformity of the facial skeleton	X		X	X	X	X	X	X	X	X	X	X		X		X	X	X
10.1 Mandibular ramus osteotomy								X		X	X			X				
10.2 Maxillary osteotomy											X	X			X			
10.3 Rhinoplasty			X															
11. Cancer of the head and neck region	X	X	X															
11.1 Excision of oral / oropharyngeal or jaw malignancy	X		X															
12. Reconstructive surgery	X	X	X	X	X	X	X	X	X	X	X	X	X		X		X	X
12.1 Pedicled flaps	X	X																
12.2 Free tissue transfer	X		X			X		X										
13. Patient requiring osseointegrated implants	X					X		X							X			
13.1 Insertion of intra-oral implants and abutment connection								X							X			

SECTION 1

Head and neck oncology

1 Complex midface reconstruction following tumour ablation

Hiba Aga, Laith Al-Qamachi and Matthew Idle

Expert commentary Nicholas Grew

Case history

A 55-year-old gentleman was referred urgently by the neurology team following initial attendance at the Emergency Assessment Unit. His presenting complaint included left facial numbness and a left temporal headache that extended to the ipsilateral occipital region. This had been worsening over the preceding five months and was not associated with any weight loss. Clinical examination revealed paraesthesia in the distribution of the left infraorbital nerve, weakness of the left facial nerve (zygomatic and buccal branches were Grade III House-Brackmann), and a 2 cm × 3 cm mass palpable over the left malar prominence.

He had a medical history of cervical spondylosis, but was otherwise fit and well. He was a retired pipe layer and had a ten-pack-year tobacco history, but was an ex-smoker for 20 years. He regularly consumed approximately 20 units of alcohol per week.

At this juncture a magnetic resonance imaging (MRI) scan (T1- and T2-weighted, FLAIR and diffusion-weighted) had already been performed by the neurologists (2 weeks previously) and demonstrated a 5.2 cm × 3.8 cm × 3.4 cm tumour in the left maxilla (Figure 1.1). It was noted that there was compression of the maxillary branch of the trigeminal nerve within the floor of the orbit.

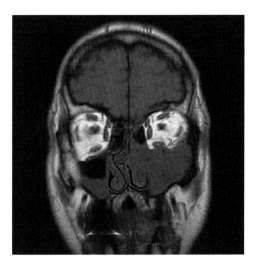

Figure 1.1 MRI (T2-weighted) in coronal section demonstrating the tumour in the left maxillary antrum with invasion of the left orbital floor (arrow). See colour plate section.

⭐ **Learning point** Imaging in head and neck cancer

There is Grade D evidence to suggest that biopsy of the primary site should be undertaken prior to scanning [2]. This is to avoid upstaging the disease, as oedema from the biopsy can give the appearance of increased primary tumour volume and also regional lymphadenopathy.

⭐ **Learning point** House-Brackmann facial nerve weakness grading system [1]

- Grade I: normal facial function in all areas.
- Grade II: slight weakness noticeable on close inspection; may have slight synkinesis.
- Grade III: obvious, but not disfiguring difference between the two sides; noticeable, but not severe, synkinesis, contracture, or hemifacial spasm; complete eye closure with effort.
- Grade IV: obvious weakness or disfiguring asymmetry and tone at rest; incomplete eye closure.
- Grade V: only barely perceptible motion; asymmetry at rest.
- Grade VI: no movement.

Based on these clinical findings an open biopsy was performed under general anaesthesia on the day following the initial presentation in clinic. An urgent computed tomogram (CT) of the head, neck, and chest was subsequently undertaken. Histopathological examination of the specimen indicated a high-grade dysplasia with features suggestive of an inverted papilloma (IP). CT confirmed the presence of a tumour causing destruction of the medial, anterior and posterior walls of the maxillary sinus and also the floor of the orbit with no evidence of involvement of the inferior rectus. There was no evidence of cervical, thoracic or abdominal metastases.

⭐ **Learning point** Inverted papilloma

This entity is also known as a Schneiderian papilloma in view of its tendency to occur in the nasal and paranasal sinuses. They are primarily benign and are locally destructive. However, they do have a propensity to recur and may undergo malignant transformation into a squamous cell carcinoma in approximately 2% of cases [2,3].

A staging system has been suggested by Krouse [4]:

- T1: IP confined to nasal cavity. No malignancy.
- T2: IP limited to ethmoid sinus and to medial and superior parts of the maxillary sinus. No malignancy.
- T3: IP extends into frontal or sphenoid sinuses or involves inferior or lateral parts of maxillary sinus. No malignancy.
- T4: IP associated with malignancy - or IP spreads outside the nose and paranasal sinuses with or without malignancy.

A week later he was discussed at the head and neck multidisciplinary team (MDT) meeting and it was decided to proceed with a left level I neck dissection, left maxillectomy, left orbital exenteration, reconstruction with a left deep circumflex iliac artery (DCIA) free flap and placement of orbital osseointegrated implants (see Box 1.1).

Box 1.1 Operative note

Initially a size 8 Portex (Smiths Medical, UK) tracheostomy tube was placed using a horizontal skin incision and a window created in the region of the third tracheal ring. The left level I nodes and submandibular gland were cleared as part of the neck access procedure. A Weber-Fergusson incision with lid preservation was then employed to gain access for tumour ablation. A left DCIA free flap was then raised with internal oblique and incorporating 10 cm x 6 cm of iliac crest (Figure 1.2). The flap inset

(continued)

was undertaken with Leibinger (Stryker, US) 2.0 mm miniplates and the internal oblique used as the oral component (Figure 1.3). Arterial anastomosis was undertaken end-to-end on the facial artery with the use of a vein graft from the external jugular vein. The venous anastomosis was performed end-to-end on the facial vein. Initially the flap failed to run but an infusion of streptokinase (calculated by body weight) rectified this complication. Two vacuum drains were placed and the neck was closed in layers. The donor site was closed meticulously with the use of a Prolene mesh (Ethicon Inc. US) supported by non-resorbable sutures and layered closure and a single vacuum drain.

❝ Expert comment

This flap failed to run after the initial anastomosis. On division distal to the anastomosis it was found to be patent and running at this location. It seems the flap had a potential problem with the circulation or microcirculation within the flap or more distally within the pedicle. I have not witnessed this previously or since. The flap was flushed gently with a solution of streptokinase calculated upon blood volume / body weight and the experience of peripheral thrombolysis. The flap was re-anastomosed and then ran perfectly on re-anastomosis.

Anastomosis in midfacial reconstruction can be difficult in the location of vessels and because of the relatively short pedicles of the flaps most appropriate for composite midfacial reconstruction.

In general terms I dissect the facial vessels as far onto the face as possible and with careful consideration of the facial nerve. I try to avoid vein grafting if possible but this may be necessary if the pedicle is short and lying high and deep within the face and when retraction means that anastomosis is not possible. The distal anastomosis of the vein graft can then be performed above the tunnel leading the pedicle to the neck and the extended pedicle then carefully passed to the neck.

❝ Expert comment

Diagnosis here was of an IP and despite repeat biopsy there was no categorical diagnosis of malignancy. This ambiguity means decisions have to be made on balance of probability assessing all clinical, radiographic, and histological evidence and recognition of the 'worst-case' pathology.

Treatment and management planning should include a full and open discussion with the patient of these issues and how any ambiguity is being addressed. This case is particularly problematic as it only gave histological evidence of a non-malignant process but features were consistent with a malignant disease process. The treatment plan was designed to address this as malignant and in so doing meant that there was no option to attempt to preserve the eye with any degree of practical function with all of the psychological, functional, and cosmetic consequences for reconstruction and rehabilitation.

⊕ Clinical tip The deep circumflex iliac artery flap

Taylor et al. [5] and Sanders and Mayou [6] first described this flap independently in 1979. It was initially employed to reconstruct the hemimandible in view of the favourable morphology, but has additionally been employed to reconstruct angle and symphyseal defects. Brown and Shaw advocate the use of this flap for restoration of Class II, III, and IV defects of the maxilla [7]. Following the work of Ramasastry et al. [8], Urken and his team showed that the use of internal oblique in these defects gave a superior oral reconstruction [9] and we would certainly agree with this. The muscle will subsequently epithelialize and provide a receptive environment for the subsequent placement of osseointegrated implants.

It is well known that the morbidity associated with this flap can be significant. Forrest et al. report that sensory changes, namely in the lateral cutaneous nerve of the thigh, can occur in 26.8% of cases with 11% experiencing gait disturbance and 10% developing a hernia [10]. It is of note that the closure of the donor site should not be undertaken lightly in view of these potential complications.

We prefer to raise this flap as a myo-osseous unit as the skin tends to be unreliable. The internal oblique is then wrapped around the iliac crest component to form the oral lining. The senior author finds that maintaining the anterior superior iliac spine helps to prevent the development of a hernia.

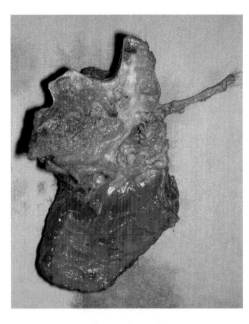

Figure 1.2 Deep circumflex iliac artery flap following contouring.

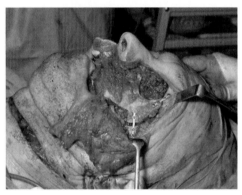

Figure 1.3 Deep circumflex iliac artery inset. See colour plate section.

The patient was transferred to the intensive care unit (ICU). He required return to theatre on day 14 for superficial debridement of the intra-oral and intra-ocular portions of the flap and this demonstrated healthy bleeding muscle underneath the slough. At outpatient review on day 20 the intra-oral component was healing appropriately but there was an area of non-viable flap in the orbit and this required debridement and a local advancement flap to cover the defect. The tumour was demonstrated to be a pT3, N0, M0, well to moderately differentiated squamous cell carcinoma in an IP. There was 2.5 mm clearance at the superficial maxillary margin with 2-4 mm of clearance at the superficial and lateral margins.

⭐ **Learning point** T-staging of maxillary tumours [2]

- T1: tumour limited to the mucosa with no erosion or destruction of bone.
- T2: tumour causing no bone erosion or destruction, including extension into hard palate and/or middle nasal meatus, except extension to posterior wall of maxillary sinus and pterygoid plates.

(continued)

- T3: tumour invades any of the following: bone of posterior wall of maxillary sinus, subcutaneous tissues, floor of medial wall of orbit, pterygoid fossa, ethmoid sinuses.
- T4a: tumour invades any of the following: anterior orbital contents, skin of cheek, pterygoid plates, infratemporal fossa, cribriform plate, sphenoid or frontal sinuses.
- T4b: tumour invades any of the following: orbital apex, dura, brain, middle cranial fossa, cranial nerves other than maxillary division of trigeminal nerve V2, nasopharynx, clivus.

The decision was then taken to refer him for post-operative radiotherapy and he began a course of 60 Gy in 30 fractions that commenced six weeks following the final surgery.

He was then followed up on a monthly basis in the head and neck oncology clinic. However, a left facial node was noted six months following his initial surgery and fine needle aspirate and subsequent resection confirmed a recurrence of papillary squamous cell carcinoma. A nuclear medicine scan in the form of a positron emission tomography (PET) CT was then performed. This demonstrated two fluorodeoxyglucose (FDG) avid areas in the left side of the face that were consistent with recurrence.

The weekly MDT was then convened and a consensus to begin chemotherapy was reached. He then underwent six cycles with cisplatin, 5-fluorouracil, and cetuximab. Further radiotherapy was given (30 Gy in 10 fractions) and cetuximab monotherapy was continued. Electron radiotherapy was also given and then methotrexate, but the disease continued to progress (Figure 1.4).

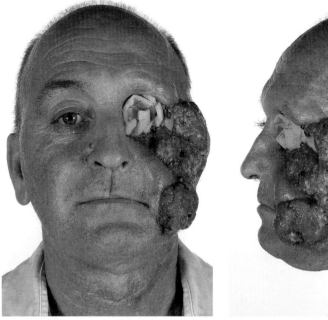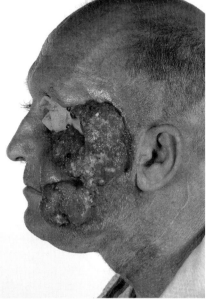

Figure 1.4 Immediate pre-operative anteroposterior and lateral views demonstrating recurrence. See colour plate section.

> **✔ Evidence base** Cetuximab-induced rash and survival [11]
>
> - Phase III randomized unblinded trial, report on 5-year data.
> - Adding cetuximab to primary radiotherapy for locoregionally advanced squamous cell carcinoma of the head and neck (LASCCHN).
> - Investigation between cetuximab-induced rash and survival.
> - LASCCHN patients of oropharynx, hypopharynx, or larynx.
> - Randomly allocated 1:1.
> - Radiotherapy alone (6-7 weeks) (n=211) versus radiotherapy plus weekly cetuximab: 400 mg/m^2 initial dose, followed by seven weekly doses at 250 mg/m^2 (n=213).
> - Primary endpoint is locoregional control.
> - Median overall survival: 49.0 months (95% CI 32.8-69.5) in the cetuximab plus radiotherapy group versus 29.3 months (20.6-41.4) in the radiotherapy alone group (hazard ratio [HR] 0.73, 95% CI 0.95; p = 0.018).
> - For patients treated with cetuximab overall survival significantly improved in those with an acneiform rash of at least Grade 2 severity compared with patients with no rash or Grade 1 rash (HR 0.49, 0.34-0.72; p = 0.002).
>
> *Source:* data from Bonner JA et al., Radiotherapy plus cetuximab for locoregionally advanced head and neck cancer: 5-year survival data from a phase 3 randomised trial, and relation between cetuximab-induced rash and survival, *The Lancet Oncology*, Volume 11, Issue 1, pp.21–28, Copyright © 2010 Elsevier Ltd.

The decision was then made to proceed with further radical resective surgery and reconstruction with a scapular/parascapular free flap. This second major resection took place 15 months following the initial surgery (Figure 1.4 and 1.5, and Box 1.2).

> **❝ Expert comment**
>
> The decision to operate at this time was taken after careful consideration on the feasibility of resection and careful analysis of available imaging. In particular, the deep resection and the need to extend the cutaneous resection to include the anterior external auditory meatus and resect all of the initial reconstruction but for a small area at the anterior margin. The request to consider further surgery was made by the oncologist because of the close understanding between oncologist and surgeon.
>
> Reconstruction in complex cases like this must first address the feasibility of resection and meaningful chance of cure. The meaningful chance of resection with this particular tumour would be the same theoretically in all patients in that it is dictated by anatomy, tumour characteristics, and location. Individual patients, however, differ in their background health, belief systems, and acceptance of such large surgery. Both resection and reconstruction require a good understanding and visualization of the likely defect and anticipation of problem areas for both.
>
> With such complex and large defects, revision surgery or additional procedures may be needed to optimize, particularly, the cosmetic result. In these defects, when structures such as the eye and orbit are lost, as well as oral continence, separation of the mouth from the face and orbit to provide an oral seal must be addressed by careful consideration of the reconstruction of the commissure and lips. The reconstruction should aim to restore facial contour. With this in mind, the surgeon should have a good understanding of the possibilities and limitations provided by individual reconstructive techniques and individual flaps. In this and in similar cases a recognition of the limitations of surgical reconstruction and the planned use of implant-retained prosthesis to obtain the best final result allows the case to be planned with the prosthetic team from the earliest preparation stages.
>
> This case demonstrates the particular flexibility of flaps harvested from the subscapular artery system. The mobility of the pedicles and the ability to isolate and rotate individual components of bone as well as the very large area of skin that can be harvested meant that this reconstruction could be achieved, although in this case the area harvested was so large that grafting was needed.

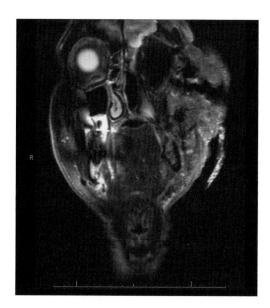

Figure 1.5 T2-weighted MRI showing the extent of the recurrence.

Box 1.2 Operative note

A size 8 Portex tracheostomy tube was placed through the existing scar employing a similar technique to that described earlier. A left selective I-IV neck dissection was then undertaken with preservation of all structures. An extensive ablation of recurrent tumour was performed by way of a left hemimaxillectomy with removal of the DCIA, cheek skin, temporalis, parotid, coronoid, and capsule of the condyle (Figure 1.6). The midface defect was noted to be a Brown Class IVb. The patient was then turned and a right scapular and parascapular flap was raised with an extensive T-shaped skin paddle (18 cm wide x 28 cm long). Closure of the donor site was not complete at this stage and a delayed skin graft was planned. Inset of the flap was then performed using the Leibinger (Stryker, US) 2.0 mm plating system and orientation of the skin paddle to reconstruct the external facial defect and also closure of the pharyngeal defect. The arterial anastomosis was performed end-to-end between the circumflex scapular artery and the ipsilateral facial artery. The venous anastomosis was performed end-to-side between the vena comitans and the internal jugular vein. Two vacuum drains were placed and the neck closed in layers.

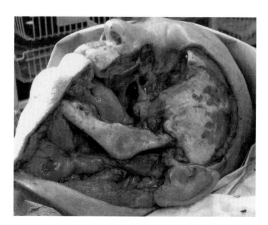

Figure 1.6 Following resection of recurrence. See colour plate section.

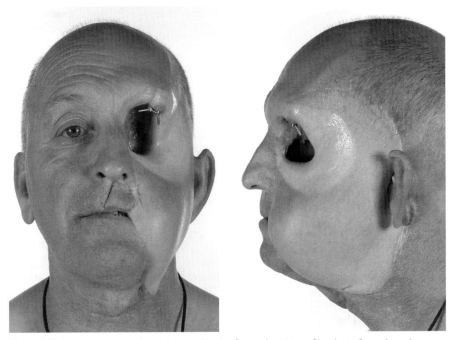

Figure 1.7 Anteroposterior and lateral views showing flap and position of implants. See colour plate section.

The patient was transferred to the ICU and made an excellent recovery with return to the head and neck ward prior to discharge home at post-operative day 15. He subsequently underwent planned surgery to debride the orbital and scapular wounds with a separate procedure to split skin graft the orbit and scapular wound from the right thigh. The back wound settled and the skin graft demonstrated adequate take. He continued to progress well with no signs of recurrence at monthly review in the head and neck joint oncology clinic (Figure 1.7).

There was, however, a degree of ptosis of the flap particularly around the left commissure and at four months post second major surgery it was deemed appropriate to perform limited flap refashioning.

Of additional note, the patient also developed an incisional hernia or weakness of the left abdominal wall from the original DCIA harvest. He recalled an event during inpatient recuperation in which he stumbled and noticed a 'tearing' sensation at the donor site wound. He was referred to the general surgeons who managed this conservatively in view of the size and difficulty in delineating the margin of the defect.

We are pleased to report that two years following the second ablation and reconstruction he remains well with no signs of local or distant recurrence. The surgical wounds have all healed well and he was further rehabilitated with an orbital prosthesis (Figure 1.8).

> ⊕ **Clinical tip** The scapular/parascapular flap
>
> The scapular flap was first successfully transferred by Gilbert and Teot in 1979 [12]. It was Nassif et al. who described the alternative skin paddle of the parascapular flap that is orientated longitudinally,
>
> (continued)

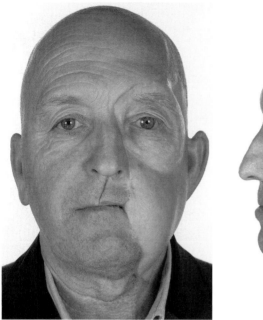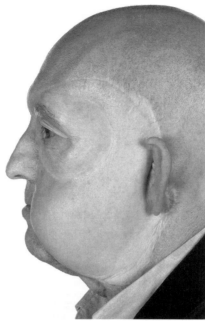

Figure 1.8 Anteroposterior and lateral views with prosthesis in position. See colour plate section.

but still based on the circumflex scapular artery (CSA) [13]. The vascular system associated with this flap is known to be of good calibre (subscapular artery = 3-4 mm [14]) and relatively resistant to arteriosclerosis when compared to other osteocutaneous free flaps such as the fibular flap.

When designing the flap we place the patient in the lateral decubitus position with the arm elevated and supported at around 60° to the long axis of the body. The flap is designed according to the triangular space (borders: teres minor, teres major, and long head of triceps). The quality and location of the CSA is assessed with the hand-held Doppler as it passes through this space.

When planning a parascapular island the skin paddle is usually orientated over the lateral border of the scapular. We harvested 28 cm in length of skin for this case and Shaw and Hidalgo reported in 1987 that up to 30 cm can be raised safely [15]. Urken states that between 10-14 cm of bone can be taken from the lateral portion of the scapular [16]. A flap based on the CSA may have a pedicle length of 7-10 cm [13] and harvesting the subscapular artery as it branches from the axillary artery may further elongate this if required.

ⓡ Expert comment

The position of the CSA is confirmed by Doppler as suggested above, but its location can be readily identified by standing behind the positioned patient and dropping your hand over the back with the palm on the scapula and with the index finger pushing gently into the posterior fold of the axilla. If you drop the middle finger you can, usually, quite readily feel it drop into the triangular space. The transverse branch lies at around 1-2 cm below the spine of the scapula in its midpoint and the descending branch around 1.5 cm in from the lateral edge of the same.

I start with the dissection from the midline proximally utilizing the plane immediately above the muscles. The surgeon needs to be aware of the subtleties of the anatomy, in particular the need to recognize how peripheral muscles belies the deltoid, trapezius, latissimus dorsi, and teres major lie

(continued)

as these can be misleading for those unfamiliar with this flap system. Similarly, the surgeon may be misled by a large perforating vessel through subscapularis around 2 cm from the lateral edge of the scapula and confuse this with the pedicle that it is often in line with. Once identified the surgeon can work around it to confirm that it is not the true pedicle and by confirmatory palpitation of the true lateral edge of the scapula. With careful proximal dissection in the correct plane one can complete the cutaneous incision towards the axilla. The anatomical triangle can then be safely exposed and the pedicle chased in the axilla by this dissection of the pedicle visualized on the deep surface of the cutaneous flap and by dissection onto teres major and deltoid to identify the other sides of the anatomical triangle. Once this is done and the top corner completed, retraction and a sweep with the finger or swab will expose the pedicle as it enters the axilla once the fascia is incised.

⊘ **Evidence Base** Brown classification, 2010 [7]

- Review of 147 cases of reconstructed midface and maxillary defects for head and neck cancer performed in the Regional Maxillofacial Unit in Liverpool, UK, since 1992 (see Figure 1.9);
- Personal view;
- Classification of maxillectomy:

Vertical
I: maxillectomy not causing an oronasal fistula
II: not involving the orbit
III: involving the orbital adnexae with orbital retention
IV: with orbital enucleation or exenteration
V: orbitomaxillary defect
VI: nasomaxillary defect

Horizontal
a: palatal defect only, not involving the dental alveolus
b: less than or equal to half unilateral
c: less than or equal to half bilateral or transverse anterior
d: greater than half maxillectomy.

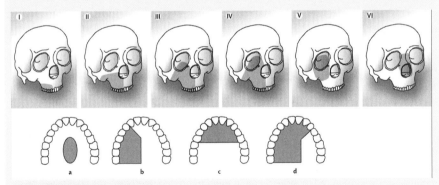

Figure 1.9 Brown classification. See colour plate section.

Classification and figure reprinted from The Lancet Oncology, Volume 11, Issue 10, Brown JS and Shaw RJ, Reconstruction of the maxilla and midface: introducing a new classification, pp.1001–1008, Copyright © 2010 Elsevier Ltd, http://www.sciencedirect.com/science/article/pii/S1470204510701133.

Discussion

Squamous cell carcinoma is the most common of this group of sinonasal tumours. Advanced disease such as this is acknowledged to have a relatively poor prognosis. The literature shows that survival rates for maxillary squamous cell carcinoma are

30-50% at five years [2]. The late presentation of these tumours has a detrimental effect on the survivability of this disease.

We are of the opinion that the excision of such tumours and reconstruction should be carried out by the same team of surgeons. The first goal should be to achieve the 'primary directive' in cancer surgery; that is ablation of the tumour with clear margins. Subsequent reconstructive challenges should not compromise this. A reconstruction of this magnitude presents a significant challenge to the head and neck surgeon. The potential for obturation should be considered by the MDT and discussed carefully with the patient. Moreno et al. reported on 113 patients following maxillectomy (43 patients reconstructed and 70 obturated). They concluded that the post-operative swallowing and speech intelligibility are improved following flap reconstruction where an extensive portion (> 50%) of the dental component of the maxilla is resected. Where defects were smaller, then these two indicators of success were comparable between the flap and obturator groups [17].

In this case an obturator may have been considered following the initial resection. However, the second surgery yielded a complex composite defect that required autogenous tissue to achieve satisfactory results.

A final word from the expert

The analysis and planning of all of these more complex oncological cases can be reduced to a few simple questions and by following general and logical principles.

Firstly, what am I hoping to achieve?

This is twofold. Surgery is performed with curative intent (with or without expected or possible adjunctive treatment). Secondly, and only after the first question is addressed: what is the objective of my reconstruction?

In relation to successful surgical ablation: What do I need to do to effectively remove this tumour? What will I be removing - hard tissue, soft tissue, and/or specialist structures (e.g. eye, nose, larynx, pharynx, facial nerve)?

Which of these structures need to be replaced to restore form, function, and aesthetics and to therefore optimize the patient's quality of life? All of these questions are asked in an attempt to rid the patient of their disease and restore them to, as near as possible, their pre-operative state and to allow them to return to society. These questions require careful but not usually ponderous thought and the details and 'difficult bits' can often be identified rapidly and thought about in more detail to identify how to overcome the challenges be it in resection or reconstruction. A good understanding of the planned defect and an artisans view of what individual flaps and techniques can achieve means that complex and large reconstructions can be performed with a degree of understanding for both the surgeon and transposed insight for the patient as to how or if to progress?

Acknowledgements

We would like to thank Mr David Ellis, Lead Maxillofacial Prosthetist at New Cross Hospital, Wolverhampton, for performing the orbital prosthetic rehabilitation.

References

1. House JW, Brackmann DE. Facial nerve grading system. *Otolaryngol Head Neck Surg* 1985: 93; 146–7.
2. Roland NJ, Paleri V(eds). *Head and Neck Cancer: Multidisciplinary Management Guidelines* 4th edition. London: ENT UK; 2011.
3. Eggers G, Mühling J, Hassfeld S. Inverted papilloma of the paranasal sinuses. *J Craniomaxillofac Surg* 2007: 35(1); 21–9.
4. Krouse JH. Development of a staging system for inverted papilloma. *Laryngoscope* 2000: 110; 965–8.
5. Taylor GI, Townsend P, Orlett R. Superiority of the deep circumflex ileac vessels as the supply for free groin flaps. *Plast Reconstr Surg* 1979; 64: 595–604.
6. Sanders R, Mayou BJ. A new vascularised bone graft transferred by microvascular anastomosis as a free flap. *Br J Surg* 1979; 66: 787–8.
7. Brown JS, Shaw RJ. Reconstruction of the maxilla and midface: introducing a new classification. *Lancet Oncol* 2010; 11: 1001–8.
8. Ramasastry SS, Tucker JB, Swartz WM, et al. The internal oblique muscle flap: an anatomic clinical study. *Plast Reconstr Surg* 1984; 73: 721–33.
9. Urken ML, Vickery C, Weinberg H, et al. The internal oblique-ileac crest osseomyocutaneous microvascular free flap in head and neck reconstruction. *J Reconstr Microsurg* 1989; 5: 203–14; discussion 215-6.
10. Forrest C, Boyd B, Manktelow R, et al. The free vascularised ileac crest transfer: donor site complications associated with eight-two cases. *Br J Plast Surg* 1992; 45(2): 89–93.
11. Bonner JA, Harari PM, Giralt J, et al. Radiotherapy plus cetuximab for locoregionally advanced head neck cancer: 5-year survival data from a phase 3 randomised trial, and relation between cetuximab-induced rash and survival. *Lancet Oncol* 2010; 11: 21–8.
12. Gilbert A, Teot L. The free scapular flap. *Plast Reconstr Surg* 1982; 69: 601.
13. Nassif TM, Vidal L, Bovet JL, Baudet J. The parascapular flap: a new cutaneous microsurgical free flap. *Plast Reconstr Surg* 1982; 69: 591.
14. Manktelow RT.*Microvascular Reconstruction*. Berlin, Heidelberg, New York : Springer, 1986.
15. Shaw WW, Hidalgo DA. *Microsurgery in Trauma*. Mount Kisco, New York: Futura, 1987.
16. Urken ML, Cheney ML, Blackwell KE, et al. (eds). *Atlas of Regional Free Flaps for Head and Neck Reconstruction: Flap Harvest and Insetting* 2nd edition. New York: Lippincott Williams and Wilkins 2012.
17. Moreno MA, Skoracki RJ, Ehab Y, et al. Microvascular free flap reconstruction versus palatal obturation for maxillectomy defects. *Head Neck* 2010; 32: 860–8.

Cutaneous malignancy

Christopher Fowell

🕕 **Expert commentary** Khaleeq-Ur Rehman

Case history: Basal cell carcinoma

A 72-year-old Caucasian male was referred by his general medical practitioner with a 4-month history of an increasing scar-like lesion on the right pre-auricular region. The patient reported the lesion to be increasing in size and although initially asymptomatic, the lesion had started to intermittently crust and ooze with a blood-stained fluid. He reported excision of a smaller, yet similar lesion some three years ago by a dermatologist at a different hospital.

The patient was a retired farmer with a history of repeated sun exposure stretching over many decades. The patient took regular amlodipine for hypertension, but no other medications.

On examination, the patient was Fitzpatrick skin type II, with blue eyes. On the right temple was a 2.5 cm × 3.0 cm pearlescent, irregular, scar-like lesion with indistinct borders (Figure 2.1). Punch incisional biopsy was completed under local anaesthetic, with histopathological analysis giving a diagnosis of morphoeic basal cell carcinoma (BCC).

✪ Learning point

BCC is the most common type of skin cancer, arising from basal keratinocytes within the epidermis. They represent over 80% of skin cancers [1]. BCCs are typically slow growing and locally invasive, with little metastatic potential unless demonstrating squamous differentiation. Regional metastasis is extremely rare, but can occur.

BCCs classically present on sun-exposed skin as pearlescent lesions that progressively increase in size and can bleed on minimal trauma. They can vary in colour from clear to deeply pigmented. Lesions may be present for months or even years, often described as a blemish that never fully heals.

Risk factors for BCC include increasing age, male gender, fair skin, and chronic sun exposure, with ultraviolet (UV) radiation (UVB 290–320 nm) being the most established aetiological factor. Patients with a history of immunosuppression, exposure to ionizing radiation, and congenital Gorlin-Goltz syndrome are at increased risk.

BCCs can be classified into differing clinical and histopathological subtypes:

- Nodular are the most common, appearing as pink, raised pearly lesions with rolled margins and central crusting depression. Approximately 90% of nodular BCCs occur on the head and neck [1].
- Superficial BCCs commonly present as well-demarcated pink lesions, often with a thread-like raised, pearlescent margin. Although common on the head and neck, they can occur with similar frequency on the trunk. As their name suggests, superficial BCCs classically develop radially, rather than demonstrating deep invasion.
- Morphoeic BCCs are the least frequently occurring subtype and present as white, grey, or yellow scar-like lesions that may be slightly raised. The limits of morphoeic lesions may be difficult to detect given their ill-defined margins. They demonstrate highly invasive features and have the potential to spread extensively.

❝ Expert comment

Morphoeic BCC is a type of infiltrating BCC histologically and commonly occurs around the most exposed part of the face, the so-called 'T' zone. It should be treated as a very high-risk lesion. These lesions have the classical appearances of flat, waxy, ill-defined edges. One has to be very cautious when reviewing cases treated previous by curettage and cautery as these scars can resemble a morphoeic BCC.

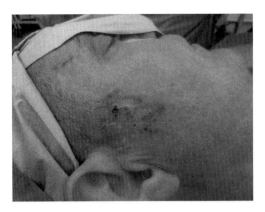

Figure 2.1 Right pre-auricular morphoeic basal cell carcinoma. See colour plate section.

There are various methods of treating biopsy-proven BCC, depending on histological subtype, anatomical location, and other clinical features (see Learning point: Surgical treatment of BCC and resection margins and Learning point: Non-surgical treatment of BCC). Tumours are typically classified as high or low risk of recurrence, dependent on the presence or absence of various prognostic factors (Box 2.1) [2].

Given the anatomical site of tumour and histological diagnosis of morphoeic BCC, the patient was referred for curative excision via Mohs micrographical surgery. Complete excision was achieved, allowing immediate reconstruction. The patient was reassured regarding the favourable prognosis of BCC, including its lack of metastatic spread and high probability of cure.

> **Expert comment**
>
> The dermatologists are very experienced in using the dermatoscope to aid diagnosis. All surgical clinicians should be aware of the common dermatoscopic findings of skin cancer lesions as this will allow proper assessment and appropriate management.

> **Expert comment**
>
> Surgical management of morphoeic BCC of the head and neck can be a little tricky because of the ill-defined peripheral margins. It is suggested that Mohs surgery should be performed in these cases but unfortunately there are not many units in the country who have trained clinicians practising this technique. As a surgical clinician I suggest obtaining the maximal margin possible at first operation, as repeat surgery can be difficult and extensive in high-risk areas of the face such as the nose, eyes, and ears.

> **Evidence base** British Association of Dermatologists (BAD) basal cell carcinoma guidelines 2008 [2]
>
> Due to the increasing prevalence of non-melanoma skin cancer (NMSC), there have been multiple studies and papers published on epidemiology, aetiology, presentation, and management. In the authors' opinions, much of the literature is best summarized in the BAD Guidelines on the management of BCC. Both surgical and non-surgical treatment options are considered and discussed. Review of the evidence has allowed the BAD to propose recommended margins for surgical excision, which currently provide the cornerstone of treatment in this patient group.
>
> Source: data from N.R. Telfer et al., Guidelines for the management of basal cell carcinoma, *British Journal of Dermatology*, Volume 159, pp. 35–48, Copyright © 2008 The Authors.

Box 2.1 Features conferring higher risk of recurrence in BCC [2]

- Tumour size >2 cm diameter
- Tumour site (eyes, nose, lips, and ears)
- Clinically ill-defined margins
- Histological subtype
- Aggressive histological features (perineural spread, perivascular involvement)
- Recurrent disease/ failure of previous treatment
- Immunosuppression

Adapted with from NR Telfer et al., Guidelines for the management of basal cell carcinoma, *British Journal of Dermatology*, Volume 159, pp. 35–48, Copyright © 2008 The Authors, reproduced with permission from John Wiley & Sons.

Review of the previous excisional biopsy histopathological report identified similar findings. The surgical margins on the previous biopsy were reported as 2 mm peripheral and 3 mm deep.

> ✪ **Learning point** Establishing a diagnosis of non-melanoma skin cancer
>
> Clinical diagnosis from history and examination may be appropriate for many skin cancer lesions, yet biopsy is often required to confirm clinical suspicion, identify and document subtype of disease, and hence guide treatment.
>
> Shave biopsy can be used on suspected superficial dermal and epidermal lesions. The recognition of pinpoint bleeding ensures the dermis is reached. This is necessary to detect invasive disease in NMSCs. As this technique does not give accurate detection of depth, it should not be used for lesions suspicious of malignant melanoma. The main complication of this technique is difficulty in definitive histopathological diagnosis due to inadequate depth of specimen.

> ➕ **Clinical tip** Techniques for skin biopsy
>
> Punch biopsy uses a cylindrical instrument with a cutting rim to obtain a plug of skin. Sizes vary from 2 mm to 8 mm in diameter. Although a full-thickness sample is obtained, the area of a lesion sampled is relatively small.
>
> Incisional biopsy is suitable for larger lesions, giving a full-thickness representation of a lesion. The sample should be taken as an ellipse across the margin of a lesion, to allow normal tissue to be compared to the pathological area.
>
> Excisional biopsy can be both diagnostic and curative. Care should be taken to include appropriate margins and also include a marker suture to allow orientation.

> ✪ **Learning point** Surgical treatment of basal cell carcinoma and resection margins
>
> The usual aim of treatment for BCC is the eradication of the cancerous cells in a manner that leads to acceptable cosmetic results for the patient. Subsequently, surgical excision is the treatment of choice for many patients, especially high-risk lesions. Non-operative treatment options may be appropriate in low-risk lesions (see Learning point: Non-surgical treatment of BCC). Tumour excision provides the highest cure rate for BCC and also provides the benefit of histopathological assessment of the entire tumour. Inclusion of a pre-determined margin of uninvolved tissue allows detection of subclinical spread and increases the probability of cure.
>
> BAD Guidelines [2] recommend excision margins of 4 mm for tumours less than 2 cm in diameter, giving a 95% confidence of complete excision. A margin of 3 mm eradicates the tumour in 85% of cases. High-risk lesions, in particular morphoeic and large (>2 cm) tumours, require increasing surgical margins to achieve cure. A 13–15 mm margin gives a 95% clearance, with 5 mm margins providing 82% clearance.

> ✪ **Learning point** Mohs micrographical surgery
>
> Mohs micrographical surgery is a specialized technique of surgical excision that utilizes real-time margin examination. Its advantages include maximum conservation of tissue and cure rates that are reported to approach 99%. The technique is recommended [2] for high-risk tumours, recurrent tumours, and in those cosmetically sensitive areas in which tissue conservation is most important.
>
> The main disadvantages of Mohs micrographical surgery remain associated to its labour-intensive nature and cost implications. Surgical time is greatly increased and several highly trained clinicians are necessary to undertake the procedural stages.

Clinical tip Mohs micrographical surgery

The procedure consists of staged excision and histopathological examination of 100% of the specimen. After excision of the clinically evident lesion and minimal peripheral tissue, the specimen is frozen, orientated on an anatomic 'map', and sectioned to allow examination by a trained pathologist or surgeon. If the lesion is deemed clear of tumour, repair of the defect can commence. If residual tumour is detected on the excised specimen, further excision occurs that can be guided precisely by the anatomical 'map'. This process is repeated until there is no further evidence of malignancy.

Learning point Non-surgical treatment of basal cell carcinoma

Superficial BCCs that do not demonstrate advanced invasion into the underlying tissues may be amenable to *topical treatments* such as chemotherapy agents (e.g. 5-fluorouracil) and immune modulators (e.g. imiquimod). To date, cure rates using these agents are inferior to those achieved with surgical excision. Although successful in the treatment of small (< 1 cm) low-risk tumours [2], the main difficulty remains that analysis of margins cannot be undertaken. Hence, it cannot be proven whether all tumour cells have been removed.

External beam radiotherapy gives high cure rates for BCC. However, a randomized trial [3] comparing surgical excision demonstrated higher recurrence rates in the radiotherapy group. Hence, radiotherapy is usually limited to elderly patients or in cases when surgical excision is likely to lead to a poor functional or cosmetic result [2].

Case history: Malignant melanoma

A 63-year-old female was referred with a pigmented lesion on the right cheek and lower eyelid that had changed in appearance over the last three months. The patient reported the recent development of a thickened, black area within a longstanding irregular, brown macular lesion (Figure 2.2). The lesion was otherwise asymptomatic, with no pain, itching or bleeding reported.

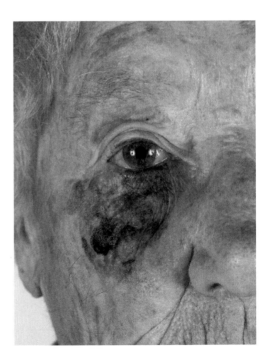

Figure 2.2 Right cheek lentigo maligna melanoma. See colour plate section.

The patient was a cleaner at a local hospital, with a medical history of gastro-oesophageal reflux and obesity. Lansoprazole was the only regular medication, with no known allergies. The patient reported smoking ten cigarettes per day.

Incisional biopsy of the lesion was completed, with histopathological examination demonstrating lentigo maligna melanoma with a Breslow thickness of 1.4 mm. The patient's case was subsequently discussed at a specialist MDT meeting and arrangements made for wide local excision and sentinel lymph node biopsy (SLNB).

> **✦ Expert comment**
>
> Research studies have shown that the incidence of malignant melanoma is on the up in the UK and have increased fivefold over the last four decades. Over 13,000 new cases are seen annually with over one-third of these cases in those under the age of 55 years. Over 2000 deaths are melanoma related accounting for 1% of all cancer deaths.

> **✪ Learning point** Melanoma: aetiology, epidemiology and risk factors
>
> Melanoma is the eighth most common malignancy in the United Kingdom with age standardized rates of approximately 17 cases per 100,000 population in 2011 [1], affecting males and females equally. Between 15% and 20% of cases reportedly affect the head and neck, although men are more at risk of melanoma in this region.
>
> Mortality rates from melanoma have increased over the last 25 years; the survival and incidence data show that men are almost twice as likely to succumb to the disease [1]. Current 5-year survival rates are 88% in males and 92% in females [1]. Mortality is highest amongst men aged over 65 who present with advanced tumours of poor prognosis. Lesions are common on the back in this patient group, making self-examination difficult. Men are also known to have a tendency to not report changing skin lesions.
>
> Melanoma is most common amongst Caucasians with fair skin, red or light-coloured hair, light eye colour, and freckles. Other risk factors include family history, regular sunbed use, and increasing numbers of benign and atypical naevi.
>
> UVB is the major cause of sunburn and skin cancer. Case-control data has demonstrated sunburn in early life as a risk factor for melanoma, with the chronic low-dose exposure typical of BCC and squamous cell carcinoma (SCC) deemed less clearly related.

> **✪ Learning point** Diagnosis and clinical subtypes of malignant melanoma
>
> Lesions suspicious of melanoma should be excised completely, with a 5 mm surgical margin and cuff of subdermal fat [4]. Shave and punch biopsies should be avoided. Sampling error and distortion can make analysis of thickness and tissue architecture difficult, compromising diagnosis and treatment planning. Full-thickness incisional biopsy should only be utilized in cases of large, multi-pigmented lesions in areas of cosmetic importance where excisional biopsy for diagnosis is deemed unsuitable.
>
> There are four clinical subtypes of melanoma, each with characteristic clinical and histopathological features:
>
> *Superficial spreading melanoma (SSM)* is the most common subtype (75% of cases) and characteristically presents as a developing pigmented lesion that expands radially over a number of months to years. Lesions may evolve and change colour over time, including various shades of brown, grey, black, and red. The development of a nodular appearance of SSM is a poor prognostic feature, representing vertical growth and invasion. These lesions are relatively uncommon on the head and neck, most commonly affecting the limbs of females and trunks of males.
>
> *Nodular melanoma* (15%) commonly presents as a rapidly increasing brown or black nodule with a propensity to bleed. Nodular melanoma is uncommon the face, usually found on the trunk. These lesions carry a poorer prognosis, demonstrated by rapid, vertical growth.
>
> *Lentigo maligna melanoma* (5–10%) is a specific type of melanoma developing from lentigo maligna (LM) in situ. It commonly develops in sun-exposed areas such as the face. LM usually develops radially over a period of many years, with 5–15% progressing to become LM melanoma. This invasive change is usually accompanied by the lesion darkening, becoming palpable, and developing a nodular or plaque-like appearance.
>
> *Acral and subungal melanomas* (< 5%) are rare, presenting on the soles, palms, and under nails.

Four injections of 0.05 ml technetium 99m antimony trisulphide colloid were injected around the primary melanoma site the day before planned surgery. Lymphoscintigraphy was undertaken immediately following injection and some three hours later. Two sentinel nodes in the submandibular region were identified and marked with dermal tattooing. The following day, the primary site was injected pre-operatively with 2 ml of patent blue-V dye. Via incisions made over the marked lymph nodes, dissection and excision of the blue-stained lymph nodes was undertaken. Due to the procedure being completed within 24-hours of radioisotope injection, a hand-held gamma probe was used intra-operatively to confirm the sentinel nodes by their high radiation counts. Wide local excision with a 2 cm excision margin of the primary lesion was completed, with local reconstruction via a cervical rotation flap to the cheek.

Histopathological analysis of the excised sentinel lymph nodes showed no features of metastatic melanoma. No further or adjuvant therapy was recommended following further MDT discussion.

The patient was formally staged using the American Joint Commission on Cancer (AJCC) staging system for cutaneous melanoma. Arrangements were made for three-monthly follow-up for the first three years post-treatment, followed by 6-monthly review for a further two years.

★ Learning point Melanoma: staging

The strongest prognostic indicators in melanoma are Breslow thickness and the presence or absence of ulceration. The Breslow thickness is the distance of the deepest part of the tumour from the granular layer of epidermis. It predicts the rate of metastasis and hence 5-year survival (Box 2.1), as well as determining the size of margin in wide surgical excision.

❝ Expert comment

Staging of melanoma is also an area of debate. From experience it has been noted that not all units treating follow the same rules. Some do a computed tomography (CT) scan, others positron emission tomography (PET) scan, yet there is guidance from the National Institute of Health and Care Excellence update document in 2011. A meta-analysis by Xing et al. 2011 concluded that ultrasound scanning was superior for detecting regional metastases and PET-CT for distant disease for staging and surveillance [5].

✓ Evidence base British Association of Dermatologists malignant melanoma guidelines 2010 [4]

As for BCC, the BAD Guidelines on the management of malignant melanoma provide the key recommendations for diagnosis, staging, and management of the condition. One of the key recommendations regards the involvement of a specialist skin cancer multidisciplinary team (SSCMDT) for many patients with malignant melanoma.

Melanoma patients who must be referred to a SSCMDT:

1. Patients with melanoma managed by other site specialist teams.
2. Patients for SLNB.
3. Patients who may be eligible for approved clinical trials.
4. Patients with multiple primary melanomas.
5. Children and young adults (< 19 years).
6. Any patient with metastatic malignant melanoma.
7. Patients with congenital giant cell naevi with clinical suspicion of malignant transformation.
8. Patients with skin lesions of uncertain malignant potential.

Surgical wider excision margins for primary melanoma:

Breslow thickness	Lateral margin
In situ:	5 mm
< 1 mm:	1 cm
1.01–2 mm:	1–2 cm
2.1–4 mm:	2–3 cm
>4 mm:	3 cm

(continued)

Adapted from Marsden JR et al., Revised UK guidelines for the management of cutaneous melanoma 2010, *British Journal of Dermatology*, Volume 163, Issue 2, pp.238-256, Copyright © 2010 British Association of Dermatologists, with kind permission from John Wiley & Sons.

✪ Learning point Sentinel lymph node biopsy in skin cancer

SLNB increases the accuracy of both staging and prognosis in melanoma. Wide local excision disturbs the anatomy and lymphatic drainage, hence SLNB should be undertaken at the same time as surgical treatment of the primary site [6].

Patients with melanoma with a Breslow thickness of 1.2–2.0 mm and a negative SLNB have a 5-year survival rate of 90%, compared with 75% in cases of a positive SLNB. Although most patients with positive SLNB usually choose to progress to completion regional lymphadenectomy, to date this has not shown to have any therapeutic value by increasing survival [6].

The application of SLNB in the management of high-risk SCC has been explored, potentially decreasing unnecessary regional lymphadenectomy. However, the overall patient benefit of the procedure is yet to be proven [7].

❝ Expert comment

Management of melanoma should be directed by a specialist MDT. Elective dissection of the neck in melanoma cases is controversial due to complex lymphatic drainage of the head and neck region. For this reason SLNB was introduced in the early nineties. This technique is well documented for other regions of the body but has not really taken off in the head and neck. Many reasons have been cited for the lower pick up in the head and neck region as compared to rest of the body. Increased vascularity, smaller lymph nodes, unpredictable pattern of lymphatic drainage (skip metastasis in SCC), and close proximity of lymph nodes to primary are some of these. More recent studies have shown positive results in favour of SLNB.

✪ Learning point Follow-up in skin cancer

Regular review of skin cancer patients allows for the prompt detection of new skin cancers and metastatic disease. It also provides an opportunity to reinforce patient education (including self-examination techniques) and offer psychological support.

Guidelines for melanoma follow-up recommend 3-monthly follow-up for all patients for three years, followed by a further two years of six-monthly follow-up in those patients originally treated for stage III or IV disease [4]. As well as the risks of recurrence and metastatic disease, 5% of melanoma patients may develop a second primary lesion.

Guidelines for SCC and BCC remain less stringent, given the decreased risk of metastasis and recurrence following effective primary treatment. Three-quarters of all local recurrent cutaneous SCC and metastases occur within two years and 95% in five years. At present there are no formal guidelines for review structure, although review for at least this time period is recommended for high-risk cancers [2,8]. Patients may be reviewed by specialists, primary care physicians, or appropriately trained clinical nurse specialists. Individual patient requirements should be decided dependent on disease risk, access to healthcare and clinician's training and interests [2,8].

❝ Expert comment

Surgery remains the mainstay of treatment for melanoma. However, pharmacological options are available in those with metastatic disease. These include inclusion in trials with ipilimumab and vemurafenib.

Case history: Squamous cell carcinoma

A 62-year-old male was referred with biopsy-proven SCC of the scalp. The patient reported a 6-month history of a painful, rapidly increasing lesion. Punch biopsy had been undertaken by local dermatology colleagues and subsequently discussed at the MDT meeting.

The patient, a semi-retired businessman and keen amateur golfer, gave a history of intermittent sun exposure without sun protection for several decades. He was systemically fit and well, with no regular medications. The patient smoked a cigar daily and drank up to 45 units of alcohol per week.

> **☀ Learning point** Squamous cell carcinoma: aetiology, epidemiology and risk factors
>
> SCC is the second most common form of skin cancer after BCC, accounting for approximately 20% of cases of NMSC. Unfortunately, NMSC is difficult to record on tumour registries, making the worldwide incidence difficult to estimate. Seventy per cent of SCCs arise on the head and neck.
>
> Sun exposure to UV radiation remains the primary aetiological factor for SCC. Pre-cancerous skin lesions such as actinic keratosis and nevus sebaceous can also predispose to SCC. A history of immunosuppression increases markedly the risk of acquiring SCC (and BCC), with subsequent disease often demonstrating more aggressive behaviour. Anti-rejection regimens for transplanted organs and immunosuppressants for autoimmune and rheumatological conditions are typically associated.

Examination revealed the patient to have Fitzpatrick skin type II. On the vertex of the scalp was a 4.0 cm × 4.5 cm red, regular, nodular lesion (Figure 2.3). The lesion had a small area of central ulceration. There were no further lesions evident on the skin of the head and neck. Cervical lymphadenopathy was not palpable.

> **☀ Learning point** Squamous cell carcinoma recurrence and metastasis: risk factors
>
> SCC tumours of the head and neck are subsequently subdivided in to low risk or high risk for recurrence and metastatic spread. Although most patients with SCC are cured by treatment of the primary lesion alone, metastasis rates of 5% are reported. Recognized risk factors for recurrence and metastasis include lesion diameter ≥2 cm, invasion depth >4 mm, recurrent tumours, poorly differentiated malignancies, and a history of immunosuppression. Different anatomical sites of primary SCC are also at higher risk of metastatic spread, with the pinna of the ear, the lip, previous scars, and non-sun-exposed sites reported [8].

Following MDT discussion, the patient underwent excision of the lesion with immediate reconstruction with local skin flaps. Histopathological analysis revealed moderately differentiated SCC with excision margins of 5 mm peripherally and 6 mm deep. A depth of invasion of 4.5 mm was reported. Features of perineural and lympho-vascular invasion were not evident in the biopsy specimen. The lesion was deemed completely excised and arrangements made for long-term follow-up.

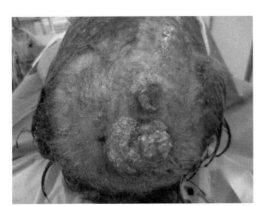

Figure 2.3 Pre-operative image of scalp squamous cell carcinoma. See colour plate section.

> ⊕ **Clinical tip** Surgical treatment of squamous cell carcinoma
>
> Surgical excision of SCC allows for assessment of completeness of excision through analysis of surgical margins, as well as histopathological assessment of the entire specimen. These benefits are not possible in non-surgical methods.
>
> Conventional surgical excision remains the mainstay of surgical treatment, being quick, safe and well tolerated by patients. For low-risk lesions, the treatment has been shown to be very effective, although this efficiency remains dependent on surgical excision margins.
>
> The BAD Guidelines state that clearance is achieved in 95% of cases when margins of 4 mm are utilized for low-risk lesions. In those patients with high-risk lesions, lesions should be removed with margins of 6 mm [8]. The use of Mohs micrographical surgery is considered the gold standard for local management of high-risk SCC, although its availability in the United Kingdom remains hampered by its cost and labour-intensive nature.

> ❻ **Expert comment**
>
> Cutaneous SCC has a metastatic rate of around 5% and to the parotid region of around 1-2%. The parotid deposits require a parotidectomy and it is often very difficult to remove all deposits due to the nature of the parotid tissue. In such cases post-operative radiotherapy is recommended. Those patients having pre-operative radiotherapy do not do as well as those receiving post-operative radiotherapy.

At outpatient review some eight months following surgical excision, the patient presented with an asymptomatic, left pre-auricular swelling of four weeks duration (Figure 2.4). Clinical examination revealed a firm, 2 cm swelling in the left parotid gland. Left-sided, firm cervical lymphadenopathy was also palpable at level II.

The patient was referred for urgent further investigation. Ultrasound examination demonstrated cervical lymphadenopathy in keeping with metastatic carcinoma. Fine-needle aspiration cytology of the parotid mass confirmed metastatic SCC. CT of the head, neck and thorax was also undertaken, revealing three unilateral metastatic nodes (<3 cm) and the absence of pulmonary metastasis. Using the tumour, node, metastasis (TNM) classification of malignant tumours, the patient was staged as T0 N2b M0.

Following MDT consideration, the patient subsequently underwent right superficial parotidectomy and elective neck dissection. After further MDT discussion the patient was offered and subsequently underwent adjuvant radiotherapy of the neck and parotid bed.

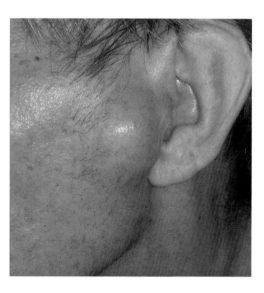

Figure 2.4 Metastatic cutaneous squamous cell carcinoma of the left parotid gland.

> ✪ **Learning point** Staging of cutaneous squamous cell carcinoma
>
> The present TNM staging for cutaneous SCC is outlined in Tables 2.1 and 2.2 [14]. The use of an internationally agreed staging system allows for better communication between healthcare professionals, standardized treatment and greater analysis of treatments and outcomes through research.

> ✪ **Learning point** Non-excisional treatment of squamous cell carcinoma
>
> Aside from localized radiotherapy, non-excisional therapies should only be utilized for the treatment of small, low-risk primary cutaneous SCC.
>
> The use of *topical and intra-lesional chemotherapy* agents has been mainly utilized for the management of BCC, although similar advantageous results have been reported in early and low-risk SCC. 5-*Fluorouracil* has been shown to give cure rates of up to 90% in cases of superficial SCC and Bowen's disease [9]. *Imiquimod*, an immune response modulator, has been used on superficial cutaneous SCC and Bowen's disease. Effectiveness has been demonstrated when used following curettage and as a preventative measure in high-risk patients presenting with dysplastic lesions such as actinic keratosis [10].
>
> *External beam radiotherapy* can be utilized for both localized, low-risk cutaneous SCC as well as advanced disease. When used in superficial SCC with favourable histology, cure rates of 90% have been reported [11].
>
> Primary radiotherapy can give better cosmetic results when compared to surgery in certain aesthetic areas of the face. These include the nose, ears and lips. However, long-term side effects such as telangiectasia, dermal atrophy and hypo- and hyper-pigmentation are well recognized. As with all localized external beam radiotherapy, the risk of in-field secondary carcinomas also exists. Hence, the BAD Guidelines for management of cutaneous SCC recommend its use as a primary modality in those patients who are poor surgical candidates or in aesthetically sensitive areas. Its use as an adjuvant therapy is recommended in locally invasive and advanced primary tumours, as well as recurrent lesions [8].
>
> *Cryosurgery*, which uses extreme cold to ablate cutaneous lesions, is predominantly used for the treatment of pre-malignant lesions such as actinic keratosis. As well as in the ablation of low-risk and superficial BCC, it can be used on SCC with proven similarly favourable clinical features. A margin of 5 mm should be used in the treatment field [12]. Side effects such as hypopigmentation and hair follicle destruction have limited its use on the head and neck.
>
> *Photodynamic therapy* has been shown to be effective in the management of superficial SCC and pre-malignant conditions, with uncertain evidence regarding invasive tumours. The procedure involves the application of photosensitizers, such as methyl aminolevulinate and 5-aminolaevulinic acid, which are converted to protoporphyrin IX once absorbed. Laser light at wavelengths 450–750 nm can then be used to activate the protoporphyrin, leading to cellular destruction. Photodynamic therapy should not be considered for thick tumours, recurrent tumours or those with aggressive histology [13].

Table 2.1 TNM staging for cutaneous squamous cell carcinoma

Primary tumour	Regional lymph nodes	Distant metastasis
Tx – Primary tumour cannot be assessed	Nx – Regional lymph nodes cannot be assessed	Mx – Distant metastasis cannot be assessed
T0 – No evidence of primary tumour	N0 – No evidence of regional lymph node metastasis	M0 – No evidence of distant metastasis
Tis – Carcinoma *in situ*	N1 – Metastasis to a single ipsilateral lymph node, ≤3 cm in greatest dimension	M1 – Distant metastasis
T1 – Tumour ≤ 2 cm with< two high-risk features(a)	N2a – Metastasis to a single ipsilateral lymph node, >3 cm but ≤ 6 cm in greatest dimension	
T2 – Tumour ≥ 2 cm or tumour with > two high-risk features(a)	N2b – Metastasis to multiple ipsilateral lymph nodes, ≤6 cm in greatest dimension	
T3 – Tumour with invasion of mandible, maxilla, orbit or temporal bone	N2c – Metastasis to bilateral or contralateral lymph nodes, ≤6 cm in greatest dimension	
T4 – Tumour with invasion of axial skeleton or perineural invasion of skull base	N3 – Metastasis to a lymph node, ≥ 6 cm in greatest dimension	

[a] High-risk features are listed in Table 2.2.
Reproduced from Compton CC et al, *AJCC Cancer Staging Atlas: A Companion to the Seventh Editions of the AJCC Cancer Staging Manual and Handbook*, Second Edition, pp 355–416, Springer, New York, USA, Copyright © 2012. With kind permission from Springer Science and Business Media.

Table 2.2 High-risk features of cutaneous squamous cell carcinoma

Depth/invasion	> 2 mm
	Clark Level IV
	Perineural invasion
Anatomic	Primary site ear/lip
Differentiation	Poor differentiation

Reproduced from Compton CC et al, *AJCC Cancer Staging Atlas: A Companion to the Seventh Editions of the AJCC Cancer Staging Manual and Handbook*, Second Edition, pp 355-416, Springer, New York, USA, Copyright © 2012. With kind permission from Springer Science and Business Media.

A final word from the expert

Skin cancer is on the rise in the UK with over 100,000 new cases per year and near 3000 deaths. Following an initial diagnosis these cases have to be discussed at the local and specialist MDTs to formulate a definitive management plan. It is very important for all those clinicians as core members of the MDT to be up to date with latest advances in order to provide a comprehensive service.

References

1. Cancer Research UK. http://www.cancerreasearchuk.org.
2. Telfer NR, Colver GB, Morton CA. Guidelines for the management of basal cell carcinoma. *Br J Dermatol* 2008; 159: 35–48.
3. Avril MF, Auperin A, Marqulis A, et al. Basal cell carcinoma of the face: surgery or radiotherapy? Results of a randomised study. *Br J Cancer* 1997; 76: 100–6.
4. Marsden JR, Newton-Bishop JA, Burrows L, et al. Revised UK guidelines for the management of cutaneous melanoma 2010. *Br J Derm* 2010; 163: 238–56.
5. Xing Y, Bronstein Y, Ross MI, et al. Contemporary diagnostic imaging modalities for the staging and surveillance of melanoma patients: a meta-analysis. *J Natl Cancer Inst* 2011; 103(2): 129–42.
6. Morton DL, Wen DR, Wong JH, et al. Technical details of intra-operative lymphatic mapping for early stage lymphoma. *Arch Surg* 1992; 127: 392–9.
7. Morton DL, Cochran AJ, Thompson JF, et al. Sentinel node biopsy for early stage melanoma - accuracy and morbidity in MSLT-1, an international multicentre trial. *Arch Surg* 2005; 242: 302–13.
8. Motley RJ, Preston PW, Lawrence CM. Multi-professional guidelines for the management of the patient with primary cutaneous squamous cell carcinoma. *Br J Derm* 2009; 146(1): 18–25.
9. Cox NH, Eddy DJ, Morton CA. Guidelines for the management of Bowen's disease. British Association of Dermatologists. *Br J Derm* 1999; 141: 633–41.
10. Ulrich C, Bichel J, Euvrard S. et al. Topical immunomodulation under systemic immunosuppression: results of a multi-centre, randomised, placebo-controlled safety and efficacy study of imiquimod 5% cream for the treatment of actinic keratosis in kidney, heart and liver transplant patients. *Br J Derm* 2007; 157 (Suppl. 2): 25–31.
11. Rowe DE, Carroll RJ, Day CL Jr. Prognostic factors for local recurrence, metastasis and survival rates in squamous cell carcinoma of the skin, ear and lip. Implications for treatment modality selection. *J Am Acad Dermatol* 1992; 26: 976–90.
12. Kufflik EG. Cryosurgery for cutaneous malignancy, an update. *Dermatol Surg* 1997; 23: 1081–7.

13. Photodynamic therapy for non-melanoma skin tumours (including pre-malignant and primary non-metastatic skin lesions). NICE interventional procedure guideline (2006). http://www.nice.org.uk/guidance/ipg155/resources/guidance-photodynamic-therapy-for-nonmelanoma-skin-tumours-including-premalignant-and-primary-nonmetastatic-skin-lesions-pdf.
14. Compton CC, Byrd DR, Garcia-Aguilar J, et al. *AJCC Cancer Staging Atlas: A Companion to the Seventh Editions of the AJCC Cancer Staging Manual and Handbook* 2nd edition. New York: Springer, 2012, pp 355–416.

3 Management of osteoradionecrosis of the mandible

Anwer Abdullakutty and Jacob D'Souza

❻ **Expert commentary** Simon Rogers

Case history

A 67-year-old male presented with a non-healing tooth extraction socket in the region of lower left second molar. The dental extraction was carried out four months prior to his presentation. Symptoms included pain, halitosis, and trismus with a maximal mouth opening of 30 mm. Despite interventions such as chlorhexidine mouth rinses and broad-spectrum antibiotics, the symptoms were progressive. Three years previously, he had undergone surgical treatment for squamous cell carcinoma of the oral cavity, followed by adjuvant external beam radiotherapy. Clinical examination confirmed radiation change involving the skin. The extraction socket had failed to heal and revealed exposed bone that appeared necrotic. There were no clinical signs of tumour recurrence. An orthopantomogram showed an area of radiolucency extending to the level of the inferior dental canal. Tissue biopsy ruled out malignancy and consequently a diagnosis of osteoradionecrosis (ORN) was made.

> ❻ **Expert comment**
>
> The history and clinical findings are suggestive of ORN. The reported incidence of ORN of the mandible varies from 2.6–22% [1,2]. More than 70% of cases of ORN have been reported to develop within the first three years of radiotherapy [1,2]. Presentation ranges from mild asymptomatic disease to progressive pain, suppuration, exposed bone, fistula and pathological fracture. Treatment strategies vary amongst clinicians and include the use of antibiotics, surgical debridement and hyperbaric oxygen therapy [3–5]. More recently, medical management with pentoxifylline, tocopherol and clodronate is gaining popularity in selected cases of established ORN [6,7]. However, the need for surgical excision of the necrotic bone is required to remove bony sequestra.

Pathophysiology

ORN preferentially affects the mandible due to its poor blood supply, especially with advancing age and in patients who have had radiotherapy. Soft tissue ischaemia mirrors bony change. The most commonly affected site is the body of the mandible.

> ➕ **Clinical tip**
>
> Surgical debridement of the necrotic bone should be conservative, with minimal stripping of the periosteum, so as to preserve blood supply to the bone. This should be supplemented with strict oral hygiene, avoidance of smoking and judicious use of antibiotics.

> ➕ **Clinical tip** Definition of osteoradionecrosis
>
> Exposed and necrotic bone associated with ulcerated or necrotic surrounding soft tissue that persists for more than three months in an area that has previously been irradiated and not caused by tumour recurrence.

> ✖ **Learning point** Diagnosis of osteoradionecrosis
>
> - Radiotherapy over a critical dose.
> - Necrotic soft tissue/bone for more than three months.
> - Radiographic change.
> - Absence of malignancy as confirmed with histopathological analysis.

⭐ **Learning point** Changing concepts

Before 1980s: trauma and infection. This formed the basis for the use of antibiotics.

1980s: Marx '3-H concept':

- hypovascularity (radiation induced thrombosis secondary to endarteritis obliterans), leading to
- hypoxia, leading to
- hypocellularity (cell death and tissue breakdown).

Current: fibroatrophic theory: 'radiation-induced fibrosis'.

➕ **Clinical tip**

Employ a system that is simple to use and helps decision making with regard to treatment and follow-up.

❝ **Expert comment**

In the past, ORN was thought to be primarily due to infection secondary to trauma in the area of radiotherapy. This formed the basis of the use of antibiotics, often on a long-term basis. Marx introduced the 3-H concept and popularized the use of hyperbaric oxygen therapy (HBOT) to vascularize the hypoxic tissue and increase the fibroblast population [4,5]. Despite gaining popularity, HBOT was not applied as per the proposed protocol universally and there were issues with compliance. In a randomized controlled trial, Annane et al. showed that HBOT is not better than placebo, and they raised concerns about its damaging effects [8]. Currently, given the equivocal evidence, there is a lack of enthusiasm amongst the surgeons in the UK to prescribe HBOT. Its use has further declined by the contemporary understanding of the pathophysiology of ORN, favouring use of drugs such as pentoxifylline, tocopherol and clodronate [7–9]. However, the need for surgical debridement to remove necrotic bone sequestra is important.

➕ **Clinical tip** Regime for medical treatment of ORN

- Pentoxifylline: 800 mg/day for 6–24 months.
- Tocopherol (vitamin E) 1000 IU/day for 6–24 months.
- Clodronate: 1600 mg/day for 6–24 months (5 days per week) [7].

Regime for patients requiring dental extractions who have previously undergone radiotherapy:

- Pentoxifylline: 400 mg twice daily.
- Tocopherol: 1000 IU once daily.

Begin this dual modality therapy one week before the procedure and continue for eight weeks.

If ORN develops then it may be worth considering the continuation of this for six months with the addition of clodronate (1600 mg/day) after three months if there is no response [10].

✔ **Evidence base** ORN96 Study Group [8]

- Efficacy and safety of hyperbaric oxygen for overt ORN of the mandible.
- Randomized, sequential, double-blind, placebo-controlled trial.
- Sixty-eight patients enrolled. The primary outcome was the number of patients who had recovered from ORN at one year.
- At second interim analysis the trial was stopped due to potentially worse outcomes in the HBO arm.
- 1 year, 19% had recovered in HBO arm and 32% in placebo arm.
- Patients with overt mandibular ORN do not benefit from hyperbaric oxygenation.

Source: data from Annane D, Depondt J, Aubert P, Villart M, Gehanno P, Gajdos P, Chevret S. Hyperbaric oxygen therapy for radionecrosis of the jaw: a randomized, placebo-controlled, double blind trial from the ORN96 Study Group, *Journal of Clinical Oncology* Volume 22, Issue 24, pp. 4893–4900 copyright © 2004 American Society of Clinical Oncology.

Classification systems for osteoradionecrosis

Various classification systems have been proposed and they differ in clinical value [4,5,11]. Some are applicable only to patients who have received hyperbaric oxygen therapy. Some systems are more suited to prospective evaluation. Systems based on clinical and radiographic involvement of the jaws have more clinical applicability.

Management of osteoradionecrosis based on Notani grading

Grade I

The clinical and radiological appearances of this early disease are demonstrated in Figures 3.1 and 3.2.

⊕ **Clinical tip** Management of Grade I osteoradionecrosis

- Lifestyle changes: avoidance of smoking, strict oral hygiene measures.
- Chlorhexidine mouth rinses.
- Judicious use of antibiotics.
- Minimal surgical debridement, avoiding unnecessary periosteal stripping.
- Consider the use of HBOT in carefully selected cases.
- Consider medical management with pentoxifylline and tocopherol. Clodronate not routinely used in early ORN.

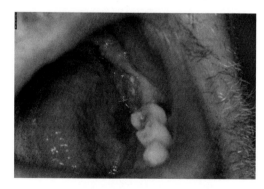

Figure 3.1 Exposed bone with surrounding erythematous oral mucosa. See colour plate section.

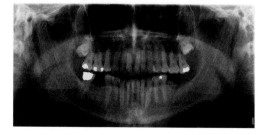

Figure 3.2 Osteoradionecrosis confined to the alveolar bone in the posterior lower left six region.

Grade II

The radiological appearance of this intermediate disease is demonstrated in Figure 3.3.

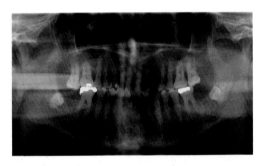

Figure 3.3 Osteoradionecrosis at the left angle of the mandible above the inferior dental nerve.

Grade III

The radiological and clinical features of this advanced disease are demonstrated in Figures 3.4 and 3.5.

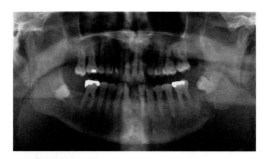

Figure 3.4 Osteoradionecrosis of the mandible resulting in full thickness involvement and pathological fracture.

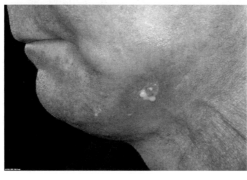

Figure 3.5 Extra-oral breach of the skin with discharge of pus and subsequent fistulation. See colour plate section.

✪ Learning point

Advanced ORN is both a clinical and social burden. Patients are often in severe pain and have difficulty in obtaining adequate nutrition. Multidisciplinary input is of the utmost importance and should include:

- Dietetics
- Speech and language therapy (SALT)
- Head and neck nurse specialist
- Pain specialist.

❝ Expert comment

Surgical reconstruction of Grade III ORN should not be underestimated. The challenges are numerous and multifactorial. Patients should have a detailed medical and anaesthetic review and often need several weeks of pre-operative optimization. The choice of free flap donor sites tends to be limited; either due to previous free flap harvest, vascular disease or lack of surgical expertise. The neck tends to be vessel depleted resulting in the need to use contralateral neck vessels, remote vessels (transverse cervical, internal mammary), or vein grafts. The surgical morbidity is therefore high; hence the need for well-informed surgical consent.

A final word from the expert

Osteoradionecrosis of the mandible is a very debilitating condition. Every effort should be made to prevent ORN. Grade I ORN can be successfully managed with conservative measures in a significant number of patients. Grade III ORN on the other hand requires radical surgery to obtain a satisfactory outcome. The decision-making process in Grade II ORN is probably the most difficult since there is often a dilemma between continued conservative management versus early radical surgery. Full cooperation of the patient is mandatory for a successful outcome in the management of all grades of ORN.

References

1. Wong JK, Wood RE, Mclean M. Conservative management of osteoradionecrosis. *Oral Surg Oral Med Oral Pathol Oral Radiol Endod* 1997; 84: 16–21.
2. Glanzmann C, Gratz KW. Radionecrosis of the mandible: a retrospective analysis of the incidence and risk factors. *Radiather Oncol* 1995; 36: 94–100.
3. Jacobson AS, Buchbinder D, Hu K, Urken ML. Paradigm shifts in the management of osteoradionecrosis of the mandible. *Oral Oncol* 2010; 46(11): 795–801.
4. Marx RE. A new concept in the treatment of osteoradionecrosis. *J Oral Maxillofac Surg* 1983; 41: 351–7.
5. Marx RE, Johnson RP. Studies in the radiobiology of osteoradionecrosis and their clinical significance. *Oral Surg Oral Med Oral Pathol* 1987; 64: 379–90.
6. Delanian S, Lefaix JL. The radiation induced fibroatrophic process: therapeutic perspective via the antioxidant pathway. *Radiother Oncol* 2004; 73(2): 119–31.
7. Delanian S, Depondt J, Lefaix JL. Major healing of refractory mandible osteoradionecrosis after treatment combining pentoxifylline and tocopherol: a phase II trial. *Head Neck* 2005; 27: 114–23.
8. Annane D, Depondt J, Aubert P, et al. Hyperbaric oxygen therapy for radionecrosis of the jaw: a randomized, placebo-controlled, double blind trial from the ORN96 Study Group. *J Clin Oncol* 2004; 22: 4893–900.
9. D'Souza J, Lowe D, Rogers SN. Changing trends and the role of medical management on the outcome of patients treated for osteoradionecrosis of the mandible: experience from a regional head and neck unit. *Br J Oral Maxillofac Surg.* 2014; 52(4): 356–62.
10. Lyons A, Ghazali N. Osteoradionecrosis of the jaws: current understanding of its pathophysiology and treatment. *Br J Oral Maxillofac Surg* 2008; 46: 653–60.
11. Notani K, Yamazaki Y, Kitada H, et al. Management of mandibular osteoradionecrosis corresponding to the severity of osteoradionecrosis and the method of radiotherapy. *Head Neck* 2003; 25(3): 181–6.
12. Shaw RJ, Dhanda J. Hyperbaric oxygen in the management of late radiation injury to the head and neck. Part I: treatment. *Br J Oral Maxillofac Surg* 2011; 49(1): 2–8.

SECTION 2

Cranio-maxillofacial trauma

4 Frontal sinus fractures

Rabindra Singh

ⓘ **Expert commentary** Lachlan Carter

Case history

A medically fit 20-year-old man presented to the Emergency Department with an injury to his forehead secondary to an assault involving multiple kicks to his face. There was no history of loss of consciousness and no nausea or vomiting.

The clinical examination revealed a noticeable depression on the right forehead. There was no evidence of paraesthesia over the forehead skin. The examination of the eyes revealed hypoglobus of the right eye with some degree of ptosis. The pupils were equal and reactive, the visual acuity on both eyes was unchanged, and there was no evidence of diplopia. He underwent orthoptic assessment, which revealed a slight restriction of elevation of the right eye possibly secondary to soft tissue oedema adjacent to the fracture. There was no evidence of cerebrospinal fluid leak.

A high-resolution computed tomogram (CT) was performed that revealed a displaced fracture of the anterior wall of the frontal bone on the right side, involving the anterior aspect of the right orbital roof (Figure 4.1). The posterior table of the frontal sinus was intact.

A detailed discussion followed on the treatment options, and the patient underwent open reduction and internal fixation of the fracture via a coronal approach 16 days post-injury to correct the forehead deformity. He made an uneventful recovery with

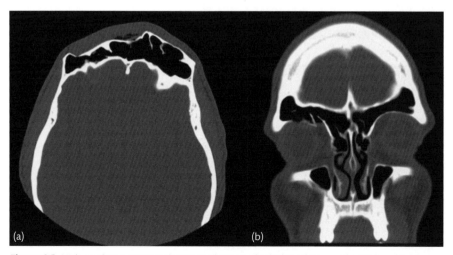

(a)   (b)

Figure 4.1 High-resolution computed tomography scan of right frontal sinus and orbital roof fractures. (a) Axial view, (b) coronal view.

good frontal bone contour and prominence. The globe position was symmetrical with a full range of movement and no diplopia. However, he had some paraesthesia over the midline of his scalp vertex behind the coronal incision (see Box 4.1).

Box 4.1 Operative note

1. A strip of hair was shaved to allow placement of a zigzag coronal incision extending from one superior aspect of the helix to the other, after injecting 8.8 ml of 2% lidocaine with 1:80,000 epinephrine.
2. The incision was deepened to the subgaleal layer and the flap was raised in a forward direction up to the superior temporal crest.
3. The right-sided incision was extended over the temporalis fascia above the level of the muscle split to facilitate access to the fracture site.
4. The flap was raised at subperiosteal level below the superior temporal crest and extended towards the superior orbital ridge, fully exposing the fracture (Figure 4.2). The intra-operative examination of the fracture revealed a comminuted anterior table fracture with intact frontonasal duct ostium.
5. The fracture was meticulously reduced and fixed with multiple 1 mm AO titanium plates and multiple 4 and 5 mm screws (Figure 4.3).
6. The closure of the wound was achieved with deep resorbable Vicryl (Ethicon Inc. US) and non-resorbable nylon skin sutures with two vacuum drains placed.
7. The patient was closely observed for any signs of post-operative retrobulbar haematoma or orbital compartment syndrome and was also prescribed broad-spectrum antibiotics, dexamethasone and nasal decongestants.

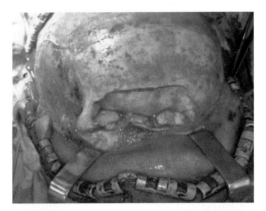

Figure 4.2 Comminuted fracture of the anterior wall of the frontal sinus and anterior orbital roof. See colour plate section.

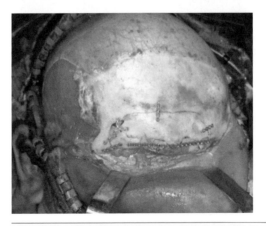

Figure 4.3 Fixation of right frontal sinus fracture with miniplates. See colour plate section.

✪ Learning point Embryology and anatomy of the frontal sinus

The frontal sinus begins to develop after two years of age and reaches the adult size at 15 years, while pneumatization continues until the age of 40 years when the final size is achieved. It becomes radiologically visible on plain films at the age of eight years. There is a wide variation in its form; it is absent in 4%, rudimentary in 5% and unilateral in 10% of the population [1–4]. The frontal sinus has one or more compartments and is lined by respiratory epithelium. It contains the foramina of Breschet on the posterior wall that are lined by the sinus mucosa and act as the path of potential intracranial spread of infection. The frontal sinus drains into the middle meatus through the frontonasal duct that is located on the posteromedial aspect of the floor of sinus. It has a variable course, and is more commonly a recess than a true duct that is only present in 15 % of the population [4]. The frontal sinus also drains indirectly into the middle meatus via the ethmoidal air cells.

✪ Learning point Management of frontal sinus fractures

The management of frontal sinus fracture is contentious as there are only a few prospective studies currently available and most series are from units analysing their data over many years. Due to the small number of cases in the studies and limited data on long-term follow-up, the quality of the current evidence is poor. Despite the lack of consensus on many aspects of frontal sinus fracture management, it is generally accepted that the aim of the management is to achieve a 'safe sinus', which means establishing normal sinus function, protecting intracranial structures and preventing complications.

Minimally displaced (<2 mm) fractures of the anterior or posterior table can be managed conservatively with nasal decongestants and long-term observation. The patients should be closely observed for the signs of sinusitis such as pain on movement and nasal discharge and also considered for a follow up with CT imaging at six weeks for signs of sinus opacification. The indications for surgical intervention are as follows:

- Anterior table displacement with significant forehead deformity.
- Frontonasal duct involvement/obstruction.
- Displacement of posterior table with underlying neurological injury.

✪ Learning point Classification of frontal sinus fractures [5]

Fracture of anterior table (displaced or undisplaced):

1. Fracture involving posterior table (displaced or undisplaced).
2. Fracture involving floor of sinus.
3. Fracture involving dural or cerebral damage.

Reproduced with permission from Bentley RP. Craniofacial trauma, including management of frontal sinus and nasoethmoidal injuries. In Langdon J PM et al. (eds), *Operative Oral and Maxillofacial Surgery*, Second Edition, Hodder and Stoughton Ltd, p. 513–530, Copyright © 2011.

✪ Learning point Complications of frontal sinus fractures

- Wound infection
- Chronic sinusitis (up to 60%) [5]
- Meningitis (6%) [6]
- Mucocoele/mucopyocoele
- Thrombosis of cavernous sinus
- Encephalitis
- Brain abscess

❝ Expert comment

The management of frontal sinus fractures is still an area of controversy that unfortunately is not aided by the poor level of current evidence. Anecdotally there is an increasing trend towards more conservative management, including cases with posterior wall fracture and/or frontonasal duct injury. Early non-surgical intervention for cerebrospinal fluid (CSF) leak with patient positioning, careful control of intracranial pressure and reduction in CSF pressure with a lumbar drain can mitigate the need for obliteration or cranialization of the frontal sinus.

✪ Learning point Anterior table fracture

If the anterior table is significantly displaced with resultant forehead deformity, an open reduction and fixation with 1–1.3 mm titanium plating system is indicated. The most common approach for the open procedure is via a coronal incision; however, an existing laceration may be used if adequate access is possible. Extending an existing laceration to expose the fracture is not recommended due to possible poor cosmetic result. Once exposed, the bony fragments may be elevated using Howarth elevators or by placing 2 mm screws into the main fragment and elevated using forceps. Occasionally, the bony fragment may need to be drilled free to allow adequate reduction. The bony fragments may be assembled on the table and transferred to reconstruct the fracture. Some authors have described endoscopic approach for reduction of the anterior table. Chen et al. [7] reported seven cases where two slit incisions were placed in the hair-bearing area, through which a 4 mm 30 degrees endoscope was inserted and subperiosteal dissection carried out to expose the fractures of the anterior table. The fractures were reduced and fixed with microplates endoscopically, achieving good aesthetic recontouring and acceptable scars. They argued that with this approach the complications of traditional coronal incision such as paraesthesia, scar and alopecia are avoided. However, this technique is only applicable in select cases where there is minimal displacement of the anterior table fracture.

Clinical tip

The diagnosis of frontonasal duct injury is therefore important and can be made using high-resolution CT pre-operatively, by an endoscopic method or by open intra-operative examination. Methylene blue dye may be used by placing it on the duct ostium on the sinus floor and checking its drainage onto the middle meatus by inserting a cotton bud to this level through the nose.

Expert comment

In terms of frontonasal duct injury, in fractures with no obvious cosmetic deficit, sinus outflow obstruction can be treated expectantly with endoscopic sinus surgery. In our practice, therefore, sinus obliteration for this type of injury is rarely undertaken. In cases with large frontal sinuses obliteration can be technically difficult to achieve and cranialization should be considered.

Learning point Frontonasal duct injury

Fracture of the floor of the sinus may result in damage to the frontonasal duct leading to impairment of the drainage system. The obstruction of the sinus may result in chronic sinusitis and formation of a mucocoele or mucopyocoele resulting in devastating consequences.

If there is a concern that obstruction of the duct is likely, then obliteration of the sinus and sealing of the duct orifice, or stenting of the duct can be considered. The stenting may be performed with tubes of different materials such as rubber, gold and silicone [8]. However, although it appears to be a simpler option, there is a concern of a high risk of long-term stenosis with this technique. We therefore recommend obliteration of the sinus cavity and sealing of the duct opening in the case of frontonasal duct obstruction. The mucosal lining is removed meticulously and the surface of the sinus is drilled over with a rotary instrument to ensure total extirpation of the sinus mucosa. The sinus cavity is then filled with a choice of variety of techniques that may include bone or fat graft, pericranial or galeal flap, temporalis muscle plug, or alloplastic materials such as Surgicel® (Ethicon Inc., US) or silicone hydroxyapatite [9–12]. We prefer a vascularized pericranial flap and autogenic bone graft due to the low risk of resorption and that it may be harvested from the calvarium which is easily accessed through the existing coronal incision. However, a significant quantity of bone may be required in the presence of a large sinus. In this instance the bone can be harvested from the iliac crest or alternative tissue utilized as mentioned previously. The previously widely used abdominal fat should be avoided due to variable levels of resorption and the potential for subsequent mucocoele formation. Keerl et al. [13] published a study of 11 patients where fat was used to obliterate the sinus cavity and post-operative magnetic resonance imaging performed from 4–24 months to assess its viability. They found that viable fat was present in only six patients. The remainder of the patients showed necrosed fat replaced by granulation and connective tissue. Weber et al. [14] also revealed over 80% fat resorption at mean follow-up of 24.1 months in over 50% of the patients.

Learning point Posterior table fracture

The most important determinants of the treatment choice in posterior table fractures are the degree of displacement, CSF leak, and the degree of comminution. The minimally displaced fractures with CSF leak are initially treated conservatively and the leak is expected to stop in approximately 50% of cases with non-surgical management [2]. Bed rest and head elevation is recommended to facilitate spontaneous resolution of the leak. If the leak persists after 5–7 days, an open approach for sinus obliteration and/or craniotomy for dural repair and cranialization are needed.

Clinical tip Posterior table fractures

The displaced fractures (greater than the thickness of posterior table or over 5 mm displacement) usually necessitate craniotomy for dural repair if a CSF leak is present. If the degree of comminution is over 30%, cranialization is preferred to obliteration of the sinus alone [15]. The cranialization involves removal of the posterior table and extirpation of the remaining sinus mucosa and creating a barrier between the intracranial structures and obliterated sinus cavity with a vascularized pericranial flap. In the long term, the frontal lobes will herniate into the space previously occupied by the frontal sinus.

Discussion

The frontal bone is extremely resilient to injury. They are a result of high-impact injury (most commonly road traffic collisions, followed by sports injuries) and represents 5–12 % of all facial fractures [1, 16, 17]. Anyone presenting with frontal sinus fractures should be viewed with a high suspicion for associated injuries. In over 75% of the patients with frontal sinus fractures neurological injuries such as closed or open head injury, cerebral contusions, pneumocephalus, haematomas, and dural tears may be present. The incidence of CSF leak is around 20% [2]. The incidences of other maxillofacial and ophthalmological injuries are 66% and 25%, respectively. Therefore, often these fractures need to be managed by a multidisciplinary team that may include maxillofacial, neurosurgical, ophthalmic surgeons and otolaryngologists. The most common type of frontal sinus fracture includes combined anterior and posterior table injury (55–67%) followed by isolated anterior table fracture in 33–39%. The least common involves posterior table fracture in isolation occurring in 6% of cases [15, 18].

> **ⓘ Expert comment**
>
> Inevitably there will be cases that require surgical correction. The case presented here highlights the need for thorough assessment and multidisciplinary management, even in the absence of brain injury or CSF leak. Although the patient had no posterior wall injury his fractures extended into the anterior orbital roof producing hypoglobus and restriction of upgaze. Orthoptic and ophthalmological assessment are important for baseline measure of globe position and motility and a significant number of periorbital bony injuries are associated with concomitant ocular injury.

Any patient suspected of frontal sinus fracture should be assessed as per the Advanced Trauma Life Support guidelines in the first instance. Loss of consciousness is common and patients suspected of head injury should have regular neurological observations. The patients commonly present with forehead laceration and any ecchymosis or haematoma on the forehead should raise the suspicion of frontal sinus injury. There may be sensory changes in the distribution of the supratrochlear and the supraorbital nerve and step deformity may be visible or palpable on the frontal bone. Any clear fluid through the nose or lacerations may suggest CSF leak and should be sampled for biochemical testing. Clear rhinorrhoea positive for beta-2 transferrin is diagnostic of a CSF leak. Apart from the CSF, only vitreous humour of the eye and the perilymph of the inner ear have been found to contain beta-2 transferrin [15]. A halo sign test may be performed that involves placing the suspected fluid on tissue paper. If any CSF is present it diffuses faster than blood, resulting in a clear halo around a bloody stain centrally. A simple glucose dipstick test may also be performed. High-resolution CT scan is the imaging of choice in suspected frontal sinus injury, providing an excellent view of the bony structures and also provides useful information to rule out any brain injury. The other investigations specific to suspected associated injuries described above may be needed.

The most controversial aspect of frontal sinus fracture management is whether or not the sinus needs to be extirpated in the case of possible frontonasal duct injury or displaced anterior or posterior table fracture. Carter et al. [19] carried out a systematic review of the literature to identify the effectiveness and safety of sinus preservation. They identified six retrospective and one prospective series (515 patients) and compared the outcome in terms of complications in patients who were treated with sinus obliteration or cranialization and patients who were treated with sinus preservation that included conservative treatment, endoscopic or open treatment with or without fixation. They found that the complications did not vary significantly between the two groups. They recommended sinus preservation in non-displaced or minimally displaced posterior table fractures with persistent CSF leak and displaced anterior table fractures with suspected frontonasal duct involvement. These scenarios would traditionally require sinus obliteration or cranialization. The limitations of this review, however, are that the level of evidence of studies included is poor. It may also be argued that the patients who received sinus preservation treatment may have sustained less severe injury, which in turn may have resulted in a decreased rate of complications, in which case the comparison between the two groups is unbalanced.

The use of antibiotics is another area of controversy in the management of frontal sinus fractures. Although empirical antibiotic regimen are frequently utilized the recent evidence is moving towards limiting antibiotic use.

⊘ **Evidence base:** Cochrane Review 2011 [20]

A recent Cochrane systematic review included five randomized controlled trials (RCTs) and 17 non-RCTs. The authors reported that there was no significant difference between antibiotic prophylaxis groups and control groups in terms of reduction of the frequency of meningitis, all-cause mortality, and meningitis-related mortality [20]. They concluded that the currently available evidence from RCTs does not support prophylactic antibiotic use in patients with basilar skull fractures, whether there is evidence of CSF leakage or not.

Source: data from Ratilal BO et al., Antibiotic prophylaxis for preventing meningitis in patients with basilar skull fractures, *Cochrane Database of Systematic Reviews* 2011, Issue 8, Art No.: CD004884, Copyright © 2011 The Cochrane Collaboration.

All patients who have sustained frontal sinus fractures require long-term follow-up regardless of whether they received conservative or surgical treatment. The duration of follow-up is again a contentious issue as complications may arise many years after the initial insult to the sinus. We recommend a CT scan a year after the injury to confirm that there is a clear sinus cavity, which will be an indication that the sinus drainage is adequate.

A final word from the expert

With the trend for more conservative management there is a need for adequate follow-up. Again this is an area of controversy as patients have been reported to develop mucocoele or mucopyocoele of the frontal sinus many years after the initial injury. A CT scan one year after injury/repair is recommended along with education of patients with respect to symptoms of frontal sinus outflow obstruction.

Frontal sinus fractures are not common and tend to be managed in major trauma centres. Excellent results can be achieved by a systematic multidisciplinary approach as described in this chapter. There is a need for collaboration between centres in order to improve the evidence base.

References

1. Rohrich RJ, Hollier LH. Management of frontal sinus fractures. Changing concepts. *Clin Plast Surg* 1992; 19(1): 219–32.
2. Yavuzer R, Sari A, Kelly CP, et al. Management of frontal sinus fractures. *Plast Reconstr Surg* 2005; 115(6): 79e–93e; discussion 4e–5e.
3. Aydinlioglu A, Kavakli A, Erdem S. Absence of frontal sinus in Turkish individuals. *Yonsei Med J* 2003; 44(2): 215–8.

4. Nambiar P, Naidu MD, Subramaniam K. Anatomical variability of the frontal sinuses and their application in forensic identification. *Clin Anat* 1999; 12(1): 16–19.

5. Bentley RP. Craniofacial trauma, including management of frontal sinus and nasoethmoidal injuries. In: Langdon J PM, Patel M, Brennan P, Ord R (eds) *Operative Oral and Maxillofacial Surgery* 2nd edition. London: Hodder & Stoughton Ltd 2011. p. 513–30.

6. Wallis A, Donald PJ. Frontal sinus fractures: a review of 72 cases. *Laryngoscope* 1988; 98(6 Pt 1): 593–8.

7. Chen DJ, Chen CT, Chen YR, Feng GM. Endoscopically assisted repair of frontal sinus fracture. *J Trauma* 2003; 55(2): 378–82.

8. Tiwari P, Higuera S, Thornton J, Hollier LH. The management of frontal sinus fractures. *J Oral Maxillofac Surg* 2005; 63(9): 1354–60.

9. Petruzzelli GJ, Stankiewicz JA. Frontal sinus obliteration with hydroxyapatite cement. *Laryngoscope* 2002; 112(1): 32–6.

10. Rohrich RJ, Mickel TJ. Frontal sinus obliteration: in search of the ideal autogenous material. *Plast Reconstr Surg* 1995; 95(3): 580–5.

11. Ducic Y, Stone TL. Frontal sinus obliteration using a laterally based pedicled pericranial flap. *Laryngoscope* 1999; 109(4): 541–5.

12. Parhiscar A, Har-El G. Frontal sinus obliteration with the pericranial flap. *Otolaryngol Head Neck Surg* 2001; 124(3): 304–7.

13. Keerl R, Weber R, Kahle G, et al. Magnetic resonance imaging after frontal sinus surgery with fat obliteration. *Journal Laryngol Otol* 1995; 109(11): 1115-9.

14. Weber R, Draf W, Keerl R, et al. Osteoplastic frontal sinus surgery with fat obliteration: technique and long-term results using magnetic resonance imaging in 82 operations. *Laryngoscope* 2000; 110(6): 1037–44.

15. Tollefson TT. Frontal sinus fractures. Medscape; 2012 [cited 201211.05.2012].

16. Gerbino G, Roccia F, Benech A, Caldarelli C. Analysis of 158 frontal sinus fractures: current surgical management and complications. *J Craniomaxillofac Surg* 2000; 28(3): 13–9.

17. Bell RB, Dierks EJ, Brar P, et al. A protocol for the management of frontal sinus fractures emphasizing sinus preservation. *J Oral Maxillofac Surg* 2007; 65(5): 825–39.

18. Rodriguez ED, Stanwix MG, Nam AJ, et al. Twenty-six-year experience treating frontal sinus fractures: a novel algorithm based on anatomical fracture pattern and failure of conventional techniques. *Plast Reconstr Surg* 2008; 122(6): 1850–66.

19. Carter KB Jr, Poetker DM, Rhee JS. Sinus preservation management for frontal sinus fractures in the endoscopic sinus surgery era: a systematic review. *Craniomaxillofac Trauma Reconstr* 2010; 3(3): 141–9.

20. Ratial BO, Costa J, Sampaio C, Pappamikail L. Antibiotic prophylaxis for preventing meningitis in patients with basilar skull fractures. The Cochrane database of systematic reviews 2011; (8): CD004884. Epub 2011/08/13.

5 Management of panfacial injuries: bottom up or top down

Richard Burnham

Expert commentary Christopher Bridle

Case history

Our patient is a healthy 34-year-old male, who, while wearing all modern protective measures fell off his motorcycle at approximately 80 mph and collided with a wooden fence. He was attended to at the scene by a first responder and the air ambulance was dispatched to manage and recover him to the Regional Level 1 Trauma Centre.

In the field the patient was intubated with an oral endotracheal tube, cervical spine triple immobilization was deployed, bilateral chest drains were placed, the long bones of the lower extremities were splinted bilaterally along with the pelvis, and he was resuscitated with intravenous fluid according to the Advanced Trauma Life Support (ATLS) algorithm.

He arrived in the emergency department resuscitation room and his primary survey was commenced. He was deemed stable enough for a computed tomography (CT) scan, which led to a decision for immediate abdominal surgery. This scan, while including his head and cervical spine, did not cover the entirety of the face, so that the full extent of his maxillofacial injury could not be ascertained.

The patient presented with the following injuries:

- head injury with cerebral contusion
- maxillofacial injuries:
  - complex and fragmented Le Fort III (total facial dysjunction)
  - bilateral comminuted condyle of mandible fractures
  - mandibular symphyseal fracture
  - soft tissue laceration overlying chin
- bilateral haemopneumothorax
- pulmonary contusion
- splenic laceration
- mesenteric artery bleed
- bilateral distal radial fractures
- fractured pelvis
- left-sided fractured femur
- bilateral tibia and fibula fractures.

These injuries required repeat life- and limb-saving surgery, and the role of maxillofacial surgery in this patient's immediate care was minimal, so as not to add to his surgical burden. The patient's condition was such that the opportunity for

> **⊕ Clinical tip** Avoiding the 'missed opportunity'
>
> This phenomenon of the 'missed opportunity' to include the facial skeleton in trauma scan when there are signs of facial fracture is well known [1]. It is helpful to remind emergency department staff of the importance of including this anatomy when appropriate. This prevents unnecessary time delays in treatment, prevents the logistical difficulty of CT scanning patients in the intensive care unit (ICU) and lowers radiation doses [2].

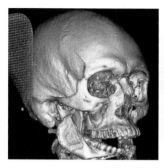 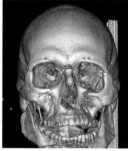 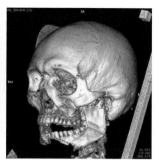

Figure 5.1 Three-dimensional reconstruction of computed tomogram demonstrating panfacial fractures. See colour plate section.

maxillofacial surgical intervention was not plausible until day ten of his ICU stay. During this time he had a repeat CT of his head, which provided his maxillofacial team the opportunity to include a fine cut CT of his facial skeleton with appropriate reformatting (Figure 5.1 and Box 5.1).

Box 5.1 Operative note

An awake fibre optic nasal intubation was employed in this case. Access was achieved via a coronal flap, which may be necessary for complex facial fractures [20], a vestibular maxillary facial degloving incision, and bilateral transconjunctival incisions with lateral cantholysis lid swing for the maxilla. A pre-existing submental laceration, which was extended to access the symphyseal fracture was employed with bilateral retromandibular approaches to access the condylar fractures.

From the pre-operative CT scans it was visualized that both the midface and mandible were grossly comminuted, and for this case either sequencing method could be utilized but a top-down method was selected. This was employed as the loss of posterior face height due to fracture of the condyles and displacement of the maxilla on the cranial base had led to a significant anterior open bite in conjunction with displacement at the symphysis. Sequential reduction of fractures at the frontozygomatic suture, zygomatic arch, frontonasal suture, orbital rims and maxillary buttresses resulted in anatomical midfacial reconstruction.

The operative technique followed the sequencing discussed and the fixation utilized titanium miniplates for support of the midfacial buttresses. The mandible fractures were addressed by intraoperative rigid MMF and miniplate fixation at the condyles for posterior mandibular height restoration. Finally, to manage the comminuted left parasymphysis, a combination of a miniplate to aid reduction and stability was used prior to placement of a load-bearing trauma plate (2.0 mm thick). The soft tissues were then carefully redraped and closed.

✪ Learning point Epidemiology of facial fractures

The incidence of complex midface fractures has decreased over the last few decades with the improvement in Health and Safety at Work [3,4] and the legislation for seat belt use, allied to advances in motor vehicle safety with crumple zone and airbags. However, we still see some impressive fractures of the midface within the specialty of oral and maxillofacial surgery.

These are usually due to significant and sustained assault, road traffic accident, industrial injury, or military action. All of these modes of injury represent high- or low-velocity transfer of significant forces to the facial skeleton, as well as the rest of the body.

✪ Learning point Classification of midfacial fractures

The face and underlying skeleton in normal patients demonstrates symmetry, which is demonstrated by the pairing of bones within the midface. There is significant support of structures and protection by solid bony pillars and columns therein [2]. The disruption patterns of these pillars form the basis of a number of midface classifications.

Le Fort Classification [5]

This classification was developed in 1901 by René Le Fort based on his work with cadaveric facial skeletons. It is divided into the well-known trio of fracture patterns. There may be disparity between the left and right regarding the level of the fracture but all will demonstrate disruption at the pterygo-maxillary junction.

- Le Fort I: horizontal fracture with separation of the alveolus of the maxilla and palate from the cranial base.
- Le Fort II: pyramidal fracture that includes the Le Fort I fragment and separation at the nasofrontal suture.
- Le Fort III: total separation of the midface from the cranial base.

The issue with the system is that these patterns are not often seen as distinct entities in clinical practice and misses other common injuries patterns e.g. zygomatic complex fractures.

This has led to the development of alternative systems, which act to encompass the full spectrum of midface trauma into one and thus tend to be cumbersome (e.g. the Buitrago-Tellez system) [6].

There has also been a drive to subdivide the midface development of more localized systems, as for the naso–orbito–ethmoid region by Markowitz [7].

Guerrissi [8] produced an inventive but slightly complex system in which injuries are classified thus:

- **Group I:** potentially life-threatening injuries.
- **Group II:** assesses functional and aesthetic severity of soft tissues and skeletal injuries in the facial region.

The final combined score gives a grade (I to III) of difficulty in treatment and evaluates long-term functional and aesthetic sequelae and probability of success of treatment.

✪ Learning point History of injury

The patient can give you valuable information about the aetiology of their injuries, which needs careful documentation. The patient's medical, social and drug history, including tetanus status, must be addressed, as these may aid in treatment planning. For example, a patient with recurrent fits may not be suitable for maxillomandibular fixation (MMF) or external fixation.

Key questions include:

- malocclusion
- reduced visual acuity
- diplopia
- pain on looking around
- paraesthesia of forehead, midface and/or mental region.

Often in polytrauma the patient is intubated, so a collateral history from the notes or ambulance crew can assist in assessment. It may be possible for the family to bring a photograph of the patient prior to their injuries, so as to visualize their true features.

✪ Learning point Examination

The examination of the patient with maxillofacial injuries forms part of the secondary survey in ATLS. While modern CT scans will guide definitive treatment, it is early assessment that elicits emergent issues, such as ocular injuries. The examination must be carried out in full on all patients and the lists below highlight some useful features.

(continued)

Soft tissues:

- Look for laceration and contusions associated with bony injuries.
- Assess for tissue loss.
- Look for facial nerve weakness.
- Look signs of parotid duct injury.

Eyes:

- Look for subconjuctival haemorrhage without posterior limit.
- Look for iris asymmetry.
- Signs of retrobulbar haemorrhage.
- Bowstring test for canthal detachment.
- Telecanthus.

Zygomatic complex:

- Look for asymmetry.
- Look for periorbital ecchymosis.

Maxilla:

- Look for bruising in the buccal vestibule and torn palatal mucosa indicating a potentially split palate.
- Palpate for movement of the maxilla and assess if this is associated with movement at the:
  - anterior nasal spine in a Le Fort I
  - frontonasal suture in a Le Fort II
  - frontozygomatic suture in a Le Fort III
  - transverse instability with a split palate.
- Percussion of the maxilla when associated with a fracture is said to produce a 'cracked cup' tone, but the practicality of this is questionable.

Nose:

- Look for loss of the frontonasal projection.
- Look for an upturned tip (piggy nose).
- Look for CSF rhinorrhoea.
- Look for septal haematoma.

Ears:

- Look for CSF otorrhoea.
- Look for Battle's sign.

Mandible:

- Look for signs of mandibular fracture:
  - sublingual haematoma
  - step deformity
  - gingival tears.

Occlusion and dentition

- Look for damage to the dentition: fractures, displacement or dento-alveolar fragments.
- Look for missing teeth and account for any acutely missing units.
- Look at the quality of the dentition. A patient with grossly decayed or periodontally involved teeth may require extractions.
- Look for steps in the occlusion.
- Look at the occlusion; often if the posterior maxilla is displaced in a caudal direction there will be anterior open bite.

➕ **Clinical tip** Immediate life saving measures with midfacial fractures: Airway

The patient with a significant facial fracture can present with a threatened or potentially at-risk airway for a number of reasons including:

- reduced level of consciousness
- bleeding
- distortion of the oropharynx due to swelling and midfacial movement.

However, the conscious patient can often place themselves in an upright position and with head down, so as to maintain a patent airway. It is vital therefore not to simply lay this patient flat and occlude their airway. Simple measures can be deployed to aid in airway management with disimpaction of the maxillary fracture and high volume aspiration. If the patient does need intubation it is wise for senior anaesthetic support to be present as an awake fibre optic nasal intubation may be the induction method of choice and surgical readiness for a surgical airway is prudent [9,10].

➕ **Clinical tip** Bleeding from the midface

Bleeding from midface fractures can be significant and difficult to control. There may be laceration of branches of the external carotid artery, but this is very rare [11]. Simple measures often have good effect on local bleeding such as:

- disimpacting the maxilla
- anterior and posterior nasal packing
- placement of bite blocks for pressure
- tacking soft tissue wounds.

In more significant and sustained bleeding it can be necessary to either tie off the external carotid artery on the affected side or more usually utilize interventional radiology to provide embolization of the bleeding vessel [12].

➕ **Clinical tip** Operative airway

The patient will need to be intubated in such a way as to allow MMF during the operative phase. However, in cases where patients are not dentate or have no meaningful occlusion, an oral tube is tolerable.

Therefore airway options include:

- Oral endotracheal intubation – where MMF is not required.
- Nasal endotracheal intubation – with a change to oral for nasal surgery at the end if MMF is required.
- Submental positioning of an oral tube [13,14].
- Surgical tracheostomy, which may be appropriate in prolonged MMF or patient whose extensive injuries will preclude from a conventional airway.

🔠 **Expert comment**

The decision to treat these fractures operatively next requires the discussion as to whether to treat the fractures with closed reduction or open reduction. With the advent of miniplate technology most midface fractures will undergo an open reduction and internal fixation, but there is still a role for closed reduction with external fixation in cases of:

- severe comminution
- wound contamination
- avulsion and loss of hard tissue at the time of injury
- significant medical history.

⭐ **Learning point** Access to the facial skeleton

The level and severity of injury will dictate the access required. However, it is imperative to ensure that the incision employed minimizes further morbidity and maximizes aesthetic outcome, while not hindering the surgical goals of treatment [15].

The methods to access the facial skeleton from cranial to caudal include:

Coronal flap [16]

Temporal/Gillies approach

(continued)

Upper eyelid:

- lateral eyebrow
- upper blepharoplasty

Lower eyelid:

- transconjuctival with or without:
  - lateral canthotomy
  - transcaruncular
- subcilliary
- midtrial
- infra-orbital

Nose:

- closed
  - transfixion incision
- open
  - transcutaneous:
  - Lynch incision
  - glabellar incision, Gull wing

Buccal vestibule/intra-oral incision

Existing laceration

Endoscopic

⊕ **Learning point** Sequencing of fracture reduction

The logical method by which complex facial fractures [17] are restored is split into two groups:

- **Bottom up:**

This sequence relies on the establishment of a normal dental occlusion as the baseline via rigid MMF. Subsequently, repair of any mandibular fractures and then maxillary fractures are undertaken. The repair then proceeds from caudal to cranial with the hopes of restoring normal anatomy. This method of sequencing still lends itself to the treatment of the patient with closed reduction.

- **Top down:**

This sequencing process requires the anatomical reconstruction of the facial pillars and columns as described by Gruss [18], from a cranial to caudal direction and finishes with the re-establishment of the dental occlusion. This method of sequencing has become increasingly widely used according to the following steps:

1. Calvarium, orbital roof, frontal bone, and sinus.
2. Zygomatic arch for anterior facial projection.
3. Zygomatic frontal suture for vertical height.
4. Inferior orbital rim for transverse facial width.
5. Zygomatic and piriform buttresses for vertical height and support of the maxilla.
6. Orbital walls.
7. Nasal bones.
8. Maxillomandibular fixation.
9. Mandibular fractures.
10. Soft tissue repair.

The issue comes in that if there is a small discrepancy at the top then the effect can be notable, resulting in a significant malocclusion.

- **Nasoethmoidal (NOE) fractures:**

This fracture pattern has caused a great deal of difficulty in its management and the sequence of NOE fracture repair is usually the end point of midfacial fracture treatment.

✅ **Evidence base** Management of NOE injuries

Ellis has described eight steps required to successfully treat these potentially difficult fractures [19].

1. Surgical exposure.
2. Identification of the medial canthal tendon / tendon-bearing bone fragment.
3. Reduction / reconstruction of medial orbital rim.
4. Reconstruction of the medial orbital wall.
5. Transnasal canthopexy.
6. Reduction of septal fractures.
7. Nasal dorsum reconstruction / augmentation.
8. Soft tissue adaptation.

Reprinted from Journal of Oral and Maxillofacial Surgery, Volume 51, Issue 5, Ellis E 3rd. Sequencing treatment for naso-orbito-ethmoid fractures, pp. 543-558, Copyright © 1993 Elsevier, with permission from Elsevier, http://www.sciencedirect.com/science/article/pii/S0278239110805129.

The patient subsequently returned to the ward. He remained as an inpatient for three weeks following his surgery for orthopaedic rehabilitation. Post-operative CT demonstrated anatomical reduction of the facial fractures (Figure 5.2).

On review at six months post-surgery he was well with normal mouth opening and an even bilateral occlusion. His vision has returned to the pre-morbid status. He has scars from the original injury and surgery, but was satisfied with his appearance.

✪ **Learning point** Secondary procedure and rehabilitation

There is a need to provide the patient the best possible care, which does not always imply the most extensive operation. An unwell patient with significant facial fractures may not be fit enough to undergo extensive maxillofacial surgery. Therefore it becomes a matter of providing a treatment plan tailored to that patient's current condition and if they survive provide secondary reconstruction.

The role of further intervention in these patients can be grouped into two categories, which affect a number of areas:

● Aesthetic:
  o Camouflage
  o Scar revision
  o Facial reanimation (static or dynamic)
  o Asymmetry correction

● Functional
  o Occlusal rehabilitation (e.g. with dental implants)
  o Improve mouth opening
  o Orbital volume correction for diplopia.

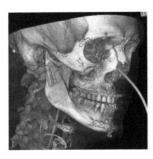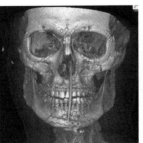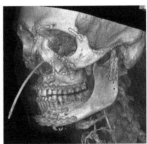

Figure 5.2 Three-dimensional reconstruction of CT illustrating the post-operative appearance. See colour plate section.

Discussion

As with all fields of medicine and surgery, the treatment of facial fractures and the evolution of treatment is often technology driven and has led to a number of advances and potential advances in patient care, which are demonstrated below:

- Stereolithic model
- Computer assisted design and manufacture (CAD/CAM)
- Computer assisted pre-operative planning
  - Mirroring for unilateral defects
  - Virtual implants for bilateral defects
  - Bespoke design for bony defects
- Bespoke and pre-bent plates [21]
- Resorbable plates
- Computer assisted surgery
- Endoscopic assistance [22]
- Navigation [23]
- Intraoperative CT.

It is hoped that with these adjuncts becoming more widely employed that complex midfacial fractures will be more successfully managed and demonstrate improved outcomes.

⊕ **Clinical tip** Management of panfacial fractures

- Obtaining a recent patient photograph from prior to the injury will tell you what you are aiming for in the patient's treatment
- Do not forget to assess the 'often overlooked' sites such as the occiput of the scalp for lacerations.
- Ensure that a high-quality fine cut (1 mm slices) CT of the facial anatomy is performed at the time of presentation. Standard reformatting should include coronal, sagittal and three-dimensional views to aid in treatment planning.
- Patients with midface fractures require pre-operative ophthalmology and orthoptic assessment prior to surgery to assess the eye and its movement, where appropriate.
- Ensure adequate exposure to the facial skeleton, so as to ensure adequate access while minimizing morbidity and maximizing aesthetic outcomes.
- It can be necessary in Le Fort injuries to ensure complete fracture on one or both sides to allow anatomical reduction to occur.
- A key point to midface correction is to assess the lateral orbital wall for adequate reduction; as if this area is not correctly reduced the rest of the facial skeleton will be misaligned [20].

✓ **Evidence base [5]**

Rene Le Fort was a French surgeon working in the 19th Century. He produced one of the first papers on midface fracture patterns that is the 'gold standard' used today.

He studied the fracture patterns produced by blunt trauma of different grades applied from a variety of directions to cadaveric heads, which he then dissected. This paper produced the seminal classification of midface fracture, although not without flaws.

Source: data form Le Fort R, Etude experimental sur les fractures de la machoir superiure: Parts I, II, III, Rev Chir, Volume 23, pp., 201, 360, 479, 1901.

> ✪ **Learning point**
>
> - The face is a 'crumple zone' to prevent transfer of significant force to the brain and skull [24].
> - High-velocity injuries are associated with potential tissue loss and the need for grafting.
> - Patients are treated along the ATLS algorithm and while maxillofacial assessment forms part of the secondary survey our skills and clinical knowledge may be required in airway management and control of haemorrhage.
> - Facial fractures are associated with 45.5% head injury and 9.7% cervical spine injury [25].
> - Patients with significant systemic injuries may not heal as predictably due to the toll of recovery from multiple operations, catabolic state and malnutrition.

✔ **Evidence base**　Complex maxillary fractures: role of buttress reconstruction and immediate bone grafting [18]

The paper was based on the surgical management of over 500 patients with midface fractures between 1978 and 1984. The basis of their treatment was the anatomical reduction and direction fixation of the facial buttresses of the skull in a vertical, horizontal and sagittal direction.

This led to a simple and standardized method of treating these patterns of fractures that could be applied to all injuries including complex cases, such as edentulous patients and those with condyle fractures. This has become the basis of sequencing for midface fractures in most units.

Source: data from Gruss JS and Mackinnon SE, Complex maxillary fractures: role of buttress reconstruction and immediate bone grafts, Plastic Reconstructive Surgery, Volume 78, Issue 1, pp. 9-22, Copyright © 1986 American Society of Plastic Surgeons.

A final word from the expert

Whatever the injury suffered in the midface, from a simple nasal bone fracture to complex panfacial fracture, it is imperative that every surgical step is taken with the forethought of maximizing the benefit while minimizing the potential morbidity. An understanding of the mechanism of injury is paramount, as this will determine the level of energy imparted to the patient and the predictability of the injuries. In complex midfacial and craniofacial trauma it is important to re-establish key anatomical landmarks. The frontozygomatic suture is more than often a pivotal landmark, together with the reconstruction of the anteroposterior length of the zygomatic arch. Once these landmarks are restored the buttresses can be addressed, with the nose and orbital rims often then being the final areas to resolve. In cases where the mandible is intact do not hesitate to utilize maxillomandibular fixation to achieve arch form and occlusion. The absolute key to panfacial injuries is to achieve good reduction and secure fixation at the first attempt. Failure to do so may result in subsequent revision procedures that will become increasingly more difficult. Access is key and good exposure of the fractures, without compromise, will facilitate reduction and fixation. Such access is readily achieved via well-hidden incisions such as the transconjunctival approach with lateral cantholysis, intra-oral incisions and a well-executed coronal flap.

References

1. Burnham R, Bhandari R, Bridle C. Review of CT imaging of the maxillofacial region in trauma cases. *Br J Oral Maxillofac Surg* Vol. 47, Issue 7, e 33.
2. Holmgren EP, Dierks EJ, Assael LA, et al. Facial soft tissue injuries as an aid to ordering a combination head and facial computed tomography in trauma patients. *J Oral Maxillofac Surg* 2005; 63(5): 651–4.

3. Boffano P, Kommers SC, Karagozoglu KH, Forouzanfar T. Aetiology of maxillofacial fractures: a review of published studies during the last 30 years. *Br J Oral Maxillofac Surg* 2014; 52(10): 901–6.

4. Ellis E 3rd, Moos KF, el-Attar A. Ten years of mandibular fractures: an analysis of 2,137 cases. *Oral Surg Oral Med Oral Pathol* 1985; 59(2): 120–9.

5. Le Fort RL. Etude expérimentale sur les fractures de la mâchoire supérieure. *Rev Chir Paris* 1901; 23: 208–27.

6. Buitrago-Tellez CH, Schilli W, Bohnert M, et al. A comprehensive classification of craniofacial fractures: postmortem and clinical studies with two- and three-dimensional computed tomography. *Injury* 2002; 33(8): 651–68.

7. Markowitz BL, Manson PN, Sargent L, et al. Management of the medial canthal tendon in nasoethmoid orbital fractures: the importance of the central fragment in classification and treatment. *Plast Reconstr Surg* 1991; 87(5): 843–53.

8. Guerrissi JO. Maxillofacial injuries scale. *J Craniofac Surg* 1996; 7(2): 130–2.

9. Ghabach MB, Abou Rouphael MA, Roumoulian CE, Helou MR. Airway management in a patient with Le Fort III Fracture. *Saudi J Anaesth* 2014; 8(1): 128–30.

10. Perry M, Morris C. Advanced trauma life support (ATLS) and facial trauma: can one size fit all? Part 2: ATLS, maxillofacial injuries and airway management dilemmas. *Int J Oral Maxillofac Surg* 2008; 37(4): 309–20.

11. Dean NR, Ledgard JP, Katsaros J. Massive hemorrhage in facial fracture patients: definition, incidence, and management. *Plast Reconstr Surg* 2009; 123(2): 680–90.

12. Yang WG, Tsai TR, Hung CC, Tung TC. Life-threatening bleeding in a facial fracture. *Ann Plast Surg* 2001; 46(2): 159–62.

13. Vidya B, Cariappa KM, Kamath AT. Current perspectives in intra operative airway management in maxillofacial trauma. *J Maxillofac Oral Surg* 2012; 11(2): 138–43.

14. Hernandes Altemir F. The submental route for endotracheal intubation. A new technique. *J Maxillofac Surg* 1986; 14(1): 64–5.

15. Ellis E, Zide MF. Surgical Approaches to the Facial Skeleton. New York: Williams and Williams 1995.

16. Zhang QB, Dong YJ, Li ZB, Zhao JH. Coronal incision for treating zygomatic complex fractures. *J Craniomaxillofac Surg* 2006; 34(3): 182–5.

17. Manson PN, Clark N, Robertson B, et al. Subunit principles in midface fractures: the importance of sagittal buttresses, soft-tissue reductions, and sequencing treatment of segmental fractures. *Plast Reconstr Surg* 1999; 103(4): 1287–306.

18. Gruss JS, Mackinnon SE. Complex maxillary fractures: role of buttress reconstruction and immediate bone grafts. *Plast Reconstr Surg* 1986; 78(1): 9–22.

19. Ellis E 3rd. Sequencing treatment for naso-orbito-ethmoid fractures. *J Oral Maxillofac Surg* 1993; 51(5): 543–58.

20. Alsuhaibani AH.Orbital Fracture: Significance of lateral wall. *Saudi J Ophthalmol* 2010; 24(2): 49–55.

21. Mustafa SF, Evans PL, Bocca A, et al. Customized titanium reconstruction of post-traumatic orbital wall defects: a review of 22 cases. *Int J Oral Maxillofac Surg* 2011; 40(12): 1357–62.

22. Kellman RM, Schmidt C. The paranasal sinuses as a protective crumple zone for the orbit. *Laryngoscope* 2009; 119(9): 1682–90.

23. Miki T, Wada J, Haraoka J, Inaba I. Endoscopic transmaxillary reduction and balloon technique for blowout fractures of the orbital floor. *Minim Invasive Neurosurg* 2004; 47(6): 359–64.

24. Morrison CS, Taylor HO, Sullivan SR. Utilization of intraoperative 3D navigation for delayed reconstruction of orbitozygomatic complex fractures. *J Craniofac Surg* 2013; 24(3): e 284–6.

25. Mithani SK, St-Hiliare H, Brooke BS, et al. Predictable patterns of intracranial and cervical spine injury in craniomaxillofacial trauma: analysis of 4786 patients. *Plast Reconstr Surg* 2009; 123(4): 1293–301.

6 Adult orbital wall fracture repair

Richard Burnham

⊕ Expert commentary Christopher Bridle

Case history

A 27-year-old medically fit and well male was intoxicated when he became embroiled in an argument and received a single blow with a fist to the right eye. He subsequently presented to the local Emergency Department two days following the injury.

He was complaining of significant orbital discomfort and irritation of the globe. At this point the emergency department staff using slit lamp examination noted a corneal abrasion. He was further investigated by means of occipito-mental plain radiographs and referred on to the department of oral and maxillofacial surgery with a provisional diagnosis of a right zygomatic complex fracture.

> **⊕ Clinical tip**
>
> Any relevant ophthalmic or medical history may lead the surgeon to tread cautiously in such scenarios. A patient with an orbital fracture who is on warfarin or other anticoagulant may warrant admission for regular eye observations. This is especially pertinent if the patient is intoxicated and history and examination prove difficult. There are a number of key symptoms to enquire about where an orbital fracture exists:
>
> - symptoms suggestive of retrobulbar haemorrhage
> - visual impairment
> - diplopia
> - pain on eye movements
> - numbness of the infra-orbital nerve
> - associated maxillofacial or ophthalmic injuries.

Following assessment by the maxillofacial team the following signs were noted:

- periorbital ecchymosis
- subconjunctival haemorrhage with no posterior limit
- paraesthesia of the infra-orbital nerve
- normal visual acuity on a Snellen chart
- discomfort on elevation of the globe
- diplopia on upward gaze.

He was diagnosed with a right orbital floor and medial orbital wall fracture in addition to a minimally displaced fracture of the superior orbital rim. He was advised to not blow his nose to prevent surgical emphysema and to sleep with the bed elevated. The team organized for him to have a fine cut computed tomogram (CT) scan of his midface with coronal and sagittal reformatting (Figure 6.1). Ophthalmology follow-up for his corneal abrasion was arranged and a request for a formal Hess chart was made. He then proceeded to operative intervention (Box 6.1).

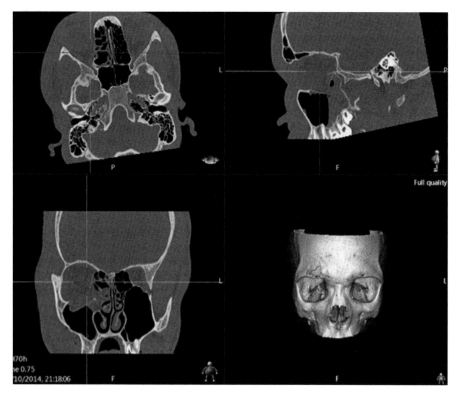

Figure 6.1 Axial, sagittal, coronal and three-dimensional reformatting of CT showing a right orbital floor fracture. See colour plate section.

> ⭐ **Learning point** Clinical anatomy
>
> The orbit is formed of two parts, the first of which is the outer frame. The outer frame is a metaphorical square of dense bone formed from the frontal, zygomatic and maxillary bones. This acts as a support and protection for the orbital contents. This outer rim is weakest at the zygomatico-frontal suture, which is a likely point of fracture and key point of fixation in zygomatic complex fractures.
>
> Secondly, within this outer ring the four bony walls of the orbit converge toward the orbital apex to form a pyramidal shape, with the medial wall and floor merging from distinct entities. The medial wall (lamina papyracea) and orbital floor are much weaker and this is where the majority of fractures occur.

> ➕ **Clinical tip**
>
> A positive Hess chart shows restriction on the affected side and over compensation of movement on the unaffected side (Herring's Law).

> ⭐ **Learning point** Orbital anatomy
>
> Knowledge of clinical anatomy of the orbit is essential to navigate this structure and in-depth description is beyond the scope of this chapter. However, some key reference points and features include:
>
> - The orbital floor has in the anterior one-third a concavity and in the posterior two-thirds a convexity, which are essential to reconstruct.
> - Position of the anterior ethmoidal artery is 10 mm from the rim.
> - Position of the posterior ethmoidal artery is 25 mm from the rim.
> - Inferior orbital fissure is 20 mm from the rim.
> - Superior orbital fissure is zygomatico-frontal suture.
> - Optic canal is 42 mm from the rim.
> - Globe volume is 8 ml.
> - Orbital volume is 30 ml.

> ⭐ **Learning point** Epidemiology
>
> Fractures of the orbit are common occurring in approximately 36% of all facial fractures [1]. They can be the result of various aetiologies, but the majority are sadly, secondary to inter-personal violence [2, 3] clustered amongst young males. They also occur in road traffic accidents, sports injuries and accidental falls, with respective decreasing frequency.

⊘ Evidence base The 'deep orbit' by Evans [4]

- If the orbit is severely disrupted then the concept of 'safe distances' (distances from the rim which are considered safe to dissect) are of limited value.
- The deep orbit begins at the anterior limit of the inferior orbital fissure.
- Anatomical landmarks are hard and soft tissue structures:
  - o infra-orbital nerve
  - o inferior orbital fissure
  - o the greater wing of the sphenoid
  - o the orbital plate of the palatine bone.
- These four landmarks are present in almost all non-penetrating orbital trauma cases.
- If the defect in the orbital wall is not fully exposed this will yield inadequate outcomes.
- It is the relationship between these structures that are of key importance rather than absolute distances.

Source: data from Evans BT, Webb AAC. Post-traumatic orbital reconstruction: Anatomical landmarks and the concept of the deep orbit. *British Journal of Oral and Maxillofacial Surgery* Volume 45, Issue 3, pp. 183–189, Copyright © 2006, The British Association of Oral and Maxillofacial Surgeons.

✪ Learning point Biomechanics of orbital wall fractures

Orbital fractures can be broadly classified into two groups:

1. Those associated with a fracture of the outer orbital rim:
   a. nasoethmoid fractures
   b. zygomatic complex fractures
   c. frontal bone fracture
   d. nasomaxillary fractures.
2. Those not associated with a fracture of the outer orbital rim
   This second group represent the true 'blow-in' and 'blow-out' fractures where a fracture occurs in isolation to the outer frame. There are two main theories to this mechanism of injury:
   a. Hydraulic theory: a blow to the globe leads to a raised intra-orbital pressure and displacement of the globe to the wall, resulting in the orbital wall giving way at its weakest point so that the globe itself is protected. This is a blow-out fracture and requires intact orbital rings. In the most extreme cases the globe can be forced from the orbit and into adjacent sites, such as the maxillary sinus [5].
   b. Buckling theory: a blow to the strong outer frame of the orbit is dissipated to the orbital floor, and while this force is not strong enough to fracture the outer frame it causes disruption and fracture of the inner frame and therefore an orbital wall fracture.

❻ Expert comment

It is imperative to have a good knowledge of the orbit's clinical anatomy, as this will lead you to success in reconstruction of any associated fracture. In addition it is essential to ensure that you are not missing an associated fracture of the outer bony rim of the orbit and most importantly to exclude an orbital compartment syndrome. If there is any doubt about this reassessment over time is crucial.

✚ Clinical tip 'Key area of Hammer'

Reconstruction of the inferomedial aspect of the floor is vital to achieve volume restoration of the orbit. The use of the infra-orbital nerve and orbital plate of the palatine bone enable localization and exposure of this region [6].

✚ Clinical tip

Permissive intra-operative hypotension allows for good haemostasis, but this must be ensured at a normotensive state and prior to extubation. This prevents post-operative complications and return to theatre for bleeding in the orbit.

Box 6.1 Operative note

The patient elected to have surgical intervention for the fractures of the orbital walls in view of the ongoing diplopia. However, he did not wish to have acute intervention for his orbital ridge fracture.

The orbit was accessed via a transconjunctival approach with a lateral canthotomy ('swinging lid'). The orbital contents were elevated free from the fracture and a solid shelf of bone was exposed around the fracture. A titanium sheet was contoured to correct the morphology and laid on solid bone, with care taken to ensure no soft tissue entrapment. The metalwork was affixed to the anterior orbital rim to prevent migration. Haemostasis was confirmed and the wound closed ensuring that the lateral canthus was repaired and that the conjunctiva was opposed, but excess blood was free to drain. Before extubation the eye's movements were accessed via a forced duction test assessing for entrapment.

Postoperatively the patient made an excellent recovery and a CT was requested to ascertain the position of the titanium plate (Figure 6.2). The diplopia in upward gaze remained following the surgery. The patient was, however, reassured and this gradually settled over the next three months.

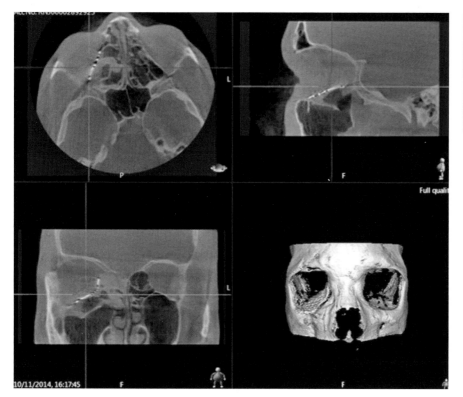

Figure 6.2 Post-operative CT demonstrating appropriate orbital reconstruction plate position. See colour plate section.

> ⊕ **Expert comment**
>
> In cases where diplopia persists it is imperative to resist the temptation to re-explore the orbit. The CT is most reassuring and demonstrates that the plate is in the correct position. In some cases it may take up to six months for total resolution of the symptoms.

> ✦ **Learning point** Ophthalmology and optometry
>
> It is essential to have a high suspicion of ocular injury in patients with orbital fractures, especially where there has been outer orbital frame disruption, high-energy injury, or penetrating injuries [7]. The rate of acute blindness as a result of these injuries is approximately 1.7% [8].
>
> The ocular injuries of note that are seen with orbital trauma include:
>
> * retrobulbar haemorrhage
> * superior orbital fissure syndrome
> * orbital apex syndrome
> * traumatic optic neuritis
> * lens dislocation
> * hyphaema
> * retinal detachment
> * direct damage to the globe.
>
> The ophthalmology evaluation will enable detailed pre-operative documentation of ocular function including visual fields and restriction of gaze. This can specifically be indicated on a Hess chart assessment that aids in the differentiation between diplopia of:
>
> * physical entrapment
> * muscular dysfunction
> * neurological defect
> * swelling.

⭐ **Learning point** Orbital compartment syndrome or retrobulbar haemorrhage

The incidence of retrobulbar haemorrhage is approximately 1% [9] and that associated with progression to blindness is 0.3% [10]. However, this is a potentially reversible cause of blindness that requires prompt surgical intervention to prevent progression and permanent damage [11].

An orbital injury without significant disruption of the orbital walls (where no drainage path exists) is at greater risk from retrobulbar bleeding. Patients with a bleeding diathesis or taking regular anticoagulants are also exposed to this increased risk. The source of this bleeding is commonly the anterior ethmoidal artery that traverses the medial orbital wall approximately 25 mm posterior to the medial orbital rim. This increase in intra-ocular volume leads to a rise in intra-orbital pressure as the hard tissue walls of the orbit and presence of intact soft tissue walls (eyelid, orbital septum and tarsal plate) prevent displacement of the contents. As the pressure increases there is a direct compression of the ophthalmic veins leading to congestion and subsequent exacerbation of the situation. As the pressure climbs above the systolic blood pressure the ophthalmic artery is occluded leading to ischaemia of the retina. After 20–30 minutes this results in permanent retinal cell necrosis.

This 'pressure kettle' effect is classic of compartment syndrome anywhere in the body. While classically due to a retrobulbar haemorrhage, this phenomenon has also been caused by air within the orbit and is thus called tension pneumo-orbitism [12, 13]. Hence, the correct term is orbital compartment syndrome.

Signs and symptoms include:

- disproportionate pain relating to the severity of the injury
- decreasing visual acuity with loss of red perception in the first instance
- ophthalmoplegia
- pupillary dilation
- loss of pupillary light reflex
- proptosis
- chemosis
- raised intra-ocular pressures.

⭐ **Learning point** Management of retrobulbar haemorrhage

This condition is an emergency and if suspected then medical treatment can be instigated to gain time until surgical intervention is feasible

Medical management [14]

Medical therapy employs drugs to reduce swelling and intra-ocular pressure. Because orbital compartment syndrome is a progressive process this is a stop-gap measure and not a definitive management.

- Mannitol 1–2 g/kg of 20% intravenously, which acts to dehydrate the vitreous humour and so reduce intra-ocular pressure.
- Acetazolamide (carbonic anhydrase inhibitor) 500 mg bolus intravenously, followed by 250 mg intravenously four times a day orally.
- Methylprednisolone 1 g intravenously as a single dose or dexamethasone 8mg intravenously three times per day.

Surgical management

There have been a number of techniques described for the surgical decompression of the orbit in compartment syndrome including [15]:

- lateral canthotomy and/or inferior cantholysis (this is the most commonly utilized).
- anterior chamber
- transantral ethmoidectomy
- transantral sphenoidectomy
- transfrontal craniotomy.

Frequent reassessment of the patient with orbital compartment syndrome post decompression is essential, as the eye remains in an 'at-risk' state.

➕ **Clinical tip** Access to the orbit

The orbit can be accessed by various approaches, each of which will allow visualization of a variety of anatomical zones within the orbit. However, each approach is associated with its own limitations and morbidities. In general, before starting surgery the level of access should have been discussed and therefore the corresponding approach accepted. The approaches include:

1. Coronal flap: roof, medial, and lateral wall.
2. Upper blepharoplasty: medial and lateral wall.
3. Transconjunctival approach with the adjuncts of transcuruncular and lateral canthotomy ('swinging lid'): floor, medial, and lateral walls.
4. Subcilliary: floor, medial, and lateral walls.
5. Midtarsal: floor, medial, and lateral walls.
6. Infra-orbital: floor, medial, and lateral walls.
7. Transantral: orbital floor.
8. Endoscopically assisted.

✖️ **Learning point** Materials for reconstruction

The reconstruction of the orbit has taken many different forms from the original autogenic bone to alloplastic materials in the reconstruction of the orbit. Recent research seems to suggest that titanium plates are superior [16, 17].

Autogenous:

• calvarium (inner and outer table)
• maxillary sinus
• mandibular cortex
• costochondral.

Alloplastic:

• Titanium
  o Mesh, average value contour and bespoke
  o Titanium with coating (e.g. Medpor)
• Porous polyethylene (e.g. Medpor)
• Silastic
• Polydioxanone.

✔️ **Evidence base** Gosau et al 2011 [18]

Retrospective study of 189 patients with fractured orbital floors.

• Surgery undertaken between 2003 and 2007.
• Mean delay to time of surgery of 2.9 days.
• Most common approach was mid lower eyelid incision.
• Materials used: polydioxanone sheets (70.5%), Ethisorb Dura (23.3%), and titanium mesh (6.2%).
• 19% complication rate.
• 3.2% had persistent diplopia.
• One patient had reduction in visual acuity and one sustained total loss of sight in the affected eye.

Source: data from Gosau M, Schöneich M, Draenert FG, Ettl T, Driemel O, Reichert TE. Retrospective analysis of orbital floor fractures–complications, outcome, and review of literature, *Clinical Oral Investigations* Volume 15, Issue 3, pp. 305-313, Copyright ©2011 Springer-Verlag.

✔️ **Evidence base** Ellis and Tan 2003 [19]

• Retrospective study covering 58 patients with pure blow-out fractures.
• All had pre- and postoperative coronal CTs.

(continued)

- Duration between date of injury and operation 7.1 days (SD, 6.3 days: range, 0–30 days).
- Orbital reconstruction with either a cranial bone graft (outer table) (26 patients) or titanium mesh (0.4 mm) (32 patients).
- One surgeon assessed the accuracy of reconstruction.
- Orbits reconstructed with titanium mesh were considered more accurate than those with bone.

Source: data from Ellis E, Tan Y. Assessment of internal orbital reconstructions for pure blowout fractures: cranial bone graft versus titanium mesh, *Journal of Oral and Maxillofacial Surgery*, Volume 61, Issue 4, pp.442–453, Copyright © 2003 American Association of Oral and Maxillofacial Surgeons.

✚ Clinical tip   Postoperative care

Postoperative eye observations

In the immediate postoperative period close eye observations (pain, visual acuity and pupil size) are required for signs of retrobulbar haemorrhage. Our protocol is:

- Every 15 minutes for 2 hours.
- Every 30 minutes for 4 hours.
- Every 60 minutes for 8 hours.

Postoperative imaging

The role of imaging is controversial with advocates on both extremes of the argument. The first option is to accept intra-operative position and image if there is an issue postoperatively. Alternatively, the patient could have a plain radiograph that will demonstrate postoperative position in a crude position. The final option is to image via CT, which will give an accurate visualization of the position of the plate in three dimensions. However, this is a relatively high radiation dose, so some advocate the use of cone beam CT [20].

General care

There are a number of immediate postoperative points of care that you and the patient may raise including:

- eye care
- no nose blowing
- suture removal
- persistent diplopia
- driving.

Discussion

The repair of an orbital wall fracture either as an isolated injury or as part of a larger facial fracture requires careful anatomical restoration of the orbital bony morphology, so as to maintain correct orbital volume and global position therein.

This can be extremely difficult to do blindly, so technology has been developed to aid in producing the best result in either primary repair, be it immediate or delayed and in secondary repair. It is exciting to see what technology has developed in the recent past and some of these novel technologies will become the norm over the next few decades as technology simplifies and the costs fall.

The technological advances include the following:

- stereolithic technology [21]
- bespoke plates:
  - ○ pre-bent for the patient [22]
  - ○ custom made for the patient

✚ Clinical tip

Orbital roof fractures ('blow-in') can present with proptosis and exophthalmos [27] as they lead to reduced orbital volume. This must be borne in mind as it may be confused with orbital compartment syndrome.

- intra-operative CT scan [23]
- intra-operative navigation [21, 24]
- endoscopic assisted and performed reduction [25, 26].

A final word from the expert

Orbital wall trauma is an area where precision is key to gaining adequate reconstruction. The maintenance of appropriate orbital volume prevents suboptimal aesthetic and functional outcomes.

Thorough preoperative assessment is a must in orbital trauma, with a thin-sliced CT of the orbits and ophthalmology assessment essential prior to any surgical intervention. The operator should ensure that appropriate and adequate surgical access is gained to allow anatomical reconstruction. When locating a reconstruction plate the orbital process of the palatine bone forms a small shelf in the posterior aspect of the orbit. This is seldom fractured and is an excellent point on which to rest a plate.

Orbital trauma is also a field in which technological advances are revolutionizing practice. Thirty years ago it was the norm to simply elevate the orbital floor fracture and provide support for healing with an antral pack, but now we have the ability to fabricate a bespoke plate of titanium designed to fit the traumatized patient and repair the fracture, which can be placed under the direction of navigation and checked with an intraoperative CT for satisfactory fit.

We hope that you will look at the technology at your disposal, so as to optimise your patient's care and outcome.

References

1. Cabalag MS, Wasiak J, Andrew NE, et al. Epidemiology and management of maxillofacial fractures in an Australian trauma centre. *J Plast Reconstr Aesthet Surg* 2014; 67(2): 183–9.
2. Eski M, Sahin I, Deveci M, et al. A retrospective analysis of 101 zygomatico-orbital fractures. *J Craniofac Surg* 2006; 17(6): 1059–64.
3. Ellis E 3rd, el-Attar A, Moos KF. An analysis of 2,067 cases of zygomatico-orbital fracture. *J Oral Maxillofac Surg* 1985; 43(6): 417–28.
4. Evans BT, Webb AAC. Post-traumatic orbital reconstruction: Anatomical landmarks and the concept of the deep orbit. *Br J Oral Maxillofac Surg* 2007; 45(3): 183–9.
5. Muller-Richter UD, Kohlhof JK, Driemel O, et al. Traumatic dislocation of the globe into the maxillary sinus. *Int J Oral Maxillofac Surg* 2007; 36(12): 1207–10.
6. Hammer B. Orbital fractures: diagnosis, operative treatment. Secondary corrections. Seattle: Hogrefe and Huber; 1995. p. 3.
7. Vaca EE, Mundinger GS, Kelamis JA, et al. Facial fractures with concomitant open globe injury: mechanisms and fracture patterns associated with blindness. *Plast Reconstr Surg* 2013; 131(6): 1317–28.
8. Magarakis M, Mundinger GS, Kelamis JA, et al. Ocular injury, visual impairment, and blindness associated with facial fractures: a systematic literature review. *Plast Resconstr Surg* 2012; 129(1): 227–33.
9. Fattahi T, Brewer K, Retana A, Ogledzki M. Incidence of retrobulbar hemorrhage in the emergency department. *J Oral Maxillofac Surg* 2014; 72(12): 2500–2.

10. Ord RA. Postoperative retrobulbar haemorrhage and blindness complicating trauma surgery. *Br J Oral Surg* 1981; 19: 202–7.
11. Popat H, Doyle PT, Davies SJ. Blindness following retrobulbar haemorrhage-it can be prevented. *Br J Oral Maxillofac Surg* 2007; 45(2): 163–4.
12. Key SJ, Ryba F, Holmes S, Manisali M. Orbital emphysema - the need for surgical intervention. *J Craniomaxillofac Surg* 2008; 36(8): 473–6.
13. Al-Shammari L, Majithia A, Adams A, Chatrath P. Tension pneumo-orbit treated by endoscopic, endonasal decompression: case report and literature review. *J Laryngol Otol* 2008; 122(3): e8.
14. Wood CM. The medical management of retrobulbar haemorrhage complicating facial fractures: a case report. *Br J Oral Maxillofac Surg* 1989; 27: 291–5.
15. Brucoli M, Arcuri F, Giarda M, et al. Surgical management of posttraumatic intraorbital hematoma. J Craniofac Surg 2012; 23(1): e58–e61.
16. Potter JK, Malmquist M, Ellis E 3rd. Biomaterials for reconstruction of the internal orbit. *Oral Maxillofac Surg Clin North Am* 2012; 24(4): 609–27.
17. Ellis E 3rd, Tan Y. Assessment of internal orbital reconstructions for pure blowout fractures: cranial bone grafts versus titanium mesh.*J Oral Maxillofac Surg* 2003; 61(4): 442–53.
18. Gosau M, Schöneich M, Draenert FG, et al. Retrospective analysis of orbital floor fractures-complications, outcome, and review of literature. *Clin Oral Investig* 2011; 15(3): 305–13.
19. Ellis E, Tan Y. Assessment of internal orbital reconstructions for pure blowout fractures: cranial bone graft versus titanium mesh. *J Oral Maxillofac Surg* 2003; 61(4): 442–53.
20. Tsao K, Cheng A, Goss A, Donovan D. The use of cone beam computed tomography in the postoperative assessment of orbital wall fracture reconstruction. *J Craniofac Surg* 2014; 25(4): 1150–4.
21. Bell RB, Markiewicz MR. Computer-assisted planning, stereolithographic modeling, and intraoperative navigation for complex orbital reconstruction: a descriptive study in a preliminary cohort. *J Oral Maxillofac Surg* 2009; 67(12): 2559–70.
22. Gordon CR, Susarla SM, Yaremchuk MJ. Quantitative assessment of medial orbit fracture repair using computer-designed anatomical plates. *Plast Reconstr Surg* 2012; 130(5): 698e–705e.
23. Hoelzle F, Klein M, Schwerdtner O, et al. Intraoperative computed tomography with the mobile CT Tomoscan M during surgical treatment of orbital fractures. *Int J Oral Maxillofac Surg* 2001; 30(1): 26–31.
24. Kim YH, Jung DW, Kim TG, et al. Correction of orbital wall fracture close to the optic canal computer-assisted navigation surgery. *J Craniofac Surg* 2013; 24(4): 1118–22.
25. Cheong EC, Chen CT, Chen YR. Broad application of the endoscope for orbital floor reconstruction: long-term follow-up results. *Plast Reconstr Surg* 2010; 125(3): 969–78.
26. Cheung K, Voineskos SH, Avram R, Sommer DD. A systematic review of the endoscopic management of orbital floor fractures. *JAMA Facial Plast Surg* 2013; 15(2): 126–30.
27. Antonyshyn O, Gruss JS, Kassel EE. Blow-in fractures of the orbit. *Plast Reconstr Surg* 1989; 84(1): 10–20.

7 Biomechanics of the mandible and current evidence for treatment of the fractured mandible

Douglas Hammond

❝ Expert commentary Ahmed Messahel

Case history

A 25-year-old male was brought to the Emergency Department (ED) following an alleged assault. A witness stated that he had been allegedly punched once and had been rendered unconscious for a period of approximately one minute. The patient had retrograde amnesia exceeding the hour prior to the event. He also had a Glasgow Coma Score of 11 on arrival in the ED. He was complaining of pain in the region of his mandible with significant deviation evident.

He had consumed approximately 15 units of alcohol during the evening prior to the event. Triple-immobilization of the cervical spine was instigated as pre-hospital care and he was transported immediately to the ED.

The patient was fit and healthy, with no past medical or surgical history. He took no regular medication and had no known drug allergies.

> **❝ Expert comment**
>
> As the patient was triple-immobilized and given that he met two of the 2014 National Institute for Health and Care Excellence guidelines for requiring an urgent computed tomogram (CT) scan to rule out a brain injury, we had little input initially. Fortunately his CT scan showed that he had sustained no radiologically significant injury to his brain. Unfortunately, however, despite requesting the CT scan to include his mandible, this was not done. The cervical spine was cleared by the ED team. His Glasgow Coma Score returned to 15 and his clinical observations were normal. After the secondary survey, no other injuries were found other than the fractured mandible and associated soft tissue laceration.

On examination he had a full-thickness laceration of his lower lip. He had obvious ecchymosis to his chin and neck. His mandible was visibly displaced, and he had an obvious anterior open bite. His temporomandibular joints were non-tender.

An orthopantomogram (Figure 7.1) and an anteroposterior mandible (Figure 7.2) radiograph were taken. These demonstrated fractures of the mandible bilaterally through the mental regions.

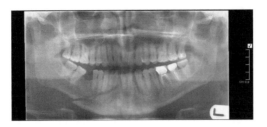

Figure 7.1 Preoperative orthopantomogram.

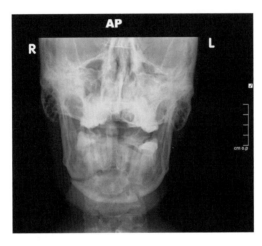

Figure 7.2 Anteroposterior view of the mandible.

Diagnoses

- Bilateral fractured mandible with a 'butterfly fragment' (or 'segmental fracture').
- Buccal luxation of 31, 32.
- Lip laceration.
- Post-traumatic concussion.

Treatment of buccal luxation of 31, 32 and lip laceration

- Infiltration from 35 to 45 and lip laceration with 10 ml 2% lidocaine with 1:80,000 epinephrine.
- Manipulation of 31, 32 into normal anatomical position.
- Placement of a bridle wire (0.45 mm stainless steel) from 43 to 33.
- Lip was debrided and closed with 3/0 Vicryl (Ethicon Inc. US).
- Skin was closed with 5/0 Prolene (Ethicon Inc. US).

Tetanus status was verbally checked. The patient was immediately started on 1.2 g co-amoxiclav intravenously three times daily and appropriate analgesia.

Treatment plan

- Open reduction and internal fixation (ORIF) of bilateral mandibular fractures with osteosynthesis miniplates and maxillomandibular fixation (MMF) via an intraoral approach (Box 7.1).

> ⊕ **Clinical tip**
>
> The patient was assessed by way of neurological observations for 24 hours, as he had a significant concussive episode. This would mean delaying his surgery for his fractured mandible until this was complete.

Box 7.1 Operative note

Technical steps for ORIF of mandible:

- Standard preparation and draping of the patient.
- 10 ml of 2% lidocaine with 1:80,000 epinephrine infiltrated from 36 to 46.
- 10 mm MMF screws were placed in the maxilla symmetrically.
- A buccal incision was made from 33 to 43 onto bone.
- Dissection was undertaken to identify the mental nerves and protect them whilst the incision was extended from 36 to 46.
- The fractures were reduced and an Erich arch bar was placed from 37 to 47. This was held with 0.45 mm stainless steel wires.
- The Erich arch bar and the MMF screws were held in the correct occlusion with 0.50 mm stainless steel wires.
- The left side was plated initially. Superiorly we placed a 2.0 mm four-hole non-spaced plate and secured with 4 mm × 6 mm screws.
- The inferior plate was initially the same plate, however, it did not provide adequate fixation, so a 2.4 mm four-hole spaced plate was employed with 4 mm × 8 mm screws.
- On the right-hand side there was a butterfly fragment present that made reduction difficult. To enable there to be at least two screws distal to the fracture, two screws medial to the fracture, and two screws in the butterfly fragment, an eight-hole 2.0 mm non-spaced plate was used; 7 mm × 6 mm screws were used and the unused hole was on the fracture line.
- Superiorly we placed a 2.0 mm four-hole non-spaced plate that was held with 4 mm × 6 mm screws.
- The incision was closed with 3/0 Vicryl and the 0.50 mm stainless steel wire MMF was released and the occlusion was checked. The occlusion was found to be correct.

✚ Clinical tip

The literature supports both the use of traditional MMF as well as the use of MMF screws to aid fixation [1–3]. The traditional MMF techniques take longer to apply and have a smaller set and rate of complications. However, there are some contraindications to its usage [4,5]. MMF screws fail more frequently and lead to more frequent damage to existing dentition. There is no definitive answer as to which is the gold standard for treatment.

Postoperative regime

- Two further doses of intravenous antibiotics leading in to oral co-amoxiclav 625 mg three times a day for five days.
- Analgesia as required.
- Place elastic bands to guide occlusion prior to discharge.
- Post-operative orthopantomogram and posteroanterior mandible (Figures 7.3 and 7.4).
- Removal of skin sutures at five days.
- Review in the outpatient department at one week.

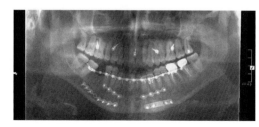

Figure 7.3 Postoperative orthopantomogram.

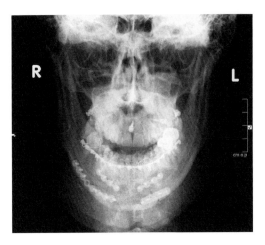

Figure 7.4 Postoperative posteroanterior view of the mandible.

Discussion

This case is interesting as the patient had two different methods of MMF. This was used in conjunction with ORIF to produce stable fixation of difficult fractures. It raises questions regarding what is the most efficacious mode of MMF.

MMF is a procedure that has been used traditionally as a sole treatment as a closed procedure, or in conjunction with ORIF. However, in the present era of miniplates, both the patient and surgeon prefer open reduction, reducing the duration of hospitalization with minimal discomfort to the patient and early return to work.

Conventional types of MMF include tooth- mounted devices such as arch bars, dental and interdental wiring and metallic and non-metallic splints. However, tooth-borne devices are always associated with problems such as poor oral hygiene, periodontal health compromise, extrusion of teeth, loss of tooth vitality, traumatic ulceration of the buccal mucosa and the risk of a sharps injury to the surgeon. Placing conventional MMF is time consuming. It is also not suitable to place wire-based MMF in patients with multiple missing teeth, grossly carious teeth, crown and bridgework, or extensively restored and periodontally involved teeth [6].

⊕ Expert comment

The use of MMF screws is not without complications. The most common include screw loosening (6.5%) and root fracture/ iatrogenic damage to teeth (4%). Fracture of the screws has also been reported. Soft tissue coverage of screws occurred in 5% of all cases.

One of the major advantages in the usage of MMF screws is the reduced operative time. The time taken to place MMF screws is between 5.7 and 10 minutes, whereas the time taken to place Erich arch bars is between 25 and 100 minutes.

To negate the issues of damage to adjacent teeth, Key stated that the angulation of the roots should be assessed radiologically [7]. He recommended placement of self-tapping screws between the canine and the first premolar region at the mucogingival junction.

⊕ **Learning point** Forces relevant to monocortical fixation

By using smaller plates with monocortical screws, the forces maintaining the stability of the treated fracture segments should be at least in excess of the critical load characteristics for the fracture fragment displacement forces. Clinically, the relevant parameters for in-vitro force application can be deduced from both the non-operated healthy individual and also the postoperative population.

The occlusal forces produced in the immediate postoperative phase in patients who have had mandibular angle fractures fixed with miniplates are much less than those recorded in both the later healing phase and in healthy patients who have not had any surgery.

Patients who have had miniplate fixation for fractures of the angle of the mandible were studied to compare their maximal occlusal forces with known norms. These patients were shown to have 31% of their expected maximal occlusal force at one week and 58% at six weeks post-surgery. The reason for this is that pain is the limiting factor in the initial stages of healing [8].

In the healthy patient, knowledge of the masticatory stresses exerted on the mandible is fundamental, because these stresses determine the rational design and positioning of osteosynthesis plates and their mechanical characteristics. The activity of the muscles of mastication can be divided into:

- temporalis forces
- masseter forces
- reactive biting forces.

The following values were obtained [9]:

- incisor region: 290 N
- canine region: 300 N
- premolar region: 480 N
- molar region: 660 N.

The interaction of these forces varies from patient to patient, and as such in each case there is a differing amount of fracture displacement that needs to be overcome by treatment. The external forces produced by the muscles of mastication results in these forces being produced. Physiologically coordinated muscle action produces forces of tension at the upper border of the mandible and compressive forces at the lower border of the mandible [10,11]. Additionally, Sustrac demonstrated that torsional forces occur anterior to the canines [12].

Every mandibular fracture that occurs causes distraction at the alveolar crest region, accentuated by the degree of trauma and by contraction of the muscles of the floor of the mouth, which may lead to displacement of the fragments. The compressive force at the lower border of the mandible is a force that is both a dynamic and a physiological force and is always exerted on the fracture fragments. This compressive force is due to the muscular tone that increases during mastication. When the fracture is adequately reduced and fixation is adequately provided, then this dynamic compression equals the physiological strains exerted on an intact mandible.

The momentums of tension, compression and torsion have been established using a mathematical model of the mandible using the formula $E = F \times L/d$, where E is the state of constraints, F is masticatory forces, L is the distance from chin to fracture line and d is the distance from plate to lower border of mandible.

In any method of fixation of a fractured bone, friction forces controlling shearing and torsion stresses are an important factor of stability. These forces between fracture surfaces exist due to interdigitation of fracture fragments and are enhanced by compressive forces [13].

⊘ **Evidence base [8,11,14]**

It was Champy's opinion that in these cases double-plate fixation is required. However, these principles are not followed today at the angle of the mandible.

If Champy's principles are followed then a fixation that is 'stable, elastic, and dynamic' will be produced.

(continued)

Fixation is stable when:

- No movement is visible between the fragments.
- After precise reduction of the fracture it provides the compressive forces with a solid support at the basilar border and ensures interdigitation and frictional forces between the contacting fracture surfaces.
- It neutralizes harmful distraction forces.
- It allows some early return to function but not complete loading.

Source: data from Champy M. et al., Mandibular osteosynthesis by miniature screwed plates via a buccal approach, *Journal of Oral and Maxillofacial Surgery*, Volume 6, pp. 14-21, Copyright © 1978 American Association of Oral and Maxillofacial Surgeon; and Champy M. et al., Mandibular osteosynthesis according to the Michelet technique I: Biomechanical basis, *Revue de Stomatologie et de Chirurgie Maxillo-faciale*, Volume 3, pp. 569–576, Copyright © 1976 Elsevier Masson SAS.

✪ Learning point Biomechanics of fixation

Fixation needs to have an element of elasticity, as rigid immobilization of the fractured bone can disrupt bone repair because it inhibits the inflammatory phase of bone healing. Elasticity is important as micro motion between the fracture surfaces enhances the healing process.

Fixation needs also to be dynamic because the adequate elasticity of the plate creates compression strains at the lower border of the mandible during masticatory activity. The interdigitation between fracture surfaces creates friction, enhancing the stability of the mechanical fixation. This compression is dynamic and physiological. It leads to a perfect contact between bone surfaces due to the adequate elasticity of the plate and at the same time, to a stimulus for bone healing. The value of micro motion is 0.5 μm. The dimension of a mandibular osteon is 60 μm. It is generally accepted that motion smaller than that of an osteon is insignificant to the healing process. If this mobility is abolished by complete rigid fixation then the inflammatory process of bone repair is shortened, which leads to impaired repair. For completeness, Cornell states that appropriate stimulus and blood supply are crucial to osteosynthesis. Controlled motion at a micromechanical level appears to optimize the physiological conditions that facilitate fracture healing [15].

✪ Learning point Rationale for fixation [11,14]

Michelet produced a monocortical fixation system, which was initially used for the fixation of midface fractures. However, Champy used this successfully for the fixation of mandibular fractures. The use of monocortical screws are required to prevent injury to the dentition and also to the inferior alveolar nerve. Champy delineates ideal lines of osteosynthesis for the fixation of mandibular fractures. He mentions three different zones (see Figure 7.5).

1. A neutral zone. This is located immediately subapical to the dentition in the lateral portion of the mandible. In this region a single plate is required for adequate fixation.
2. A two-level zone. This is between the mental foramina. In this region two plates are required to resist the tensional and torsional forces.
3. The angle of the mandible. Fixation can be adequately achieved either cranially, or buccally to the external oblique ridge with a single plate.

The treatment of fractures of the angle of the mandible is controversial, as there have been few prospective, randomized controlled trials. Even when these studies are published the exclusion criteria are not well defined, especially in regard to the vertically or horizontally favourable or unfavourable nature of fractures. The in-vitro experimentation regarding monocortical fixation of mandibular fractures should reveal clinical evidence justifying plating patterns; however, it does not [16–19].

Champy suggested that a single 2 mm thick four-hole spaced plate with four monocortical non-compression screws (normally of 6 mm length) is adequate for the fixation of a mandibular angle fracture when placed either cranial or buccal to the external oblique ridge. In spite of this there are advocates of biplating in biplanar fashion (one plate on the superior border and one plate on the

(continued)

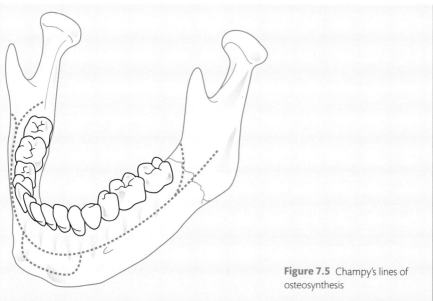

Figure 7.5 Champy's lines of osteosynthesis

lateral aspect of the mandible) and also of biplating in a monoplanar fashion (superior and inferior on the buccal aspect of the mandible). This is a contentious issue and there is a debate as to the biomechanical stability of each method and the amount of either lingual or lower border gaping post fixation and whether it is relevant [11,14].

Final word from the expert

The Cochrane Review of Mandibular Fractures states 'This review illustrates that there is currently inadequate evidence to support the effectiveness of a single approach in the management of mandibular fractures without condylar involvement'. This necessitates the ability to be adaptable and coherent in different methods of fixation and be able to use different methods of fixation in a single case [20].

The increase in research into biomechanics is leading to development of further scientific evidence in the field of fracture treatment. Hopefully the production of higher level evidence is not too far off in the future with regards to the treatment of mandibular fractures.

References

1. Arthur G, Berardo N. A simplified technique of maxillomandibular fixation. *Br J Oral Maxillofac Surg* 1989; 47(11): 1234.
2. Coletti DP, Salama A, Caccamese JF Jr. Application of intermaxillary fixation screws in maxillofacial trauma. *J Oral Maxillofac Surg* 2007; 65(9): 1746–50.
3. Holmes S, Hutchison I. Caution in use of bicortical intermaxillary fixation screws. *Br J Oral Maxillofac Surg* 2000; 38(5): 574.
4. Hashemi HM, Parhiz A. Complications using intermaxillary fixation screws. *J Oral Maxillofac Surg* 2011; 69(5): 1411–4.

5. Majumdar A. Iatrogenic injury caused by intermaxillary fixation screws. *Br J Oral Maxillofac Surg* 2002; 40(1): 84–8.

6. Sahoo NK, Mohan R. IMF screw: An ideal intermaxillary fixation device during open reduction of mandibular fracture. *J Oral Maxillofac Surg* 2010; 9(2): 170–2.

7. Key S, Gibbons A. Care in the placement of bicortical intermaxillary fixation screws. *Br J Oral Maxillofac* 2001; 39(6): 484.

8. Champy M, Lodde JP, Schmitt R, et al. Mandibular osteosynthesis by miniature screwed plates via a buccal approach. *J Oral Maxillofac Surg* 1978; 6: 14–21.

9. Gerlach KL, Schwarz A. Bite forces in patients after treatment of mandibular angle fractures with miniplate osteosynthesis according to Champy. *Int J Oral Maxillofac Surg* 2002; 31: 345–8.

10. Gerlach KL, Schwarz A. Load resistance of mandibular angle fractures treated with miniplate osteosynthesis. *Mund-Kiefer-Heilkunde* 2003; 7: 241–5.

11. Champy M, Lodde JP, Jaeger JH, Wilk A. Mandibular osteosynthesis according to the Michelet technique I: Biomechanical basis. *Rev Stomaol Chir Maxillofac* 1976; 3: 569–76.

12. Sustrac B, Villebrun JP. Biomechanique des osteosyntheses par plaques vissees miniaturisees des fractures du corps de la mandibule. Etude. Strasbourg: Ecole Nat. Sup. Art. Ind; 1976: 134.

13. Ewers R, Harle F. Biomechanics of the midface and mandibular fractures: Is a stable fixation necessary? In :Hjorting-Hanson E (ed.) *Oral and Maxillofacial Surgery*. Chicago: Quintessence; 1985a: pp. 207–11.

14. Champy M, Wilk A, Schnebelen JM. Treatment of mandibular fractures by means of osteosynthesis without intermaxillary immobilisation according to F.X. Michelet's technique. *Zahn Mund Kieferheilkd Zentralbl* 1975; 4: 339–41.

15. Cornell CN, Lane JM. Newest factors in fracture healing. *Clin Orthop Relat Res* 1992; 277: 197–311.

16. Ellis E. Treatment methods for the fixation of the mandibular angle. *J Cr-Maxillofac Tr* 1997; 2: 28–36.

17. Siddiqui A, Markose G, Moos KF, et al. One miniplate versus two in the management of mandibular angle fractures: A prospective randomised study. *Brit J Oral Maxillofac Surg* 2007; 45: 223–5.

18. Ellis E, Waler L, Shafer D. Treatment of mandibular angle fractures using two noncompression miniplates. *J Oral Maxillofac Surg* 1994; 52: 1032–7.

19. Schierle HP, Schmelzeisen R., Rahn B., Pytlik C. One or two plate fixation of mandibular angle fractures. *J Craniomaxillofac Surg* 1997; 25: 162–8.

20. Nasser M, Pandis N, Fleming PS, et al. Interventions for the management of mandibular fractures. *Cochrane Database Syst Rev 2013* July 8: 7; CD006087.

SECTION 3

Military maxillofacial trauma

8 High-energy ballistic injuries to the face

John Breeze

Expert commentary Sat Parmar and Andrew Monaghan

Case history

A UK soldier was on foot patrol in Iraq when he was struck by two high-velocity bullets. The first projectile was stopped by his body armour, knocking him to the floor. The second bullet ricocheted from the ground, hitting the soldier in the upper arm and the face. Battlefield first aid was immediately instigated by his patrol with a haemostatic dressing packed into the arm wound and a first field dressing applied directly above to provide pressure. A wound was seen in the soldier's right cheek but little bleeding was noted and he was talking to the members of his patrol throughout his evacuation to the deployed field hospital. Two other soldiers in his patrol had been wounded in the same firefight, both more seriously and were immediately taken to theatre.

In the emergency department of the field hospital the arm wound was superficially cleaned and dressed. The patient was still happily talking to the nurses as his cheek wound was examined and exposed mandible clearly seen. The deployed oral and maxillofacial surgeon was called and immediately examined the mouth and remaining face, noting a large sublingual haematoma and a probable exit wound in the left cheek. The decision was made to take the patient to theatre to debride his arm wound. A computed tomography scan of his head and neck region was performed, which demonstrated a wound tract that passed across his mandible through the base of his tongue.

The patient was evacuated by military critical care air transport to the Role 4 medical facility at the Royal Centre for Defence Medicine, based at University Hospital Birmingham. Following a thorough secondary survey, the patient was taken to theatre, which was approximately three days after initial injury. His arm was again debrided and a vacuum-assisted dressing applied. The patient was placed in maxillomandibular fixation and an external fixator was applied to the mandible enabling stabilization of the comminuted fragments (Figure 8.1). The external fixator was removed six weeks later and stability of the mandible was noted.

The patient returned to his unit and was very pleased with his progress but was keen to have prosthodontic rehabilitation of his dentition. A free bone graft from the iliac crest was raised and plated in situ (Figure 8.2), followed by dental implant placement four months later (Figure 8.2b). However, after the transmucosal abutments were fitted it was clear that the extent of bone loss meant that insufficient depth of vestibule was present in conjunction with a lack of attached keratinized gingiva (Figure 8.3). A split skin graft was raised from the patient's thigh and inset

Learning point

The conflicts in Iraq and Afghanistan have seen the development of haemostatic dressings that can be poured as a powder, or packed as thickened ribbon into the open wound. These dressings have now been introduced into the ambulance services and have in certain instances been used to arrest haemorrhage from penetrating neck injury.

Expert comment

The airway remains the primary cause of death in patients with maxillofacial ballistic injuries. Consideration should be made to performing a surgical tracheostomy at the time of damage control surgery should any concern be highlighted.

Clinical tip

It is essential to attempt to visualize the path that the projectile has taken through the tissues. However, even with knowledge of entry and exit wounds, as well as utilizing cross sectional imaging, this is difficult. A low threshold for suspecting occult vascular and aerodigestive injury must be adopted for all patients wounded by high-velocity projectiles.

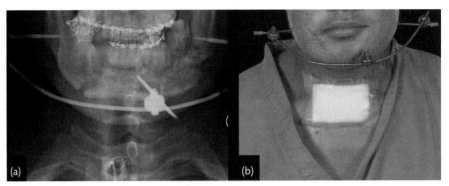

Figure 8.1 An external fixator applied to a grossly comminuted mandible in conjunction with upper and lower arch bars.

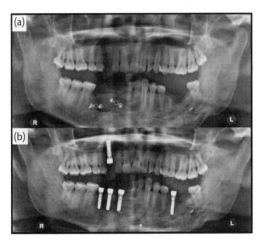

Figure 8.2 An iliac crest free bone graft was inset and plated to the mandible (a), enabling subsequent osseointegrated dental implant placement (b).

into the tissues buccal to the implants (Figure 8.3b), with increased vestibular depth noted at review three months later (Figure 8.3c).

Discussion

The incidence of maxillofacial injuries sustained by UK soldiers in Iraq and Afghanistan is higher than that found in previous conflicts, primarily reflecting improvements in body armour in conjunction with increased use of explosive devices [2]. High-velocity bullets are currently responsible for one in five wounds to the face and neck [2] and are characterized by the high energy that they impart to the tissues within the wound tract. Although military bullets generally have a full metal jacket reducing the energy transmitted by limiting deformation, the temporary cavity can be considerable in size. The permanent wound tract comprises those tissues irreversibly destroyed by the projectile passage and is greatly increased in size when bone is hit or when bullets have ricocheted prior to impact [3]. This has a number of important implications when managing these wounds. The vitality of the tissues

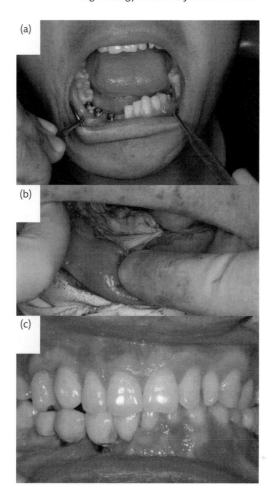

(a)

(b)

(c)

Figure 8.3 When the second stage abutments were applied insufficient vestibular depth was noted (a). A vestibuloplasty utilizing a split skin graft (b) provided increased depth to enable proper function (c).

around the wound tract is often not known, so that wounds to the extremities are debrided on consecutive occasions perhaps for up to a week until consistent healthy tissue is found [4]. This same concept of serial debridement until viability is assured should also be applied to the maxillofacial region, despite our knowledge that this region has an inherently better blood supply [5]. Great care should be made to preserve the periosteal attachment of any of the comminuted fragments and only completely avulsed tissue and foreign bodies should be excised [6].

Evidence base

Tan et al. [7] experimentally fired fragment simulating projectiles at the faces of dogs, noting thrombosis in facial vessels up to 3 cm from the macroscopic wound edge. They attributed this to the effect of the temporary cavity and remarked that this will have to be accounted for in any future vascular anastomosis. Interestingly, they stated that repair started within seven days and at ten days there was resolution of all the microvascular changes. The healing after anastomosis of the small vessels is characterized by necrosis of the tunica media and a slow repair of the endothelium.

Source: data from Tan YH, Zhous S, Liu Y, et al. Small vessel pathology and anastomosis following maxillofacial firearm wounds: an experiment study, *Journal of Oral and Maxillofacial Surgery*, Volume 49, Issue 4, pp. 348–352, ©1991 Elsevier Inc.

A small series of US soldiers injured in Iraq in whom their fractures were treated definitively whilst still on operations was published in 2007. However, limited conclusions can be made as the mechanism of injury was not described (high-velocity bullet injury was mixed in with blunt trauma from road traffic accidents) and limited follow-up data was provided [8]. It has been the experience of those maxillofacial surgeons whom have deployed on operations as well as their colleagues who have managed those soldiers evacuated to the UK, that conventional methods of fracture fixation are often inappropriate [9,10]. An external fixator can provide anatomical reduction and fragment stability and can be used with arch bars as used in the case above. In the early stages of the Iraq conflict no specific external fixator was available for the maxillofacial skeleton and surgeons often utilized ones used for wrist fractures [4,6,10]. However, later Synthes® introduced an external fixator that has been utilized both on operations and in the UK [6,11]. In some cases direct methods of fixation can be utilized to stabilize fragments in close proximity to one another. Thicker profile (reconstruction) plates should be used that utilize load-bearing osteosynthesis, in conjunction with as limited stripping of the periosteum as possible. The use of custom-made plates pre-bent on stereolithographic models enables larger bony defects to be spanned, but are not suitable for gross comminution and still rely on periosteal stripping to provide direct bone contact.

🍀 Expert comment

Vascular injury to the face is often accompanied by significant bleeding. Control of facial vascular injuries should progress from simple wound compression for minor bleeding to possible vessel ligation for more significant bleeding. Vessel ligation should only be performed under direct visualization and after careful identification of the bleeding vessel. Blind clamping of bleeding areas should be avoided because critical structures, such as the facial nerve or parotid duct, are susceptible to injury. Wound packing with a pressure dressing may control active craniofacial bleeding. Haemostatic gauze may also be used [1].

✪ Learning point

Protective equipment worn by soldiers in current conflicts is very effective in stopping low-velocity ballistic projectiles such as explosively propelled fragments. It should be remembered that only the ceramic plates worn in the body armour vests are designed to retard high-velocity bullets, the remainder is to prevent penetration of explosively propelled fragments. Currently UK soldiers wear the following items that may potentially protect against fragments penetrating the tissues in the maxillofacial region: a combat helmet, ballistic glasses and a detachable neck collar. The effectiveness of these items often means that the outline is clearly demarcated, with the remaining exposed skin peppered with small fragments and discoloured by soil debris. Great care must be taken to thoroughly debride the exposed skin and remove any visible fragments. Clinical experience would suggest that removal of all fragments is futile and there is no proven clinical benefit. Consideration to removing larger fragments lying close to the great vessels or vertebral arteries [12] should be made once the patient is stabilized in the UK, but this should be an elective procedure with radiological assistance available.

➕ Clinical tip

With the exception of fractures that compromise the airway or impair haemostasis, repair may be delayed for up to ten days after injury, especially if a high-energy transfer mechanism is suspected. Open fractures should be debrided, irrigated and closed temporarily to prevent infection [1].

The long-term maxillofacial rehabilitation of these patients with gross bony injury likely revolves around provision of enough bone to enable placement of dental implants [10]. The amount of bone will usually necessitate grafts originating from the iliac crest, tibia, or fibula. However, great care must be made in the use of vascularized flaps as evidence exists that the temporary cavity produced by these high-velocity bullets can cause non-macroscopic vascular damage [7], placing the anastomosis at increased risk. In this case an iliac crest graft was taken, which provided substantial bone to enable implant placement. However, with such a block graft it can be difficult to reproduce the vestibular anatomy, with subsequent difficulty in mastication and cleaning. This can be facilitated by the insetting of a split skin graft taken from the thigh or less commonly from the arm due to the extensive leg injuries that some of these soldiers have sustained.

✪ Learning point

No objective clinical research exists to compare the outcomes of immediate versus delayed repair of facial fractures sustained in the military setting. However, experience from both UK and US authors would suggest that delayed repair should be chosen in any wound in which the vitality of surrounding tissues is not known. Methods that do not interrupt the soft tissue envelope such as external fixators and arch bars should be utilized. If direct plates are utilized, they should be rigid and of a thickened profile to ensure load-bearing osteosynthesis.

In current conflicts the burden of maxillofacial injuries directly sustained from conflict far outweighs that sustained outside of battle or secondary to disease, in direct contrast to every conflict our country has ever experienced in history. Penetrating injuries due to bullets and explosively propelled fragments are responsible for 96% of combat injuries sustained by UK soldiers on operations [2]. A small proportion (4%) of battle injuries are thought to be from blunt trauma, primarily from the force of the explosive blast wave throwing the soldier against an object. Blunt injury due to interpersonal assault or road traffic accidents is responsible for most non-battle maxillofacial injuries, with patterns reflective of that seen in normal civilian practice. Most bullet wounds are from high-velocity rifles, usually resulting in significant energy transfer and tissue cavitation. Low-velocity bullet wounds are rare on the modern battlefield but this has the potential to change were more urban conflicts to occur. Explosively propelled fragments may be formed from grenades (including those propelled by rockets), mines, or mortars [13]. However, the most common cause of these fragmentation injuries currently is from improvised explosive devices. By their nomenclature they are heterogeneous group of home-made devices capable of explosively propelling any kind of debris. They are generally buried and therefore end up propelling soil debris and its associated microbiological flora into any wounds produced [13].

⊕ Clinical tip

Preservation of tissue is key to managing high-velocity injury to the facial tissues as knowledge of which tissues will survive is not always clear [5]. Surgeons should strongly consider antibiotic coverage for *Pseudomonas* and *Staphylococcus* organisms when exposure of the cartilage of the nasal and auricular regions has occurred and minimize the use of sutures and compression bandages that may cause further necrosis.

A final word from the expert

Experience gained in treating high-velocity injuries has resulted in the re-learning of many principles utilized by our surgical predecessors. Serial debridement and tension-free direct closure, where possible in conjunction with surgical tracheostomy to produce a definitive airway, remains the cornerstone of initial management. Conventional methods of fracture fixation such as miniplate osteosynthesis are often inappropriate due to periosteal stripping resulting in bone devitalization. An external fixator can provide anatomical reduction and fragment stability and can be used in conjunction with arch bars.

References

1. Cubano MA, Lenhart MK. Face and neck injuries. In: *Emergency War Surgery*, 4th Revision 2013. Borden Institute, Fort Sam Houston, TX: US Department of Defense USA. ISBN 13: 9780160921971.
2. Breeze J, Gibbons AJ, Shieff C, et al. Combat-related craniofacial and cervical injuries: a 5-year review from the British military. *J Trauma* 2011; 71(1): 108–13.
3. Breeze J, Sedman AJ, James GR, et al. Determining the wounding effects of ballistic projectiles to inform future injury models: a systematic review. *J R Army Med Corps* 2014; 160(4): 273sw .
4. Powers DB, Will MJ, Bourgeois SL, Hatt HD. Maxillofacial Trauma Treatment Protocol. *Oral Maxillofacial Surg Clin N Am* 2005; 17: 341–55.
5. Will MJ, Goksel T, Stone CG Jr, Doherty MJ. Oral and maxillofacial injuries experienced in support of Operation Iraqi Freedom I and II. *Oral Maxillofac Surg Clin North Am* 2005; 17(3): 331–9.
6. Gibbons AJ, Mackenzie N, Breederveld RS. Use of a custom designed external rotocol. models: a systematic review. steal stripping result. *Int J Oral Maxillofac Surg* 2011; 40(1): 103–5.
7. Tan YH, Zhous S, Liu Y, et al. Small vessel pathology and anastomosis following maxillofacial firearm wounds: an experiment study. *J Oral Maxillofac Surg* 1991; 49(4): 348–52.
8. Lopez MA, Arnholt JL. Safety of definitive in-theater repair of facial fractures. *Arch Facial Plast Surg* 2007; 9(6): 400–5.
9. Gibbons AJ, Mackenzie N. Lessons Learned in Oral and Maxillofacial Surgery from British Military Deployments in Afghanistan. *J R Army Med Corps* 2010 Jun; 156(2): 113–6.
10. Monaghan AM. Maxillofacial ballistic injuries. InBrooks A, Clasper JC, Midwinter MJ, Hodgetts TJ, Mahoney PF (Eds)*Ryan's Ballistic Trauma* 3rd edition, 2011. New York: Springer.
11. McVeigh K, Breeze J, Jeynes P, Martin T, Parmar S, Monaghan AM. Clinical strategies in the management of complex maxillofacial injuries sustained by British military personnel. *J R Army Med Corps* 2010 Jun; 156(2): 110–3.
12. Fox CJ, Gillespie DL, Weber MA, Cox MW, Hawksworth JS, Cryer CM, Rich NM, O'Donnell SD. Delayed evaluation of combat-related penetrating neck trauma. *J Vasc Surg* 2006; 44(1): 86–93.
13. Goksel T. Improvised explosive devices and the oral and maxillofacial surgeon. *Oral Maxillofac Surg Clin North Am* 2000; 17(3): 281–7.

9 Reconstructive challenges following blast injuries to the facial soft tissue and skeleton

Kevin McMillan

⑥ Expert commentary Tim Martin

Case history

A 23-year-old fit and well soldier was injured in a detonation of an improvised explosive device in Afghanistan. He was evacuated from the point of injury to a field hospital setting by helicopter where he received emergency care. The primary goal of this was to ensure safe repatriation to the UK.

At the field hospital he was noted to be suffering from severe injuries. These included bilateral traumatic amputations of his lower limbs. His upper limbs had bilateral shrapnel injuries but no fractures. The patient had been wearing full torso and abdominal body armour as well as a peroneal protective garment. As such, there were no significant injuries to his trunk. He had a large shrapnel injury to his chin area with an extensive comminuted fracture of the mandible. There was a soft tissue defect of 6 cm × 5 cm in the chin area with bone fragments exposed. As part of his mandibular fracture, he had several teeth damaged and a significant amount of debris in the wound and oral cavity.

From a physiological point of view, the patient was unwell due to hypovolaemic shock. He underwent trauma resuscitation according to local protocols. He was taken to the operating theatre and underwent damage control surgery. This involved a surgical tracheostomy, debridement of all wounds and placement of negative-pressure dressings (V.A.C.® KCI, US) to the open peripheral wounds. The facial wound was washed out, carefully debrided and packed with povidone-iodine soaked gauze held in place with sutures. The patient was administered with empirical broad spectrum antimicrobial drugs and repatriated by air to the Role 4 Hospital in the UK. This process took less than 48 hours from the point of injury.

Upon arrival at the Role 4 Hospital, the patient underwent a first-look procedure in theatre. Given the unstable nature of his physical state the procedure time was very limited. His leg dressings were changed and his oral wounds were debrided (Figure 9.1). The oral pack was also changed at this point.

A further 24 hours later, the patient was returned to theatre for a second look. At this time an external fixator was placed on the mandible to stabilize the main bony segments. The exposed bone was covered by mobilizing local soft tissue. The wound in the chin was washed and the pack changed. Stock arch bars were placed and the patient was put into maxillomandibular fixation (MMF) (Figure 9.2).

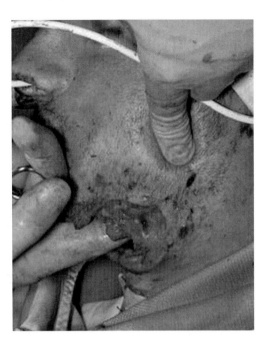

Figure 9.1 First-look procedure demonstrating the submental soft tissue defect.

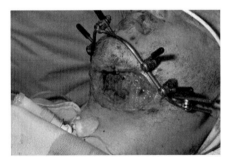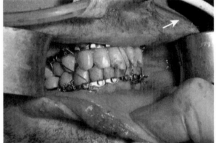

Figure 9.2 Second-look procedure following placement of external fixator and MMF.

⑥ Expert comment

This patient was managed in a Role 4 Hospital that was the sole receiving hospital for all UK military casualties. Concentration of these complex casualties facilitates reflection of learning experiences within the clinical team. Management of ballistic mandibular injuries has evolved from open reduction and internal fixation to simpler MMF and external fixation for all but the simplest of fractures. This case ultimately demonstrates the effectiveness of this treatment strategy.

★ Learning point Options for fixation of the blast injured mandible

Maxillomandibular fixation

Advantages:

- simple
- no stripping of periosteum required
- no specialist equipment required.

Disadvantages:

- lack of teeth for fixation can be a problem
- long-term fixation can prolong need for nasogastric feeding.

(continued)

Open reduction internal fixation (ORIF)

Advantages:

- direct visualization of fracture enabling good bony reduction
- open soft tissue injury may allow easy access
- can allow earlier return to oral intake.

Disadvantages:

- requires periosteal stripping which can lead to avascular necrosis of comminuted fragments.
- metalwork can serve as source of infection.

External pin fixation

Advantages:

- no stripping of periosteum required
- rigid fixation.

Disadvantages

- can be technically challenging to position
- pin site infection
- potential for malocclusion.

The patient was managed in the intensive care unit over the following days. He received nutrition via nasogastric tube. The chin wound was debrided and the dressing changed on a regular basis. At that time the patient remained in a systemic inflammatory response state and reconstruction was delayed for this reason. Additionally, the challenges of reconstructive surgery in terms of donor site selection made the decision to operate difficult.

❻ Expert comment

Although this patient had a comminuted fracture of the mandible and submental soft tissue loss, intra-oral mucosal soft tissue loss was minimal. The patient did have some soft tissue loss of the floor of the mouth and a consequent small orocutaneous fistula. The use of a V.A.C. dressing had been proposed; however, in the presence of an orocutaneous fistula this would have been inappropriate. In defects resulting in a significant orocutaneous fistula or involving aesthetic facial units where failure to reconstruct would result in significant aesthetic compromise, early reconstruction may have been prompted.

Over the following weeks, the patient improved physically and underwent multiple orthopaedic procedures to revise his leg stumps. At three weeks post injury, the MMF was released revealing a stable occlusion in the external fixation device. The patient was commenced on a soft diet and tolerated this well. The soft tissue defect had begun to contract and now measured 4 cm × 3 cm. The wound bed looked healthy. Given the improvement in the wound, reconstruction was delayed further to observe the extent of healing.

At six weeks post injury, the external fixator was removed from the fixation pins. The mandible was stable and showed clinical and radiographic evidence of healing. The fixation pins were removed and the patient increased the repertoire of his diet with no complications.

Three months following the injury, the chin wound had completely healed with some scarring and contracture. His occlusion was stable and he had good mouth opening and jaw function. He was discharged from hospital to a rehabilitation facility to continue his post-traumatic rehabilitation (Figure 9.3).

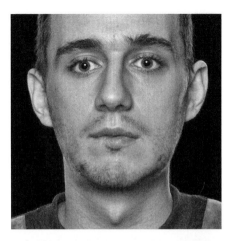

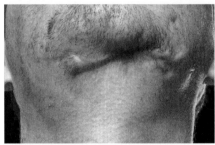

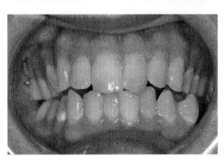

Figure 9.3 Post-treatment images demonstrating complete healing of the submental defect with an even bilateral occlusion of the dentition.

Discussion

This case illustrates some of the key issues in managing severe traumatic maxillofacial injuries caused by ballistic and explosive trauma. The types of blast injury are presented in Table 9.1. The patient sustained multiple injuries in an austere setting. The initial management of the patient should be entirely focused on life-saving procedures and stabilization. Patients who are involved in these scenarios are typically physically fit, but this is not certain. They display a rapid acute systemic inflammatory response and have significant problems with temperature homeostasis [1]. The austere environment and contaminated shrapnel ensure that wounds sustained are dirty and require meticulous washout and decontamination. Sepsis is common and empirical broad spectrum antimicrobial use should be instigated. The presence of atypical and antimicrobial resistant microbes is also a commonly encountered problem [2,3].

Table 9.1 Types of blast injury. Note that the effect of the quinary blast injury is potentially profound and can delay operative management of maxillofacial wounds.

Type of blast injury	Effect
Primary blast injury	Blast overpressure causes tissue damage
Secondary blast injury	Debris displaced by blast cause penetrating of blunt tissue trauma
Tertiary blast injury	Physical displacement of person by blast
Quaternary blast injury	Follow on effects of the injury (e.g. burns)
Quinary blast injury	Hyper-inflammatory state

When managing maxillofacial injuries in the initial setting, the extent of treatment is debatable. In our experience, a very conservative approach is most sensible. It is useful to remember that the excellent facial blood supply means that debridement of facial soft tissue does not need to be as aggressive as in the limbs. Removal of obviously necrotic and heavily contaminated tissue should be the focus. Stabilization of fractures in the austere environment is not usually recommended. If the patient is not actively bleeding, has undergone initial decontamination and has a secure airway then no further management is usually required prior to repatriation.

Within the first few days of injury, the polytrauma patient will require intensive care support. The frequency with which post-traumatic inflammatory response is encountered means that this problem should be anticipated. Management of maxillofacial injuries will frequently be delayed as a result of the patient not being fit for prolonged surgery. In these instances, a pragmatic approach to keep wounds decontaminated and fractures stabilized in the initial days is best.

In terms of traumatic fracture management, it is well regarded that ORIF can be problematic in these cases. The high degree of comminution as well as contamination of soft tissues can result in frequent infection of metalwork. Additionally, the blood supply to the bone is at risk and a serious complication of avascular necrosis can occur. The use of MMF for fracture stabilization is certainly valid in this type of case. It offers the benefit of closed reduction and no stripping of the periosteum is required. This ensures that blood supply to comminuted fragments is preserved where possible. One challenge of using MMF is the lack of available teeth for fixation. However, transmucosal screw fixation can alleviate this concern.

The use of external fixation devices is also advocated. This has the advantage of allowing good bony reduction of the main fracture segments without the need for extensive disruption to the soft tissues. Pin site infection can be problematic with the external fixator but rarely causes deep-seated infection. It is vital that any exposed bone should be covered with soft tissue if possible as any exposed fragments will desiccate and can become problematic. Any exposed loose bony fragments should be judiciously removed but the surgeon should aim to be very conservative in their approach to debridement [4,5].

⭐ **Learning point**

The injuries caused by blast trauma can be multifocal and heterogeneous. There may be elements of penetration, avulsion and burn injury

The nature and anatomical distribution of fractures associated with blast and penetrating trauma is frequently different to that of more mainstream trauma (i.e. interpersonal violence and other common non-military causes).

✅ **Evidence base [4]**

There is no globally accepted 'landmark paper' relating to ballistic and blast-related trauma. This reflects the fact that these cases are rare in civilian life and case series numbers tend to be low. As a result, there tends to be conflicting opinions on the management of these complex patients and injuries. Particular sources of controversy relate to:

- timing of primary surgery
- the type fixation used for fracture fixation (particularly so in mandibular fractures)
- the timing and donor site for advanced reconstructive techniques.

(continued)

💬 **Expert comment**

In this case bone fragments that had been assessed carefully for potential vascularity were left exposed extra-orally. With appropriate wound management and careful monitoring granulation tissue eventually covered the bone.

This paper describes the challenges and evolution of management of military maxillofacial injury. In particular it focuses on the challenges of mandibular injury management. This paper is written based upon a high volume of experience in a modern warfare setting.

Key points identified in the paper include

- External pin fixation and closed reduction of mandibular fractures still have a role in management of complex mandibular injury.
- When managing complex injuries:
  o Small, devitalized fragments of bone should be removed;
  o Larger fragments should be reduced and fixated;
  o Use inter-maxillary fixation (IMF) to align dentoalveolar fragments;
  o Cover exposed bone when possible;
  o Delayed grafting with a healthy, infection-free tissue bed if necessary;
  o Consider osseous free flap for defect greater than 6 cm;
  o Open fractures of the mandibular body are difficult to treat. Disruption of blood supply in this area is common and necrosis is frequently seen.

(These principles are very much in keeping with our experience and ethos)

  o Complications of these injuries are frequently encountered and should be anticipated.

Source: data from Tucker DL et al., Characterization and management of mandibular fractures: lessons learned from Iraq and Afghanistan, *Atlas of the Oral and Maxillofacial Surgery Clinics of North America*, Volume 21, Issue 1, pp.61-68, Copyright © 2013.

The reconstruction of soft tissue defects in the polytrauma patient is complex. A decision to perform reconstruction using either pedicled or free flaps should not be taken lightly. In a patient who has sustained limb loss, the prospect of donor site morbidity should not be understated. A patient in these circumstances would become more dependent upon their upper body for mobility (wheelchair etc.). Any pedicled or free flap procedure taken from the upper limb or the trunk may impact on upper body function and the risk of loss of function warrants careful consideration [6,7].

⭐ **Learning point** Options for reconstruction of defects following ballistic trauma [8]

(Note 1: in the polytrauma patient a number of these flaps may not be suitable or advisable. Consideration of donor site and effect on patient mobility and function is paramount)

(Note 2: multiple flaps may be required in order to reconstruct the defect)

Soft tissue only

Pedicled flap:

- Pectoralis major
- Deltopectoral

Free flap:

- Radial forearm
- Lateral arm
- Latissimus dorsi
- Thoracodorsal perforator
- Scapular
- Anterolateral thigh
- Rectus abdominis

(continued)

Bone only

Free bone graft:

- Cranium
- Iliac crest
- Rib

Free flap

- Radial forearm
- Deep circumflex ileac artery (DCIA)
- Scapular
- Fibular

Composite flap (likely to be required and most useful)

- Radial forearm
- DCIA
- Fibula
- Scapular

A further consideration in free flap surgery is the prospect of poor vessel availability making anastomosis a potential challenge. Trauma to the head and neck region could reduce the number of vessels available for anastomosis. Additionally, the prospect of intimal damage to the vessels as a result of the injury can further increase the risk of flap failure. For this reason, a CT angiogram should be performed to exclude subclinical vascular injury. Additionally, consideration of overall operative time in the acute setting should be openly discussed with other specialities involved in the patient's care. Prolonged operative time in an acutely ill patient should be avoided.

It should also be noted that coagulopathy is frequently encountered in polytrauma patients. Embarking upon free flap surgery in the presence of abnormal coagulation carries significant risk of free flap failure. This should be avoided [9].

As this case demonstrates, fairly extensive defects of the head and neck region can close with appropriate dressings and management. Frequently, a delayed approach to reconstruction can reap benefit as well as reduce the potential morbidity of further surgery.

✪ **Learning point** Treatment algorithm for blast injury and ballistic injury patients

Point of injury:

- Focus on acute stabilization of patient.
- Secure airway.
- Ventilatory and circulatory support.
- Thorough debridement of wounds (conservative debridement of head and neck wounds).
- Secure dressings.
- Antimicrobial agents.
- Repatriation.

Initial management:

- Focus on intensive care unit management.
- Reduce operative time to minimum.

(continued)

- Delay extensive procedures.
- Stabilize fractures avoiding ORIF if possible.
- Ensure exposed bone is covered with soft tissue if possible.

Delayed management:

- Focus on reconstruction and rehabilitation management.
- Ensure patient physiologically and nutritionally able to manage treatment.
- Discuss extensive procedures planned with other clinicians and rehab staff.
- Extensively consider reconstructive options to minimize donor site morbidity.

A final word from the expert

Serious consideration was given to early microvascular reconstruction of the submental defect of this patient, only the patient's physiological status prevented such an approach. Had microvascular reconstruction been conducted the cutaneous reconstruction would have been of significantly different colour and texture to the surrounding skin. If soft tissue microvascular reconstruction were to be considered then a soft tissue scapular flap gives a superior skin match to the more commonly used radial or anterolateral thigh free flaps. Relatively straightforward submental scar revision for this patient will undoubtedly result in a superior aesthetic outcome compared to flap reconstruction; a valuable learning point.

References

1. Hawksworth JS, Stojadinovic A, Gage FA, et al. Inflammatory biomarkers in combat wound healing. *Ann Surg* 2009; 250: 1002–7.
2. Davis KA, Moran KA, McAllister K, Gray PJ. Multidrug resistant *Acinetobacter* extremity infections in soldiers. *Emerg Infect D*is 2005; 11: 1218–24.
3. Murray CK, Roop SA, Hospenthal DR, et al. Bacteriology of war wounds at the time of injury. *Mil Med* 2006; 171: 826–9.
4. Tucker DL, Zachar MR, Chan RK, Hale RG. Characterization and management of mandibular fractures: lessons learned from Iraq and Afghanistan. *Atlas Oral Maxillofac Surg Clin North Am* 2013; 21(1): 61–8.
5. Title SM, Gwinn DE, Andersen RC, Kumar AR. Soft tissue coverage of combat wounds. *J Surg Orthop Adv* 2010; 19: 29–34.
6. Sardesai MG1, Fung K, Yoo JH, Bakker H. Donor-site morbidity following radial forearm free tissue transfer in head and neck surgery. *J Otolaryngol Head Neck Surg* 2008; 37(3): 411–6.
7. Moukarbel RV, Fung K, Franklin JH, et al. Neck and shoulder disability following reconstruction with the pectorals major pedicle flap. *Laryngoscope* 2010; 120: 1129–34.
8. Stanec Z, Skrbic S, Dzepina I, et al. High energy war wounds: Flap reconstruction. *Ann Plast Surg* 1993; 31: 97–102.
9. Kumar AR, Harshbanger R, Martin B. Plastic surgery challenges in war wounded. In: Sen CK (ed) Advances in Wound Care vol. 1. New Rochelle: Mary Ann Liebert; 2010, pp. 65–9.

10   Low-energy explosive fragmentation injuries to the neck and face

John Breeze

Expert commentary   Andrew Gibbons and Ian Sharp

Case history

A 23-year-old UK soldier was on foot patrol in Afghanistan when he stood on a pressure plate improvised explosive device. This resulted in traumatic amputations of both legs and extensive fragmentation wounds to the arms, neck and face. Care under fire was instigated by his colleagues and tourniquets applied to both legs to arrest haemorrhage. The medical emergency response team within a Chinook helicopter was able to land and pick up the soldier in less than 20 minutes. The doctor on board intubated the patient and was able to provide blood products including factor VII concentrates using both intravenous and intraosseous access. Upon arrival to the UK Role 3 field hospital in Camp Bastion the patient was placed through the computed tomography (CT) scanner before being taken to the operating theatre. Utilizing a 64-slice scanner in conjunction with a tailored scanning algorithm, the scan took less than 30 seconds and resuscitation continued throughout. Gross comminution to the right side of the mandible was noted (Figure 10.1). In total it had taken 45 minutes since initial wounding to the first incision being made on the operating table.

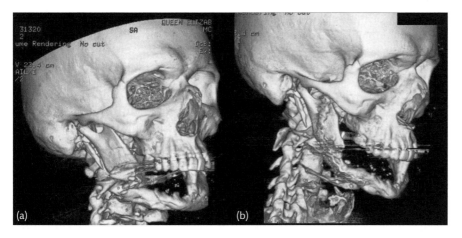

Figure 10.1 Three-dimensional CT reformats of the original comminuted mandibular fracture (a) and following application of a custom-made pre-bent reconstruction plate (b). See colour plate section.

❝ Expert comment

Explosively propelled fragments were responsible for 79% of face and neck injuries sustained by UK soldiers during the recent Iraq and Afghanistan conflicts. The improvised explosive device became the signature weapon, with most being laid in the ground and victim operated [1]. The explosive fragments usually produced significant lower limb and genital injuries, but the direction of threat and effectiveness of thoraco-abdominal body armour resulted in higher numbers of degloving injuries to the anterior mandible and nasal tip regions than seen in previous conflicts [2].

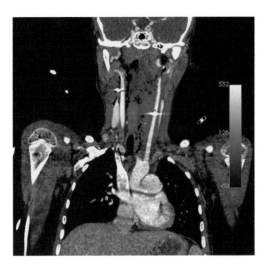

Figure 10.2 A coronal reformat of a computed tomography angiogram demonstrating two metallic fragments in close proximity to the carotid vessels.

In polytrauma cases such as this, both the surgical teams as well as the anaesthetists work in pairs with either two general surgeons or orthopaedic surgeons on each leg. The oral and maxillofacial surgeon performed a surgical tracheostomy and superficially debrided the face and neck wounds. CT angiography demonstrated that although a number of explosively propelled fragments lay in proximity to the cervical vasculature (Figure 10.2), no direct vessel damage could be seen and therefore no surgical exploration was undertaken. Vacuum-assisted dressings were applied to each leg and the patient was taken to the intensive care unit.

Within ten hours of injury, the patient was on a specially outfitted aircraft incorporating critical care facilities en route to the UK. The patient arrived at the Role 4 military medical facility based at the Queen Elizabeth Hospital Birmingham approximately 24 hours after injury. The on-call oral and maxillofacial surgery consultant had been contacted by the military registrar responsible for coordinating care. The patient required multiple visits to theatre to debride the leg wounds, and at one of these theatre sessions, four days post injury a custom-made preformed titanium reconstruction plate was placed. This had been made from a three-dimensional printed model generated from CT DICOM (Digital Imaging and Communications in Medicine) data. Periosteal stripping was kept to a minimum and the plate enabled mandibular arch width and to a lesser degree vertical facial height to be restored.

The patient spent three months on the ward in Birmingham during which he underwent multiple surgical procedures. Despite careful antimicrobial chemoprophylaxis, one of his legs developed a wound infection, necessitating further debridement. He was discharged from Birmingham to Headley Court, the UK military's centre for rehabilitation. Although the patient's primary focus was on trying to gain independence, eating had become a considerable problem and he was troubled by the aesthetics of his lack of teeth and also had a vertical mandibular bone defect. A bone graft would enable dental implant placement but the usual donor sites such as the tibia, iliac crest or scapula were either not available or contraindicated. For example the patient had both legs traumatically amputated but needed both his hips and arms to use his wheelchair. The mandible was therefore

Expert comment

The ability to be able to arrest haemorrhage from the neck is a core skill required of oral and maxillofacial surgeons in the deployed setting [3].

Clinical tip

- Clinical 'hard signs' of penetrating neck injury warranting surgical exploration can be divided into vascular and aerodigestive [4].
- Vascular: ongoing bleeding from the neck region that is not amenable to pressure, an expanding haematoma and a bruit or thrill in the neck.
- Aerodigestive injury: crepitus or subcutaneous emphysema, dyspnoea or stridor, air bubbling from the wound, tenderness or pain over the trachea, hoarse or abnormal voice, haematemesis or haemoptysis.

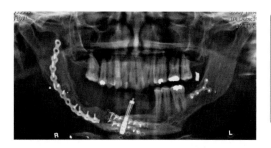

Figure 10.3 An orthopantomogram demonstrating the custom reconstruction plate with good bony union and an internal osteodistraction device. Note some small radiopaque explosive fragments still in situ.

> ✪ **Learning point**
>
> Military polytrauma patients are sometimes so badly injured that less life-threatening injuries can be initially missed. A thorough secondary survey of the neck and craniofacial region is essential following initial stabilization.

osteotomized at the site of the defect and an internal distractor placed (Figure 10.3). After a short latent period this was activated and over the course of three weeks sufficient bone height was achieved to enable placement of implants and subsequent oral rehabilitation.

> ✚ **Clinical tip**
>
> Utilizing a custom-made titanium reconstruction plate that is pre-bent using a three-dimensional printed stereolithographic model provides the surgeon with the confidence of reproducibly restoring mandibular or maxillary shape without having to bend it at the time of operation. Location tags enable correct seating and these can be cut off when drill holes have been made. Bone grafts can be attached to bridge gaps and plate shape can also accommodate the likely position of any vascular pedicle if required so that it might be protected.

Discussion

Maxillofacial wounds are currently present in approximately 21% of all injuries sustained by UK soldiers in combat, higher than the mean of 16% experienced in conflicts from the twentieth century [2]. Evidence of isolated blow-out orbital fractures without surrounding rim fractures have been described, suggesting a directly compressing effect of the blast wave itself on the globe, although such an injury is likely to be rare in survivors [5].

> ✪ **Learning point**
>
> Terminal ballistics is the study of the effects of ballistic penetration and a basic understanding of its principles is fundamental to correctly managing such injuries. It involves the complex interaction of three variables: the projectile, the target tissue and any ballistic protective elements including clothing. High-velocity bullets generally deposit more energy than explosively propelled fragments, which is increased if tumbling occurs such as with a ricochet prior to impact or deflection off a bone within tissues.

> ✪ **Learning point**
>
> The speed in which UK soldiers are usually evacuated from the theatre of operations is rapid, with many being back in the UK within 24 hours of initial injury. Although stabilized, these patients are often incredibly unwell and require multiple trips to theatre (e multiple t) in which their wounds are extensively debrided until healthy tissue is found.

Penetrating neck injury (PNI) and its sequelae have become one of the signature injuries of the Afghanistan conflict, reflecting the explosive weaponry used, inherent anatomical vulnerability and a lack of body armour worn to protect the area [6]. The initial management of face and neck injuries on the battlefield itself is slightly different from established Advance Trauma Life Support protocols in that the control of catastrophic, life-threatening haemorrhage is dealt with first [7]. Immediate

⊕ Clinical tip

In the future interventional radiology may potentially be able to embolize bleeding from many penetrating neck injuries without having to resort to surgical exploration to either ligate or more rarely graft the damaged section.

mortality from PNI is primarily due to exsanguination from carotid or vertebral artery damage, with a smaller contribution from airway compromise, especially from explosive fragments [6]. Modern battlefield haemostatic agents may be useful, but unfortunately most bleeding sources in maxillofacial injuries are often inaccessible [8]. Oesophageal injury is difficult to diagnose and is the most common cause of morbidity in PNI if missed [9]. The shearing effects from the temporary cavity produced by high-velocity projectiles predisposes to oesophageal injury, potentially resulting in mediastinitis and intractable sepsis. Concurrent cervical spine injury is believed to be less common in ballistic injury than with blunt trauma, but should be suspected in soldiers exposed to blast injury who may have been thrown against objects by the blast wave as this may cause blunt trauma.

Division of the neck into three zones, in combination with clinical 'hard signs' necessitating mandatory surgical exploration, remain the most practical method of aiding decision making in military PNI [4,8]. Serial physical examination and non-operative management, with mandatory surgical exploration only in the presence of clinical hard signs, is analogous to current management of PNI in a civilian setting. However, explosive fragmentation injury differs in that the blast wave in conjunction with large numbers of small fragments may cause both vascular injury as well as aerodigestive damage in patterns that may not provide these hard signs in such a reproducible manner [9,10]. CT angiography is essential for demonstrating subclinical vascular damage in these cases and outweighs the risks of any delays in resuscitation that may be incurred. Currently the facilities for interventional radiological techniques in the deployed setting do not exist, but it is likely that those clinicians capable of performing selective intravascular embolization will deploy in more established medical facilities in the future. However, the ability to perform surgical exploration of the cervical vasculature remains one of the core skills of an oral and maxillofacial surgeon in the deployed setting [3,8]. It is traditionally taught that vascular access to the carotid and jugular systems should be through an incision along the anterior border of the sternocleidomastoid muscle. Although such an approach provides excellent access to these vessels along their whole length, enabling ligation or venous interposition grafting, it limits access to other structures in the neck. It has been the experience of deployed maxillofacial surgeons to raise neck flaps analogous to those used in oncological neck dissection in certain situations [8]. They can be cosmetically superior and provide access to the lower border of the mandible for contemporaneous bony fixation.

Infection in patients wounded by explosively propelled fragments is common, primarily reflecting the severity of their injuries in conjunction with the impregnation of foreign material from within the device and within the soil. In particular the bacterium *Acinetobacter baumannii* was found in large numbers of US and UK soldiers evacuated home, resulting initially in small outbreaks in non-military patients treated at these hospitals and demonstrated multiple antibiotic resistance [11]. The origin of this organism was debated initially but evidence emerged that it was found in the soil in both Iraq and Afghanistan, resulting in the increased prevalence in those soldiers injured by buried explosive devices. Invasive fungal infections have also emerged as an important cause of morbidity and mortality among US military personnel who have suffered combat-related traumatic injuries [12]. The most common features among these patients are lower extremity amputation with perineal or pelvic injury and receipt of massive blood transfusions following blast injuries incurred while on foot patrol in southern Afghanistan. Treatment of these wounds by meticulous low-pressure irrigation and debridement is essential as the thrombosed blood vessels from the blast wave itself results in poor tissue penetration of antifungal and antimicrobial agents [13]. Serial debridement occurs approximately every 48 hours with wound closure often only considered a week after initial injury and only in the presence of wound contraction and healthy non-infected-appearing granulation tissue. The use of vacuum-assisted drainage has significantly reduced wound exudate and thereby reducing super infection by bacterial and fungal species.

> ✪ **Learning point**
>
> Ballistic injuries sustained in wartime often result in avulsion of soft and hard tissues that necessitates grafting at a later date. This case demonstrates the use of distraction osteogenesis to create new bone at the site of injury that alleviates the requirement for a donor site and therefore additional potential morbidity. Distraction also allows stretching of the soft tissue envelope, histogenesis of soft tissues, and reduction in potential scarring.

Final word from the expert

The effectiveness of modern body armour has changed the distribution of injuries sustained by soldiers on current operations. The fragmentation vest and combat helmet provide excellent protection to the head and thoraco-abdominal regions, such that the extremities including the face and neck have a higher proportion of injuries [2,3]. There has also been an increase in the speed at which soldiers are evacuated from the battlefield as well as advances in resuscitative techniques including the re-emergence of the tourniquet. Thus, soldiers who would not have survived ten years ago, prior to recent conflicts in Iraq and Afghanistan, are now progressing to comprehensive medical care. These present new challenges to oral and maxillofacial surgeons working in the theatre of war and when the soldier is evacuated back to the UK [8].

References

1. Ramasamy A, Hill AM, Clasper JC. Improvised explosive devices: pathophysiology, injury profiles and current medical management. *J R Army Med Corps* 2009; 155(4): 265–72.
2. Breeze J, McVeigh K, Lee JJ, et al. Management of maxillofacial wounds sustained by British service personnel in Afghanistan. *Int J Oral Maxillofac Surg* 2011; 40(5): 483–6.
3. Gibbons AJ, Mackenzie N. Lessons learned in oral and maxillofacial surgery from British military deployments in Afghanistan. *J R Army Med Corps* 2010; 156(2): 113–6.
4. Hale RG, Hayes DK, Orloff G, et al. Maxillofacial and neck trauma. In Savitsky E, Eastridge B (eds) *Combat Casualty Care: Lessons Learned from OEF and OIF*. Washington DC: Office of the Surgeon General Department of the Army, Borden Institute; 2012.
5. Breeze J, Opie N, Monaghan A, Gibbons AJ. Isolated orbital wall blowout fractures due to primary blast injury. *J R Army Med Corps* 2009; 155(1): 70.
6. Breeze J, Allanson-Bailey LS, Hunt NC, et al. Mortality and morbidity from combat neck injury. *J Trauma Acute Care Surg* 2012; 72(4): 969–74.
7. Hodgetts TJ, Mahoney PF, Russell MQ, Byers M. ABC to <C>ABC: redefining the military trauma paradigm. *Emerg Med J* 2006 October; 23(10): 745–6.
8. Monaghan AM. Maxillofacial ballistic injuries. In Brooks A, Clasper JC, Midwinter MJ, Hodgetts TJ, Mahoney PF (eds) *Ryan's Ballistic Trauma* 3rd edition, 2011. New York: Springer.

9. Asensio JA, Chahwan S, Forno W, et al. Penetrating esophageal injuries: multicenter study of the American Association for the Surgery of Trauma. *J Trauma* 2001; 50(2): 289–96.

10. Brennan J. Experience of first deployed otolaryngology team in Operation Iraqi Freedom: the changing face of combat injuries. *Otolaryngol Head Neck Surg* 2006; 134(1): 100–5.

11. Turton JF, Kaufmann ME, Gill MJ, et al. Comparison of *Acinetobacter baumannii* isolates from the United Kingdom and the United States that were associated with repatriated casualties of the Iraq conflict. *J Clin Microbiol* 2006; 44(7): 2630–4.

12. Warkentien T, Rodriguez C, Lloyd B, et al. Invasive mold infections following combat-related injuries. *Clin Infect Dis* 2012; 55(11): 1441–9.

13. Petersen K, Colyer MH, Hayes DK, et al. Prevention of infections associated with combat-related eye, maxillofacial, and neck injuries. *J Trauma* 2011; 71(2 Suppl 2): S264-L 9.

SECTION 4

Craniofacial surgery

11 Cranial vault reconstruction following decompressive craniectomy

Luke Williams and Francine Ryba

Expert commentary Robert Bentley

Case history

A fit and well 30-year-old presented to the Emergency Department with sudden onset speech problems, right-sided weakness and altered sensation in the right arm. An urgent head computed tomogram (CT) demonstrated a left subarachnoid haemorrhage. A CT angiogram demonstrated a right middle cerebral artery (MCA) aneurysm. The aneurysm was embolized using n-butyl cyanoacrylate glue. However, during the procedure there was inadvertent extrusion of material into the surrounding vasculature that resulted in embolization and infarction of the right MCA. The patient was transferred to the neurosurgical intensive care unit for monitoring. The patient's Glasgow Coma Scale (GCS) deteriorated from 10 to 5 with a fixed and dilated left pupil. A repeat CT head showed significant secondary infarction of the left MCA territory and resultant mass effect. An emergency left fronto–temporo–parietal decompressive hemicraniectomy with durotomy and duroplasty was carried out (Figure 11.1).

> **Learning point** Decompressive craniectomy
>
> Decompressive craniectomy and durotomy is removal of a significant portion of the cranium and opening of the dura to improve cerebral perfusion in situations of intractable raised intracranial pressure (ICP). This allows oedematous brain to swell beyond the normal confines of the cranial cavity, reducing ischaemic neuronal injury and limiting compression of brain parenchyma against the rigid intracranial structures such as the falx, tentorium and sphenoid ridge (Figure 11.2).

> **Expert comment**
>
> In cases of intracranial haemorrhage, a large bone flap is resected comprising portions of the frontal, temporal, parietal and occipital bones on the ipsilateral side to the stroke. A bifrontal craniectomy is used in cases of diffuse cerebral oedema following head trauma. The relevance of this to craniofacial surgeons is the design of the soft tissue flap, ideally situated over the residual bone, carefully placed to preserve adequate blood supply.

> **Evidence base** Decompressive craniectomy versus medical management in MCA infarct
>
> Several retrospective case series suggested decompressive craniectomy decreased mortality at the expense of increased and severe neurological morbidity amongst survivors. The DESTINY [1], DECIMAL [2] and HAMLET [3] trials have been carried out to assess survival and functional outcome of decompressive craniectomy versus best medical management alone in the setting of raised ICP following MCA infarct.
>
> **Inclusion criteria:**
>
> - DESTINY: age 18–60 years, < 36 hours before surgical intervention, unilateral MCA infarction. Trial stopped at 32 patients (188 projected sample size).
> - DECIMAL: age 18–55, < 30 hours before surgical intervention, unilateral MCA infarct. Trial stopped at 38 patients.
> - HAMLET: age 18–60 years, < 96 hours before surgical intervention, unilateral MCA infarct. Trial included 64 patients.

(continued)

Results: DESTINY and DECIMAL trials were ended early due to significant reductions in mortality at one month with surgical decompression and the possibility of a meta-analysis of the pooled data from the three trials. HAMLET showed significant reduction in mortality at one month but no significant difference in outcome at six months between surgical versus medical management.

Conclusions: The pooled analysis of these studies included 93 patients under the age of 60 randomly assigned to medical or surgical therapy within 48 hours of onset of symptoms [4]. The pooled results showed a reduction in mortality at one year from 78% in the medically treated group to 28% in the surgically treated group. Good functional outcomes were seen in 43% of the surgical group compared to 21% of the medical group.

Source: data from Juttler E et al., Decompressive surgery for the treatment of malignant infarction of the middle cerebral artery (DESTINY): a randomized, controlled trial, Stroke, Volume 38, Issue 9, pp. 2518–2525, Copyright © 2007 American Heart Association; Vahedi K. et al., Sequential-design, multicenter, randomized, controlled trial of early decompressive craniectomy in malignant middle cerebral artery infarction (DECIMAL Trial), Stroke, Volume 38, Issue 9, pp. 2506–2517, Copyright © 2007 American Heart Association; and Hofmeijer J. et al., Surgical decompression for space-occupying cerebral infarction (the Hemicraniectomy After Middle Cerebral Artery infarction with Life-threatening Edema Trial [HAMLET]): A multicentre, open, randomised trial, The Lancet Neurology, Volume 8, Issue 4, pp. 326–333, Copyright © 2009 Elsevier Limited.

One week after decompressive craniectomy, a surgical tracheostomy was required due to fluctuating GCS and slow wean from mechanical ventilation. When stable, the patient was transferred to a neurological rehabilitation centre with a gastrostomy

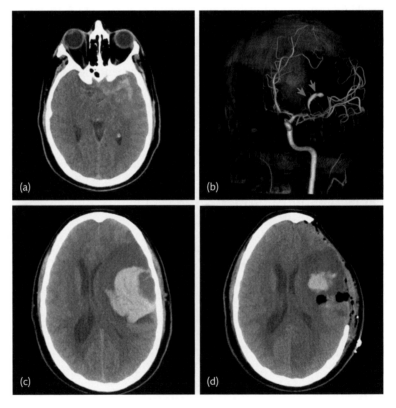

Figure 11.1 (a) Presenting scan demonstrating subarachnoid haemorrhage in the left parietal region (arrows). (b) Computed tomogram angiogram demonstrating right MCA aneurysm (arrows). (c) Middle cerebral artery infarct, effacement of ventricles, midline shift. (d) Appearance following decompressive craniectomy with reduction of mass effect on left side.

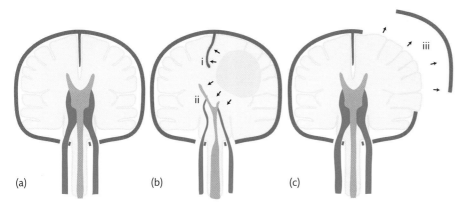

Figure 11.2 (a) Within the fixed volume of the skull are three components: brain, blood and cerebrospinal fluid (CSF). (b) An increase in volume of one of these components must be at the expense of the other components to prevent extreme rises in intracranial pressure – the Monro-Kellie doctrine. Cerebral oedema causes midline shift and compression of brain against fixed structures such as the falx (i). Compression of the ventricles leads to CSF flowing out of the cranium and decreased cerebral blood flow (ii). (c) Decompressive craniectomy (iii) creates space to allow cerebral oedema to occur preventing mechanical damage from compression and ischaemic damage from reduced cerebral blood flow.

to facilitate feeding and referred for reconstruction of the calvarial defect. Several days post transfer, the patient appeared unresponsive with decrease in GCS and a tense and bulging craniectomy site.

Magnetic resonance imaging (MRI) scan showed secondary external hydrocephalus. The patient returned to high dependency unit for insertion of a lumbar-peritoneal drain that resolved the tense bulging craniectomy defect and improved the neurological status to baseline. A repeat MRI demonstrated an unexpected intraventricular haemorrhage with associated obstructive hydrocephalus. A CT angiogram failed to demonstrate a source for the haemorrhage and an external ventricular drain (EVD) was inserted to relieve the hydrocephalus.

> ✪ **Learning point** Management of shunts
>
> Hydrocephalus is common following cerebral infarction and decompressive craniectomy. It can lead to significant bulging of the skin flap resulting in increased technical difficulty of dissecting the scalp from the dura and insufficient space for cranioplasty insertion [5]. With small volume hydrocephalus excess CSF can be drained using a temporary lumbar tap or drain. With larger volume hydrocephalus a shunt (lumbar-peritoneal or ventriculo-peritoneal) is required. These can be placed prior to cranioplasty or at operation. Evidence suggests that shunts placed at the same time of cranioplasty are associated with increased complications so the recommendation is to carry out shunt insertion and ensure hydrocephalus is resolved prior to cranioplasty [6].
>
> Over shunting will result in a significant dead space beneath a cranioplasty implant that can lead to haematoma or seroma formation and increased risk of infection. This can be addressed by temporarily occluding the shunt to allow CSF to accumulate or alternatively, as in this example, if a programmable shunt valve is present this can be adjusted to allow the slow accumulation of CSF preoperatively and then reset postoperatively to optimize CSF drainage.

The patient developed lower right limb swelling and a duplex ultrasound confirmed thrombus formation of the right common femoral vein. An inferior vena cava (IVC) filter was inserted.

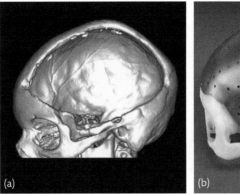
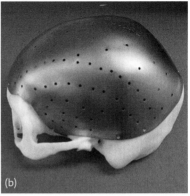

Figure 11.3 (a) Three-dimensional reformatting of cranioplasty protocol CT scan shows extent of craniectomy defect. (b) Completed titanium reconstruction in situ on model.

Three weeks later the EVD was clamped and this resulted in bulging of the skin flap indicating CSF accumulation. A ventriculo-peritoneal shunt with a variable flow magnetic valve was inserted and the EVD was removed. The patient returned to the neurological rehabilitation unit.

❝ Expert comment

The usual situation following MCA infarction is anticoagulation with dual antiplatelet therapy and a bridging plan of low molecular weight heparin is required to maintain appropriate anticoagulation in the perioperative period. In this case, the risk of further intracranial haemorrhage is too great to allow conventional management of venous thrombosis, hence the need for an IVC filter.

A fine-cut CT scan of the head (0° gantry angle, 0.5 mm slice) was obtained and a stereolithographic model generated using additive manufacturing. The model was used to reconstruct the defect in plaster and a hydraulic press used to form 0.8 mm thick titanium sheet to accurately reconstruct the contour of the skull (Figure 11.3).

❝ Expert comment

Calvarial grafts have a role in smaller calvarial defects. However, the large defects created by decompressive craniectomy are better reconstructed with a biomaterial. Preserved bone flaps have a higher failure rate than biomaterials. Titanium is the most widely used material although polyetheretherketone (PEEK) is gaining in popularity. Engineered tissues are still in early stages of development.

✪ Learning point Materials for cranioplasty

The choices for cranioplasty are either autologous bone or a biomaterial. Autologous bone grafts act as an osseoconductive scaffold to allow eventual replacement with normal vital bone in a process termed creeping substitution and is the obvious choice in terms of biocompatibility. In situations of large full-thickness calvarial defects, sources of autologous bone can be either the patient's preserved craniectomy bone flap or a split calvarial graft. The craniectomy bone flap can be cryopreserved and stored extracorporeally or can be stored in a subcutaneous pocket surgically created on the abdomen of the patient prior to reinsertion. Infection and resorption account for failure rates of up to

(continued)

50% using a preserved bone flap [7]. Split calvarial grafts have the advantage of being harvestable in the proximity of the defect eliminating a donor site and having low infection and resorption rates, but are disadvantaged by limited quantity of suitable bone for large defects and the diploic space is poorly formed before the age of five resulting in technically challenging bone harvest.

There are several biomaterials currently used in reconstruction of large calvarial defects. Polymethymethacrylate (PMMA) is widely used and can be shaped freehand and molded in situ or prefabricated and inserted as a solid implant. The principle advantage of PMMA is low cost; however, disadvantages include high infection and implant exposure rates of up to 80% and implant fracture [8].

Polyetheretherketone (PEEK) is a thermoplastic polymer that is increasingly used in cranioplasty. PEEK is used exclusively as a prefabricated implant and has been widely used in hip and spinal prostheses. It is biocompatible, similar in mechanical properties to bone, radiolucent and can be adjusted with a bur at the time of insertion to optimize fit, unlike metallic implants [9].

Hydroxyapatite (HA) ceramics have been widely reported in craniofacial reconstruction, usually in combination with titanium mesh for large defects [10]. HA is osseoconductive and eventual replacement of the material with bone has been demonstrated for small material volumes but complete bony replacement does not occur for large reconstructions. Significant foreign-body tissue reactions have been reported with HA cements, resulting in progressive erosion and thinning of the overlying skin, material fragmentation and exposure [11].

Titanium is widely used for cranioplasty and is supported by several large case series demonstrating the lowest infection and failure rates. Titanium is available as a mesh for intraoperative contouring or in sheet form as a prefabricated custom-made implant. It is biocompatible, sufficiently radiolucent to not create artefact on imaging and is associated with rates of infection and failure of approximately 10% [12].

At the time of admission for the cranioplasty, the defect was noted to be significantly endophytic. In close cooperation with the neurosurgeons, the lumbar-peritoneal drain was clamped and the ventriculo-peritoneal shunt adjusted to allow accumulation of CSF and re-expansion of the scalp.

The patient was admitted to the ward and noted to be febrile, hypoxic, tachycardic and tachypnoeic with radiographic evidence of chest sepsis. A diagnosis of a lower respiratory tract infection was made and the patient was started on intravenous piperacillin sodium / tazobactam sodium on the advice of microbiology and the cranioplasty delayed until resolution of the infection.

⊗ **Learning point** Minimizing complications

Infection is the leading cause of implant removal in cranioplasty. The success of calvarial reconstruction is ultimately dependent on the vascularity of local tissue and the characteristics of the implant material itself. Incisions to expose the defect should be carefully planned and wherever possible should utilize existing scars and lie directly over bone. Continuity of the frontal sinus with the cranioplasty implant is associated with increased risk of infection and obliteration of an involved sinus is necessary. Care should be taken with screw fixation that there is no inadvertent frontal sinus breach. Late versus early timing of cranioplasty has no effect on failure rates.

The patient underwent insertion of the titanium implant eight months from craniectomy and was discharged to the rehabilitation unit eight days later. A postoperative CT scan showed significant improvement of cerebral compression and restoration of the normal cranial contour (Figure 11.4).

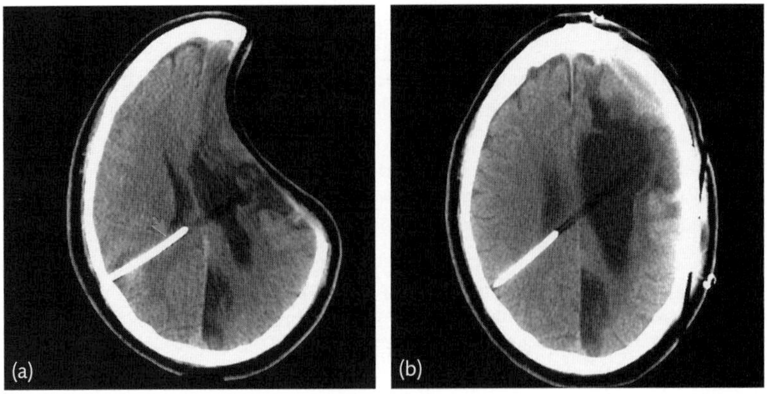

Figure 11.4 (a) Preoperative computed tomogram (CT) showing ventriculo-peritoneal shunt (arrow), endophytic craniectomy defect and compression of brain parenchyma. (b) Postoperative CT showing restoration of intracranial volume and improvement in ventricular/ midline appearance.

❻ Expert comment

Any concurrent sepsis should be managed aggressively and evidence of infection eliminated prior to definitive reconstruction. Reducing the time from craniectomy to reconstruction should not be at the expense of increasing risk of future infection and failure.

The patient was reviewed in the outpatient clinic one month following discharge. A small seroma was noted at the cranioplasty site without evidence of any other complications. The patient had been making good neurological progress and was able to roll independently, swallow liquids (although still gastrostomy dependent), engage in limited communication with his family and perform tasks including tooth brushing and basic writing skills.

⊕ Clinical tip Neurological improvement

The 'syndrome of the trephined' and 'sunken skin flap syndrome' describe several symptoms including neurological impairment, extreme fatigue, headaches and depression. The pathophysiology of these phenomena is not well understood but it is proposed that a calvarial defect leads to atmospheric pressure displacing the unsupported scalp inwards which leads to direct pressure on the cortex, reduction in cerebral blood flow and disruption of cerebrospinal fluid flow dynamics [13,14]. Improvements in cerebral perfusion, glucose metabolism and neurological functional following cranioplasty occur, with favourable outcome associated with younger patients and early reconstruction. The current recommendation is to undertake cranioplasty at the earliest opportunity.

Discussion

Previously controversial, decompressive craniectomy has been shown to have significant benefits in reduction of mortality and improvement in neurological outcome and will continue to provide craniofacial surgeons with challenging defects mandating reconstruction. The principle reasons for reconstruction of full-thickness calvarial defects are protective and cosmetic, although there is increasing evidence that cranioplasty has a significant functional benefit in a subset of patients. The subset of patients who will benefit the most is an interesting and important field of continuing research. In the future, tissue-engineering approaches to reconstruction may become feasible but until then biomaterials such as titanium and PEEK will remain the gold standard for extensive full-thickness calvarial defects. Careful surgical planning to minimize the potential for infection, the leading cause of reconstruction failure and a multidisciplinary team approach including neurosurgeons, craniofacial surgeons, maxillofacial prosthetists, neurologists and rehabilitation specialists are prerequisites for success in this complex group of patients.

A final word from the expert

This case demonstrates several important issues surrounding cranioplasty management. When a bone flap is not available or appropriate, extensive defects should be reconstructed with a prefabricated implant made of biomaterial such as titanium or PEEK.

In cases such as this one where the defect is endophytic, close cooperation with the neurosurgeons is required to effectively manage the potential dead space. With the aid of CT scans and clinical assessment the neurosurgeons will advise on any shunt adjustments both before and after placement of the cranioplasty.

Neurological improvement is sometimes seen following cranioplasty and this case illustrates this very well. This patient presented with a ruptured MCA aneurysm and malignant MCA infarction syndrome that has an associated mortality rate of 80%. Despite these poor odds the patient survived. Although still highly dependent for activities of daily living, after the cranioplasty the patient's baseline function improved so that they were able to communicate with their family and carry out basic tasks. This is a quantum leap from preoperative status in quality of life terms and is directly attributable to cranial reconstruction.

References

1. Juttler E, Schwab S, Schmiedek P, et al. Decompressive Surgery for the Treatment of Malignant Infarction of the Middle Cerebral Artery (DESTINY): a randomized, controlled trial. *Stroke* 2007; 38(9): 2518–25.
2. Vahedi K, Vicaut E, Mateo J, et al. Sequential-design, multicenter, randomized, controlled trial of early decompressive craniectomy in malignant middle cerebral artery infarction (DECIMAL Trial). *Stroke* 2007; 38: 2506–17.
3. Hofmeijer J, Kappelle LJ, Algra A, et al. Surgical decompression for space-occupying cerebral infarction (the Hemicraniectomy After Middle Cerebral Artery infarction with Life-threatening Edema Trial [HAMLET]): a multicentre, open, randomised trial. *Lancet Neurol* 2009; 8: 326–33.
4. Vahedi K, Hofmeijer J, Juettler E, et al. Early decompressive surgery in malignant infarction of the middle cerebral artery: a pooled analysis of three randomised controlled trials. *Lancet Neurol* 2007; 6: 215–22.
5. Li G, Wen L, Zhan RY, et al. Cranioplasty for patients developing large cranial defects combined with post-traumatic hydrocephalus after head trauma. *Brain Inj* 2008; 22: 333–7.
6. Heo J, Park SQ, Cho SJ, et al. Evaluation of simultaneous cranioplasty and ventriculoperitoneal shunt procedures: clinical article. *J Neurosurg* 2014; 121(2): 313–8.
7. Grant GA, Jolley M, Ellenbogen RG, et al. Failure of autologous bone-assisted cranioplasty following decompressive craniectomy in children and adolescents. *J Neurosurg Pediatr* 2004; 100: 163–8.

8. Marchac D, Greensmith A. Long-term experience with methylmethacrylate cranioplasty in craniofacial surgery. *J Plast Reconstr Aesthet Surg* 2008; 61: 744–52.

9. Hanasono MM, Goel N, DeMonte F. Calvarial reconstruction with polyetheretherketone implants. *Ann Plast Surg* 2009; 62: 653–5.

10. Ducic Y. Titanium mesh and hydroxyapatite cement cranioplasty: a report of 20 cases. *J Oral Maxillofac Surg* 2002; 60: 272–6.

11. Moreira-Gonzalez A, Jackson IT, Miyawaki T, et al. Clinical outcome in cranioplasty: critical review in long-term follow-up. *J Craniofac Surg* 2003; 14: 144–53.

12. Eufinger H, Rasche C, Wehmoller M,*et al*. CAD/CAM titanium implants for cranioplasty-an evaluation of success and quality of life of 169 consecutive implants with regard to size and location. *Int Congr Ser* 2005; 1281: 827–31.

13. Joseph V, Reilly P. Syndrome of the trephined. *J Neurosurg* 2009; 111: 650–2.

14. Winkler PA, Stummer W, Linke R, et al. The influence of cranioplasty on postural blood flow regulation, cerebrovascular reserve capacity and cerebral glucose metabolism. *Neurosurg Focus* 2000; 8: e 9.

Distraction osteogenesis: a reconstructive option

Matthew Idle

ⓘ **Expert commentary** Andrew Monaghan

Case history

A 27-year-old male was referred to the Oral and Maxillofacial Surgery Outpatients with a bony discontinuity in his right mandible, resulting in pain and mobility of the hemi-mandible segments. He had been the victim of an alleged assault in a jail in Iraq 15 years ago and sustained a fracture to the right angle of the mandible. The injury was initially managed by wire osteosynthesis, but there was a malunion and subsequent osteomyelitis. This resulted in a bony defect ranging from the lower left 1 to the lower right 7. Prior to his referral several non-vascularized autogenous free bone grafts to the area had been unsuccessful.

His initial work-up included a computed tomogram (CT) with three-dimensional reconstruction and this demonstrated the scale of the defect requiring restoration (Figure 12.1). A distance of 35 mm was noted between the lower right 7 and the lower left 1. The initial treatment plan involved extraction of the lower right 6 and the patient, requesting reconstruction, was offered the following two options:

1. Application of distraction osteogenesis (DO) technique with bone transport of the proximal fragment (bifocal distraction [1]) with subsequent placement of a titanium mandibular reconstruction plate.
2. Immediate reconstruction with a fibular free osteocutaneous flap.

Both of these options would allow for the subsequent rehabilitation with osseointegrated Straumann dental implants and a prosthesis borne on this substructure.

ⓘ **Expert comment**

Creation of new tissue using distraction obviates the morbidity associated with the use of a free flap and the donor site. In this case the risks associated with a fibular flap are: 5–10% risk of flap failure, risk of vascular compromise to the foot, common peroneal / sural nerve injuries and compartment syndrome. An alternative consideration would be an autogenous free bone graft as the width of the defect is less than 5 cm. However, this has been attempted unsuccessfully in the past and as such would not be the first option. The ultimate aim in this case is composite reconstruction of the mandible and dentition with the return to normal mastication, speech and swallowing in the absence of pain, mobility and infection.

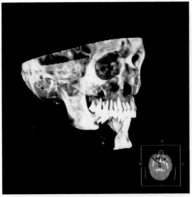
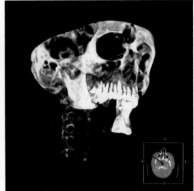
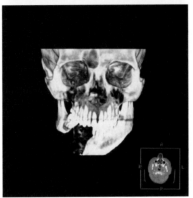

Figure 12.1 Computed tomogram with three-dimensional digital reconstruction demonstrating the right hemi-mandibular defect.

⭐ **Learning point** The history of distraction osteogenesis

The procedure was initially introduced in 1905 by Codivilla for use in orthopaedic surgery, namely lower limbs [2]. In 1951 Ilizarov discovered, by chance, that new bone was formed when the osteotomy site was placed under tension. Ilizarov described a tension-stress model in which 'slow steady traction of tissues causes them to become metabolically activated, resulting in an increase in the proliferative and biosynthetic functions' [3]. The new bone produced achieves 90% of normal bony architecture and is able to resist normal functional loading.

Transport distraction osteogenesis of the mandible

The process of transport DO to reconstruct defects of the mandible was first described by Constantino et al. in canine models [4]. It was subsequently described in humans with hemi-facial microsomia by Cohen et al. [5].

Types of distractor

- Intra-oral / extra-oral
- Single-vector / multi-vector
- Alveolar
- Curvilinear
- Horizontal / ramus
- Sub-mucosal / extra-mucosal.

The patient elected to proceed with distraction and the procedure was carried out approximately a decade following the initial assault (Figure 12.2). Under general anaesthetic he underwent linear corticotomy at the right angle of the mandible and had placement of a Synthes titanium single-vector mandibular distractor (DePuy Synthes, Johnson & Johnson, US).

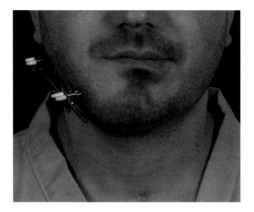

Figure 12.2 Postoperative view (following commencement of distraction) with the distraction device in place demonstrating the Synthes transcutaneous single-vector device. See colour plate section.

⊗ **Learning point** Indications for mandibular osteodistraction

- Bilateral hypoplasia (Treacher-Collins, Pierre-Robin sequence)
- Unilateral hypoplasia (hemi-facial microsomia)
- Severe non-syndromic hypoplasia
- Obstructive sleep apnoea
- Trauma
- Post-surgical segmental resection (neoplasia / cyst)
- TMJ ankylosis
- Inadequate alveolar height (pre-prosthetic)

⊗ **Learning point** Contraindications to osteodistraction

There are no absolute contraindications to distraction osteogenesis, but the relative contraindications are:

- poorly compliant patients
- inadequate native bone
- irradiatiated tissue
- older patients with reduced healing potential due to a reduction in mesenchymal stem cells
- metal allergies
- epilepsy.

Activation of the device was initiated seven days post-operatively at a rate of 1 mm per day (rhythm of 2 mm × 0.5 mm activations per day). Distraction was terminated after 12 weeks, after which time the gap was reduced to 10 mm (Figure 12.3) with the creation of 25 mm of new mandible.

⊗ **Learning point** Phases of distraction

There are three distinct phases:

Latency phase. This represents the time between the corticotomy and the beginning of activation of the distractor. During this period a callus forms and it is vital for subsequent osteogenesis that it is of appropriate volume.

Distraction phase. The device is activated to create tension across the callus and this leads to new bone formation in the presence of an intact periosteum. The rate is usually between 0.5 mm and 2 mm per day with a *rhythm* of either one or two activation(s) per day to achieve this distance. However, Ilizarov has described up to four 0.25 mm activations per day, but this requires dedicated patient and/ or carer cooperation.

Consolidation phase. Following an appropriate period of distraction the device is locked and the new bone is allowed to consolidate. This is usually for a minimum of eight weeks. It will take approximately eight months for the new bone to reach 90% of the strength of surrounding native bone.

❝ **Expert comment**

In this case the patient presented with total interruption of the right inferior dental nerve. However, where the nerve is intact the corticotomy must be carried out with care to avoid injury to this structure. We advocate the use of buccal, superior and inferior osteotomies with a reciprocating saw and then completion of the lingual portion of the corticotomy using a Tufnol Handled Chisel in a rotational fashion (greenstick fracture). This gives adequate protection of the neurovascular bundle.

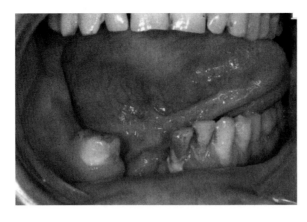

Figure 12.3 Intra-oral view following termination of distraction.

⊕ **Clinical tip** Duration of latency phase

McCarthy states in his report on ten years of experience in DO of the mandible that he employs a latency phase of five days in all cases [6]. Glowacki et al., however, demonstrated in porcine models that a latency period of either zero or four days showed no difference in bone stability [7]. Shorter latency periods have been proposed in the craniofacial skeleton due to an excellent vascular supply when compared to the remainder of the skeleton. Times of greater than seven days, especially in neonates and infants, are likely to lead to premature consolidation of the corticotomy site.

⊕ **Clinical tip** Distraction rates

The most commonly adopted rate is 1 mm per day [8]. Slightly increased rates of 1.5–2 mm may be employed in neonates and infants as early consolidation is more likely. McCarthy proposes a rate of 1.5 mm per day in patients younger than three [6]. More than 2 mm of distraction per day is considered too fast and leads to poor quality bone. The callus does not have adequate time to form and thus does not have suitable osteogenic potential. Distraction rates of less than 0.5 mm per day may lead to premature consolidation.

⭑ **Learning point** Types of distraction [1]

- **Monofocal:** new bone created by a single osteotomy with a device attached across this gap.
- **Bifocal:** this uses unilateral bone transport to close a pre-existing defect.
- **Trifocal:** this incorporated a bilateral osteotomy and transport until the segments meet. This is usually undertaken to close symphyseal defects.

The newly formed bone was allowed to consolidate for four weeks. A secondary procedure to remove the distraction device was undertaken, with bone harvested from the left retromolar region and grafted to the residual cleft and removal of the transported lower right 7. In conjunction with this procedure a 2.4 mm / 3.0 mm locking reconstruction plate (LRP) (16 hole, DePuy Synthes, Johnson & Johnson, US) was placed to reinforce the mandible. Radiologically there was evidence of sound new bone formation in the right mandible (Figure 12.4).

The case was subsequently reviewed in a multidisciplinary clinic including: an oral and maxillofacial surgeon, a restorative dentist and a specialist head and neck prosthetist, with the following conclusions being drawn:

1. A bony union had occurred between the independent portions of the mandible.
2. Limited vertical space was noted in the mandibular right quadrant.
3. Lower centre line shift of 2 mm to the right.
4. There was good dental interdigitation on the left side.
5. Evidence of generalized tooth wear.

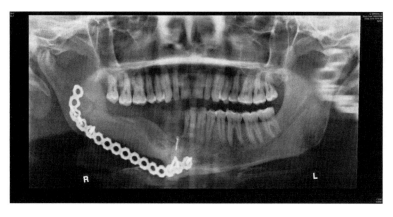

Figure 12.4 Postoperative orthopantomogram following removal of distraction device, left retromolar bone graft, and placement of a locking reconstruction plate.

Following this assessment he underwent a general anaesthetic for placement of four Straumann (Ch) implants and sectioning of the LRP leaving the proximal five holes of the plate in situ (Figure 12.5). The subsequent prosthetic rehabilitation was undertaken at the affiliated regional dental hospital (Figure 12.6).

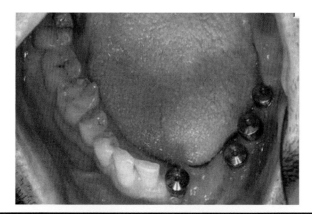

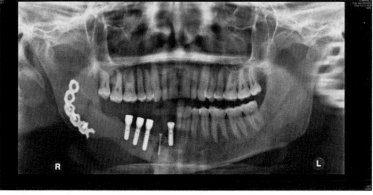

Figure 12.5 Following placement of four Straumann osseointegrated implants in the right neomandible.

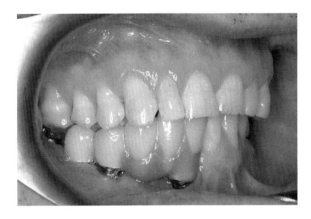

Figure 12.6 Following prosthetic rehabilitation.

❛❛ Expert comment

In this scenario a single-vector extra-oral distractor was used, but with the advent of new designs it may be worth considering a multi-vector device, or an intra-oral curvilinear device that will more favourably reproduce the shape of the mandible. Ultimately, close follow-up and good patient cooperation are of the utmost importance when such a sizeable and complex distraction is attempted. The quality of this neomandible is demonstrated in the receptiveness to osseointegrated implants and its ability to withstand normal masticatory forces.

✪ Learning point Histology of bone formed by distraction [9]

1. Fibrous central zone: longitudinally orientated fibrous bundles.
2. Transition zone: osteoid formation within collagen framework.
3. Remodelling zone: significant osteoclast activity.
4. Mature bone zone: compact cortical bone with an appearance similar to the adjacent non-distracted bone.

At one month there is continuity of bone between the corticotomy sites and at two months this bone is mineralized with subsequent remodelling (see Figure 12.7).

Reproduced from Karp NS et al., Membranous bone lengthening: a serial histological study, *Annals of Plastic Surgery*, Volume 29, Issue 1, pp.2–7, Copyright © 1992 Wolters Kluwer Health Inc., with permission from Lippincott, Williams, and Wilkinson.

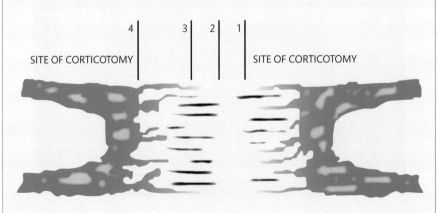

Figure 12.7 Histology of bone formed by distraction.

✅ **Evidence base** Karp 1990 - Canine trial [10]

- Principles of bone lengthening applied to the craniofacial skeleton.
- Growing mandible of dogs used as a model.
- Six mongrel dogs aged five months.
- Unilateral, periosteal-preserving osteotomy.
- External device at a right angle to the corticotomy.
- Latency phase: ten days of external fixation.
- Distraction phase: 1 mm/day for 20 days.
- Consolidation phase: 56 days (8 weeks).
- Dogs were euthanased.
- Histology confirmed new bone formation.

Source: data from Karp NS, et al., Bone lengthening in the craniofacial skeleton, *Annals of Plastic Surgery,* Volume 24, Issue 3, pp.231–237, Copyright © 1990, Wolters Kluwer Health Inc.

✅ **Evidence base** McCarthy 1992 - Human trial [12]

- Lengthening of the mandible by gradual distraction.
- Increase ranged from 18–24 mm.
- Four patients (average age 78 months).
- Consolidation period of nine weeks using an external distractor.
- Follow-up between 11 and 20 months.
- Trial represents introduction of technique.

Source: data from McCarthy et al., Lengthening the human mandible by gradual distraction, *Plastic and Reconstructive Surgery,* Volume 89, pp.1–8, Copyright © 1992, American Society of Plastic Surgeons.

> ❂ **Learning point** Tension-stress / -strain effect [8,11]
>
> The application of tensile stress across a fracture that is undergoing healing causes the production of new bone. Tensile strain is the relative elongation of an object when subjected to tension. Thus a distraction of 1 mm/day when the defect is 1 mm results in a tensile strain of 100%. Higher levels of tensile strain (> 15%) result in bone resorption, whereas lower levels of tensile strain are required for bone formation (2–8%). Therefore bone formation will not begin for several weeks following the commencement of distraction.

Discussion

Distraction osteogenesis of the mandible has gained in popularity since the original work by McCarthy and co-workers in 1990. It is safe, quick, reliable and does not require an extensive access procedure. The study by Tuinzing et al. also suggests a predictable degree of stability with DO of the mandible [13]. The avoidance of donor site morbidity is also a notable benefit. In addition, the new bone has neovascularity that seems to have a protective effect against infection when compared with free bone grafts [14]. The technique can be applied in infants with micrognathia and can assist in early decannulation where there is upper airway obstruction. There does not appear to be an upper age limit for this procedure and McCarthy reports the eldest patient from their series was 42-years-old. It has also been noted that inpatient time is reduced for this group when compared with free bone grafting from distant sites or composite free tissue transfer.

✅ **Evidence base** Tuinzing 2004-Stability following distraction osteogenesis of the mandible [13]

- Study of 50 patients (mean age, 14.7 years; range 11.2–37.3 years) with mandibular hypoplasia.
- Divided into high-angle (14 cases) and low/normal angle (36 cases).
- Bilateral single-vector submerged distraction device.
- Latency phase: 6 days.
- Distraction schedule: 1 mm/day (0.5 mm every 12 hours), no overcorrection.
- Cephalometric analysis just before operation, immediate post distraction, six months and one year.
- 8/14 (57%) high-angle cases showed a degree of relapse.
- 3/36 (8.3%) low- / normal-angle cases showed relapse.
- Concluded that DO is safe and predictable in low- / normal-angle cases.

Source: data from van Strijen PJ et al., Stability after distraction osteogenesis to lengthen the mandible; results in 50 patients, *Journal of Oral and Maxillofacial Surgery,* Volume 62, Issue 3, pp.304–307, Copyright © 2004 Elsevier Inc.

Several potential complications are associated with this technique, notably failure of distraction, pin tract infections, loosening of pins/device, hypertrophic scars, marginal mandibular nerve injuries, inappropriate vectors of distraction, malocclusion, relapse and injury to developing tooth germs. There is also the possibility of compressive forces on the condylar head which may result in symptoms or remodelling of the condylar head or potentially condylar resorption.

> ★ **Learning point** 'Molding of the regenerate' [7,15]
>
> This is a concept whereby the regenerate zone can be 'molded' by angulation of the device, digital manipulation or the use of interdental maxillomandibular wiring. It has been described in patients with hypoplastic mandibles as a way of closing an anterior open bite. The studies on canines show that 'molding' can be carried out once there is 10 mm of bony regenerate [16]. However, this technique while performed in the late distraction phase can also be successfully achieved in the early consolidation phase. The canine studies also demonstrated histologically that there was no evidence of a fibrous union following 'molding' and that bony union had occurred. From a technical point of view it necessitates removal of the distraction device about two to four weeks following the termination of distraction and instigation of elastic orthodontic therapy until the consolidation phase is complete.

In such complex reconstructive cases the final goal should be to restore pre-morbid coherent mandibular form, enabling a pain-free range of motion and subsequent dental rehabilitation. There should be close follow-up during the treatment process and liaison with the multidisciplinary team so that complications during treatment can be identified early and dealt with appropriately. It is very common to make adjustments to the treatment plan during the three phases of distraction osteogenesis. The restorative dentist will coordinate the positioning of the implants taking the subsequent prosthetic rehabilitation into account. This will also ensure occlusal harmony, thereby optimizing mastication and swallowing. The holistic care of the team will also take the aesthetic expectations of the patients to ensure that they can be met.

A final word from the expert

This chapter has advocated the benefits of DO as a method for the generation of new bone, but it will also enable associated enlargement of the soft tissues (distraction histiogenesis) and this seems to aid in the reduction of relapse. Distraction histiogenesis will allow, as seen in this case, the formation of keratinized mucosa that proves ideal for the placement of implants. With a complex distraction such as this, the positioning of the correctly selected device to achieve the appropriate vectors is the crucial step. There is some scope to correct any occlusal discrepancy that may develop during the distraction phase with the 'molding of the regenerate' technique described above. This was, however, not necessary in the case that we have described as the patient achieved good interdigitation of the existing dentition on the left-hand side. In such a case the 'norm' appears to be the use of autogenous ileac crest graft or a fibula free osseocutaneous flap. This demonstrates the great potential and reliability of using distraction osteogenesis in such cases.

Acknowledgements

We would like to thank Mr. Stephen Dover, Consultant Oral and Maxillofacial Surgeon at University Hospitals Birmingham, for placing the implants and Dr Kathy Warren, Consultant Restorative Dentist at Birmingham Dental Hospital for undertaking the subsequent restorative work.

References

1. Costantino PD, Friedman CD. Distraction osteogenesis. Applications for mandibular regrowth. *Otolaryngol Clin North Am* 1991; 24(6): 1433–43.
2. Codivilla A. On the means of lengthening in the lower limbs, the muscles, and tissues which are shortened through deformity. *Am J Orthop Surg* 1905; 2: 353–69.
3. Ilizarov GA. *The Transosseous Osteosynthesis: Theoretical and Clinical Aspects of the Regeneration and Growth of Tissue.* New York: Springer-Verlag; 1992, p. 800.
4. Costantino PD, Shybut G, Friedman CD, et al. Segmental mandible regeneration by distraction. *Arch Otolarygol Head Neck Surg* 1990; 116: 535–45.
5. Cohen SR, Rustrick RE, Burstein FD. Distraction osteogenesis of the human craniofacial skeleton: initial experience with a new distraction system. *Craniofac Surg* 1995; 6: 368–74.
6. McCarthy JG, Katzen JT, Hopper R, Grayson BH. The first decade of mandibular distraction: Lessons we have learned. *Plast Reconstr Surg* 2002; 110: 1812–27.
7. Glowacki J, Shusterman EM, Troulis M, et al. Distraction osteogenesis of the porcine mandible: histomorphic evaluation of bone. *Plast Reconstr Surg* 2004; 113: 566–73.
8. Ilizarov GA. Clinical application of the tension-stress effect for limb lengthening. *Clin Orthop Rel Res* 1990; 250: 8–26.
9. Karp NS, McCarthy JG, Schreiber JS, et al. Membranous bone lengthening: a serial histological study. *Ann Plast Surg* 1992; 29(1): 2–7.
10. Karp NS, Thorne CH, McCarthy JG, Sissons HA. Bone lengthening in the craniofacial skeleton. *Ann Plast Surg* 1990; 24(3): 231–7.
11. Gang L. New development and insights learned from distraction osteogenesis. *Curr Opin Orthop* 2004; 15: 325–30.
12. McCarthy JG, Schreiber J, Karp N, et al. Lengthening the human mandible by gradual distraction. *Plast Reconstr Surg* 1992; 89: 1–8.
13. van Strijen PJ, Breuning KH, Becking AG, Tuinzing DB. Stability after distraction osteogenesis to lengthen the mandible; results in 50 patients. *J Oral Maxillofac Surg* 2004; 62(3): 304–7.
14. Walker D. Buried bidirectional telescopic mandibular distraction. In: Samchukov M, Cope J, Cherkashin A (eds) *Craniofacial Distraction Osteogenesis.* St. Louis: Mosby; 2001, pp. 313–22.
15. McCarthy JG, Hopper RA, Hollier LH Jr, et al. Molding of the regenerate in mandibular distraction: clinical experience. *Plast Reconstr Surg* 2003; 112(5): 1239–46.
16. Luchs JS, Stelnicki EJ, Rowe NM, et al. Molding of the regenerate in mandibular distraction, part I: Laboratory study. *J Craniofac Surg* 2002; 13: 205.

Posterior calvarial osseodistraction for syndromic craniosynostosis

Neil Opie

Ⓒ **Expert Commentary** Martin Evans

Case history

A two-month-old male child born to non-consanguineous parents was referred to the craniofacial unit with a number of marked dysmorphisms.

He was brachycephalic, had marked hypertelorism (Figure 13.1), and a number of digital anomalies including extra-terminal digits, flexion deformities and webbing of both the hands and feet [1]. Pfeiffer's syndrome was clinically diagnosed and confirmed by genetic testing.

He was seen on the Multidisciplinary Craniofacial Clinic at approximately six months of age. His bicoronal synostosis was confirmed as the cause of his brachycephaly. He was noted to be hyperteloric and also to have a high arched palate.

At this stage there was no clinical evidence of raised intracranial pressure (ICP), but it was felt that this was highly likely to develop in the future. Recent literature suggests that up to 67% of syndromic craniosynostosis cases do go on to develop this complication [2].

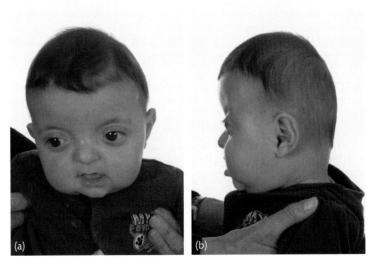

Figure 13.1 Frontal and lateral photographs showing features of brachycephaly.

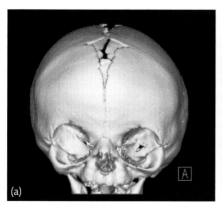
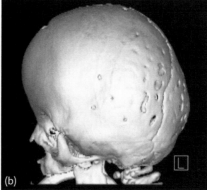

(a)   (b)

Figure 13.2 Three-dimensional reconstruction of cross-sectional imaging showing premature fusion of the coronal sutures and 'thumb-printing' in the occipital region.

Investigations were organized in the form of high-contrast computed tomogram (CT) and magnetic resonance imaging (MRI) scans (Figure 13.2). He also underwent ophthalmic review, speech and language assessment and he was also assessed by a hand surgeon due to his accessory digits, broad thumbs and webbing.

The patient underwent posterior calvarial osseodistraction under general anaesthesia at age nine months to avoid the complications related to raised ICP (Box 13.1).

⊕ **Learning point** Pfeiffer's syndrome

Pfeiffer syndrome is a rare autosomal dominant genetic disorder believed to affect approximately 1 in 100,000 live births. It is named after RA Pfeiffer who described a list of characteristics that included a coronal synostosis, turribrachycephaly, midface hypoplasia, exorbitism and the hallmark broad thumbs and great toes with variable soft tissue syndactyly [3,4]. Other features include hypertelorism, strabismus, downslanting palpebral fissures, class III malocclusion and a beaked nasal deformity. Approximately 86% of children with Pfeiffer syndrome have conductive hearing loss [5]. Pfeiffer syndrome is strongly associated with mutations of fibroblast growth factor receptor 1 and 2 (FGFR-1/-2), important receptors for normal bone development. Although the majority of cases involve FGFR-2, the approximate 5% of patients who express an FGFR-1 mutation are known to demonstrate a less severe phenotype [5–8].

⊕ **Learning point** The craniofacial multidisciplinary team and diagnostic work-up

The multidisciplinary team comprises maxillofacial, plastic, neuro and ophthalmic surgeons, as well as speech and language therapists and specialist nurses. The patients are seen in a combined clinic by all team members and other specialist teams are also utilized depending on the individual child's specific problems. Hearing is assessed at six months and an ear, nose and throat surgical opinion may be sought, as well as the opinions of other specialists (such as the congenital hand surgeon in this case).

Typical 'work-up' prior to surgery for a Pfeiffer's syndrome case such as this would be an initial assessment in clinic, height and weight charting (plus head circumference measurements), high-contrast CT scanning and MRI scanning, plus an ophthalmological assessment for the presence of raised ICP. The purpose of this assessment stage would be to identify current or impending raised ICP and calvarial expansion surgery would typically be planned.

Box 13.1 Operative note: posterior calvarial osseodistraction [9,10]

The patient is placed in the prone position. A standard coronal approach is utilized, with a *sine wave* or *wavy line* incision placed anterior to the calvarial osteotomy site. The bony cuts with a craniotome extend from the vertex laterally on each side to then continue horizontally through the occipital bone below the estimated position of the torcula, typically within 2–3 cm of the foramen magnum. It should be noted that the transverse occipital osteotomies are widened to create a 5 mm bone gap, thus preventing premature fusion of this bone whilst actively distracting. The calvarial bone flap created with the osteotome is not elevated from the dura and this in addition to the placement of the calvarial osteotomies avoiding any trans-osseous communicating veins is thought to reduce intra-operative bleeding thereby reducing morbidity from haemorrhage and dural tears.

Two internal 30 mm titanium single vector distractors (Synthes/Stryker) are positioned in a horizontal vector parallel to the Frankfort plane and fixed with at least four 4 mm screws per footplate. The incision is then closed in a standard fashion. A Biopatch™ chlorhexidine-impregnated sponge dressing (proven to reduce central-line associated infections) is placed over the skin port sites, and the operative site is covered with a head bandage. It is not our practice to place a suction drain in these cases.

In this case an operative time of 3.5 hours was recorded and 487 ml of blood loss documented. The patient was observed as an inpatient for 7 days prior to discharge.

⊕ Clinical tip Postoperative management

The latency period utilized in our unit is 72 hours, followed by a distraction rate of 1 mm/day with a frequency of 0.5 mm every 12 hours. Our short latency period reflects our experience in syndromic infants that with longer periods, premature bone fusion can occur and this can lead to failure of distraction.

This patient was distracted for 29 days after which his head circumference had increased from 45.3 cm pre-surgery to 50.4 cm (Figure 13.3 and 13.4).

Our unit's preferred consolidation period is three months and our patient had his distraction apparatus removed under general anaesthesia at approximately three months post surgery (Figure 13.5) as a combined procedure with the congenital hand surgeon treating him, who addressed his accessory digits and flexion contractures.

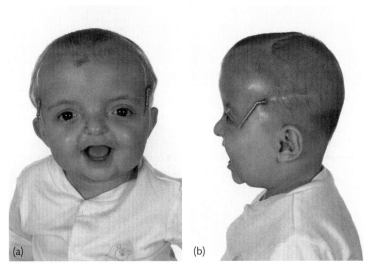

(a)   (b)

Figure 13.3 Postoperative photographs demonstrating the position of the coronal incision and exit ports for the distractors.

Reproduced courtesy of Birmingham Children's Hospital NHS Trust.

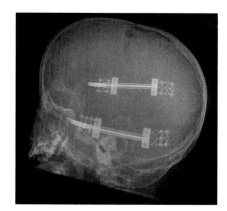

Figure 13.4 Plain film radiograph demonstrating the position of the distractors (at termination of distraction).

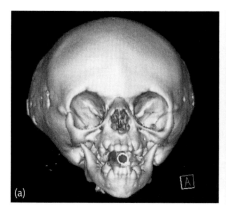

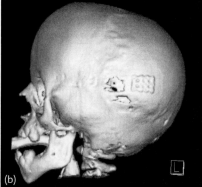

Figure 13.5 Three-dimensional reconstruction of cross-sectional imaging showing skull morphology at the termination of distraction.

⬤ Expert comment

The procedure has evolved since first being undertaken at our unit in 2006. The bone flap size and position has been modified, the number of distractors has varied (maximum four, minimum two distractors) and there is a suggestion that a consolidation period of 90 days is too long and shorter periods are acceptable.

Also during the learning curve, some complications have arisen. Footplate loosening has been eradicated by modifications to the distractor position and fixation, but cerebrospinal fluid (CSF) leak from dural tear either intraoperatively or during the distraction period is an ever-present concern.

✪ Learning point The terminology of distraction osteogenesis

- **Latency phase:** time between the osteotomy and activation of the distractor.
- **Distraction phase:** period during which the bone ends are being separated, with a rate of 1 mm/day (0.5 mm / 12 hourly) being employed.
- **Consolidation phase:** period allowing for bone maturation during which no further active expansion takes place.

✪ Learning point Complications

- CSF leak
- Distractor trauma
- Footplate loosening
- Wound dehiscence
- Cerebritis

> ⭐ **Learning point** Comparison of conventional posterior calvarial augmentation surgery, spring-assisted cranioplasty and posterior calvarial osseodistraction [11]:
>
> | | Advantages | Disadvantages |
> | --- | --- | --- |
> | Posterior calvarial augmentation | Not appliance dependent
No second procedure required | Relapse
Problematic soft tissue closure |
> | Spring-assisted cranioplasty | Short operating time | Lack of control over expansion distance/vector
Expansion dependent on sutural position
Second procedure required |
> | Posterior calvarial osseodistraction | Control over expansion distance/vector
Large and predictable volume gains
Accommodation of the soft tissue envelope
Maintenance of bone vascularity
Limited production of dead space (reduced infection / relapse risk) | Percutaneous hardware- a potential route for infection
Second procedure required
Device-related complications
Prolonged treatment time
Expensive |

Discussion

Craniofacial growth generally follows a craniocaudal pattern with an initial rapid calvarial growth during the first two years of life, followed by midface growth until approximately ten years of age and mandibular growth thereafter into adulthood. In the first two years, the brain rapidly grows and an increase in calvarial size to accommodate the expanding brain is the result. The infant calvarium reaches 77% of its adult volume by age two years and 90% by age five years. There is also a corresponding increase in head circumference. During the first year of life, the greatest gains in volume of the infant skull occur in the posterior half of the cranial vault. This is not the case in syndromic craniosynostosis, where the posterior fossa is often underdeveloped (short cranial base). It is this underdevelopment of the posterior fossa, due to skull base and lambdoid suture premature fusion, that is thought to account for the association between Chiari I malformation (cerebellar tonsillar herniation) and syndromic craniosynostosis. The incidence of Chiari I malformation is known to be as high as 70% for Crouzon syndrome, 82% for Pfeiffer syndrome, and 100% for Kleeblattshadel. Untreated Chiari I malformation can lead to non-communicating hydrocephalus as a result of obstruction of CSF outflow and venous hypertension [5,12].

The aetiology of the craniosynostoses is still not fully understood, but the resulting characteristic patterns of restricted and compensatory growth are well recognized. Although these compensatory growth patterns can be significantly disfiguring, the most significant consequence of craniosynostosis is insufficient skull growth resulting in cephalocranial disproportion, which is known to be a major factor (but not the only one) in the development of raised ICP. In syndromic craniosynostoses, the risk of intracranial pressure is known to be further increased by intracranial venous congestion, hydrocephalus and upper airway obstruction [13].

Surgery for craniosynostosis dates from the nineteenth century, but was associated with both high morbidity and mortality. Paul Tessier revolutionized cranial vault reconstruction in the late 1960s when he introduced his intracranial approach that allowed for accurate osteotomy, mobilization and repositioning of the forehead and supraorbital regions. Since that time several significant advances have taken place, including earlier surgical intervention, increasingly advanced imaging modalities and the development plating systems and appliances. However, the goals of treatment remain the same: expansion of intracranial volume to prevent or reduce raised ICP and improving head shape.

The techniques most commonly employed for the initial cranial vault expansion in craniosynostosis are fronto-orbital advancement with anterior cranial vault remodelling or posterior cranial vault expansion (fixed augmentation) [14]. Alternative techniques for expansion have also been reported and may be utilized in certain circumstances [15]. Expansion of the posterior vault provides a larger volume increase per millimetre of advancement than anterior expansion [2,16,17]. However, surgery in the posterior fossa can be technically difficult because of the anatomical constraints of the area as well as the need to operate on the prone patient [18]. Scalp closure in posterior calvarial augmentation can be under tension leading to wound breakdown and scarring. Postural forces leading to relapse are also known to be significant. The use of distraction osteogenesis for posterior calvarial vault expansion has therefore become an increasingly adopted alternative to posterior calvarial augmentation surgery.

✔ **Evidence base** White, Evans, Dover et al. [19]

- Six patients undergoing posterior cranial vault distraction to manage raised intracranial pressure.
- Introduction of technique.
- Four patients with Apert syndrome and two patients with Crouzon syndrome.
- Age range: 9 to 19 months.
- Mean distraction period of 28 days (range 24–1 days).
- Mean consolidation period of 49 days (range 0–115 days).
- Single distraction vector devices.
- Five patients completed distraction period.
- Three patients completed consolidation period.
- Significant calvarial expansion was achieved in all six cases.
- Safe and more efficient than conventional techniques with a shorter operating time.

Source: data from White N et al., Posterior calvarial vault expansion using distraction osteogenesis, *Child's Nervous System*, Volume 25, Issue 2, pp.231–236, Copyright © 2009 Springer International Publishing AG.

Distraction osteogenesis has been applied to the cranial vault, midface and mandible in order to achieve bony growth over the past 20 years. The technique's advantages include the maintenance of bone vascularity, the production of vascularized bone and the reduction of the volume dead space produced. Disadvantages include the need for a second procedure to enable device removal, device-related complications and prolonged treatment time.

An interesting benefit of distracting the posterior calvarium is the improvement observed in the cerebellar anatomy of patients with syndromic craniosynostosis and Chiari malformation, which, as stated above, is frequently found in syndromic craniosynostosis [12]. It has also been observed in that series that posterior distraction also has an anterior effect and significant anterior cranial fossa expansion has been observed during posterior calvarial osseodistraction cases. It is postulated that this is due the calvarial plasticity in infants less than two years of age as well as the horizontal direction of the distraction vectors [19].

Despite this anterior affect, posterior calvarial osseodistraction leaves the anterior cranial fossa surgically untouched so that future procedures (such as fronto-orbital or monobloc advancement) are not compromised by prior surgery. This is an important consideration as there is a significant need for further surgery to the anterior skull base and midface in this group of patients for aesthetics, function and for potential upper airway compromise [20].

A final word from the expert

Maxillofacial surgeons have a considerable experience of using distraction osseogenesis as a treatment modality.

Posterior calvarial osseodistraction is a technique for addressing posterior calvarial growth insufficiency that has been performed for eight years in Birmingham, UK. Since our initial paper (Childs Nervous System 2009), the technique has been adopted in the worldwide craniofacial community as a treatment modality to achieve permanent posterior calvarial expansion safely with few complications.

There have been promising results in the treatment of some non-craniosynostotic patients with Chiari I malformation and we await further novel uses for this technique.

References

1. James W, Berger T, Elston D (eds). *Andrews' Diseases of the Skin: Clinical Dermatology* 10th edition. London: WB Saunders; 2001.
2. Derderian C, Seaward J. Syndromic craniosynostosis. *Semin Plast Surg* 2012; 26(2): 64–75.
3. Pfeiffer RA. Dominant hereditary acrocephalosyndactylia. *Zeitschrift für Kinderheilkunde* 1964 (in German) 90: 301–20.
4. Vogels A, Fryns JP. Pfeiffer syndrome. *Orphanet J Rare Dis* 2006; 1: 19.
5. Fearon JA, Rhodes J. Pfeiffer syndrome: a treatment evaluation. *Plast Reconstr Surg* 2009; 123(5): 1560–9.
6. Chan CT, Thorogood P. Pleiotropic features of syndromic craniosynostoses correlate with differential expression of fibroblast growth factor receptors 1 and 2 during human craniofacial development. *Pediatr Res* 1999; 45(1): 46–53.
7. Cornejo-Roldan LR, Roessler E, Muenke M. Analysis of the mutational spectrum of the FGFR2 gene in Pfeiffer syndrome. *Hum Genet* 1999; 104(5): 425–31.
8. Muenke M, Schell U, Hehr A, et al. A common mutation in the fibroblast growth factor receptor 1 gene in Pfeiffer syndrome. *Nat Genet* 1994; 8(3): 269–74.
9. Derderian CA, Bastidas N, Bartlett SP. Posterior cranial vault expansion using distraction osteogenesis. *Childs Nerv Syst* 2012; 28(9): 1551–6.
10. Steinbacher DM, Skirpan J, Puchala J, Barlett SP. Expansion of the posterior cranial vault using distraction osteogenesis. *Plast Reconstr Surg* 2011; 127(2): 792–801.
11. Sgouros S, Goldin JH, Hockley AD, Wake MJ. Posterior skull surgery in craniosynostosis. *Childs Nerv Syst* 1996; 12(11): 727–33.
12. Ahmad F, Evans M, White N, et al. Amelioration of Chiari type 1 malformation and syringomyelia following posterior calvarial distraction in Crouzon's syndrome - a case report. *Childs Nerv Syst* 2014; 30(1): 177–9.

13. Taylor WJ, Hayward RD, Lasjaunias P, et al. Enigma of raised intracranial pressure in patients with complex craniosynostosis: the role of abnormal intracranial venous drainage. *J Neurosurg* 2001; 94(3): 377–85.

14. Wall SA, Goldin JH, Hockley AD, et al. Fronto-orbital re-operation in craniosynostosis. *Br J Plast Surg* 1994; 47(3): 180–4.

15. Czerwinski M, Kolar JC, Fearon JA. Complex craniosynostosis. *Plast Reconstr Surg* 2011; 128(4): 955–61.

16. Goldstein JA, Paliga JT, Wink JD, et al. A craniometric analysis of posterior cranial vault distraction osteogenesis. *Plast Reconstr Surg* 2013; 131(6): 1367–75.

17. Nowinski D, Di Rocco F, Reiner D, et al. Posterior cranial vault expansion in the treatment of craniosynostosis. Comparison of current techniques. *Childs Nerv Syst.* 2012; 28(9): 1537–44.

18. Lauritzen CG, Davis C, Ivarsson A, et al. The evolving role of springs in craniofacial surgery: the first 100 clinical cases. *Plast Reconstr Surg* 2008; 121(2): 545–54.

19. White N, Evans M, Dover MS, et al. Posterior calvarial vault expansion using distraction osteogenesis. *Childs Nerv Syst* 2009; 25(2): 231–6.

20. Siddiqi SN, Posnick JC, Buncic R, et al. The detection and management of intracranial hypertension after initial suture release and decompression for craniofacial dysostosis syndromes. *Neurosurgery* 1995; 36(4): 703–8.

SECTION 5

Orthognathic surgery

14 The anterior open bite

Barbara Gerber

ⓘ **Expert commentary** Andrew Currie

Case history

A 14-year-old boy was referred by his orthodontist due to an increased overjet, crowding in the upper maxilla with mandibular retrognathia and retrogenia. The patient requested treatment as he wanted 'his teeth to be straighter and for his chin to be brought forward'. He mentioned some adverse comments at school in the preceding years and desired a more favourable appearance of his teeth.

He had no previous orthodontic or dental treatment and only suffered with occasional asthma for which he used a salbutamol inhaler. His family history was unremarkable.

On examination, it was immediately apparent that he had an anterior open bite (AOB) with incompetent lip seal at rest. It was also noted that he had retrognathia and retrogenia. Notably he had antegonial notching and features of an unfavourable clockwise growth pattern of the mandible.

✪ **Learning point** Mandibular growth

The mandible has the most postnatal growth of all the facial bones. The right and left bodies of the mandible unite at the midline of the mental symphysis during the first year of life. The primary sites of growth are at the condylar cartilages, posterior rami and alveolar ridges [1].

Mandibular growth is highly dependent on the functional demands placed on it and has a capacity to adapt. Numerous functional matrices including the muscles of mastication, facial soft tissues and the tongue ultimately all influence the size and shape of the mandible [1].

Deep antegonial notching has been associated with a smaller increase in total mandibular length, corpus length and less displacement of the chin in a horizontal direction than those with shallow notches [2,3]. The clinical presence of a deep mandibular antegonial notch is indicative of a diminished mandibular growth potential and a vertically directed mandibular growth pattern [3]. It is often associated with a steeper mandibular plane, smaller chin and greater anterior facial height with the mandible having a more backward and downward growth.

Several cephalometric features have been indicated with abnormal growth rotations to include the backward inclination of the condylar head, a reduced inter-incisal and inter-molar angle, a straight mandibular canal, an antegonial notch, retrogenia and an increased lower face height [4].

Various quantitative predictors have been suggested to include the anterior face height ratio [5] and the overbite depth indicator [6], with varying degrees of validity.

At this time it was discussed with the patient that it was likely he would need an orthodontic and surgical approach to his AOB, as it was likely that his AOB would worsen with age and orthodontic treatment alone could not camouflage this discrepancy.

⚖ Expert comment Orthodontic treatment alone

Non-surgical treatment for AOB can be difficult and prone to relapse and is often limited to selected cases or when the patient declines a combined surgical/orthodontic approach. Early intervention can include the use of numerous methods and appliances ranging from deterrent appliances, high-pull headgear, vertical chin cup, various types of bite blocks, active vertical corrector and the Frankel IV appliance to skeletal anchorage with miniplates or screws [7].

Camouflage treatment of milder AOBs aim to address the AOB by dental movement without correcting the skeletal profile. Methods with fixed appliances can be extraction/non-extraction approach to reduce the inclination of the both lower and upper incisors to decrease the open bite (OB), or extract molars to compensate for the over eruption that led to the AOB.

A Multi-loop edgewise archwire technique aims to correct the occlusal plane, align the maxillary incisors relative to the lip line and make the posterior teeth upright. Its main effect is by retraction and extrusion of anterior teeth. This has limited value in those patients that already have adequate or excessive dental display prior to treatment [7]. This approach has also been shown to have significant relapse [8].

Skeletal anchorage devices have been described since 1985 and are secured into the mandibular or maxillary bone and used as immobile intraoral anchors to achieve molar intrusion. Once molar intrusion has occurred, fixed appliance therapy can commence to complete the closure of the AOB. The advantages of this approach are that the undesirable effects of anterior tooth extrusion and root resorption are avoided. It has been shown that up to 5 mm intrusion can occur whilst also achieving counter-clockwise rotation of the mandible. Relapse of intrusion has been shown to be approximate, therefore 30% overcorrection has been advocated [8].

These devices have been used and advocated for the use in mild to moderate AOB cases; however, the clinician must be mindful that the overall skeletal aesthetics will not be addressed and clear goals should be discussed with the patient.

He was then seen again in a combined orthognathic clinic at age 16 whereupon he had further assessment. At that time he had an extensive AOB that spanned the arch from 16 to 24 and 34 to 46, with incompetent lips at rest. It was also noted that he had increased vertical facial proportions, with pronounced retrognathia and retrogenia. Extra-orally he had a skeletal Class II base with no signs of cranial base abnormality. He appeared to have an average lower face height with his chin point to the right.

His upper incisor show was 2 mm at rest and 6 mm smiling with no gingival exposure. His nasolabial angle was approximately 90–110°. He also had deviation of his chin point to the right that was co-incident with a centre line shift of his lower incisors.

★ Learning point Aetiology of anterior open bite

It is defined as no contact or vertical overlap between the maxillary and mandibular incisors [9]. The incidence ranges from 1.5% to 11% and varies between races and with dental age [10]. It has been noted that the incidence of AOB is four times higher in the Afro-Caribbean population than that of the Caucasian population [11]. Reasons for this are not entirely clear, but are often based on the skeletal pattern.

This is a multi-factorial process and its outcome can often be dependent of the age of presentation. AOB is a complex phenotype and can be attributed to a combination of factors:

• **Skeletal:** associated with an increased lower anterior face height (LAFH) often described as 'long face syndrome' with vertical maxillary excess, usually with an increase in the Frankfort-mandibular plane angle (FMPA). This is often linked to a shortened mandibular ramus and opening rotation of the mandibular ramus [10].

(continued)

- **Dentoalveolar:** there is no change to the skeletal pattern with no increase in the LAFH or FMPA. The AOB is purely at the dentoalveolar level. Deficient eruption of the anterior teeth contribute to the AOB.
- **Soft tissues:** Tongue thrusting or forward posture of the tongue may interfere with incisor eruption and lead to an AOB. Tongue thrusting is primary or secondary (adaptive). Secondary tongue thrusting is when the tongue moves to contact the lips to form an anterior seal (usually where the lips are incompetent) [12]. This is often not seen as being as important as the resting tongue position. A forward position exerts a low continual force to interrupt tooth position and produce a reverse curve of Spee [13]. Macroglossia has also been implicated in the development of an AOB and could be part of a syndrome or growth disturbance (e.g. Beckwith-Wiedemann or acromegaly).
- **Habitual:** digit sucking is dependent on frequency and duration and commonly presents in the primary dentition. Those that suck for more than six hours a day often develop a significant malocclusion and is often asymmetrical co-incident with the region of the digit [12,13]. It can also be associated with a transverse constriction of the maxilla and bilateral crossbite [14]. Often resolution occurs if the habit is not prolonged.
- **Progressive condylar resorption (PCR):** this is a rare condition of unknown aetiology that leads to a potential Class II relationship from dysfunctional remodelling of the condyles. It is has been theorized to occur in the adult patient after growth is complete and hence the mandible recedes and in the juvenile patient to lead to diminished mandibular growth [15]. The juvenile form has not been proven, whilst the adult form has been clinically documented.

  Many theories as to the aetiology and associated factors that lead to PCR have been postulated. The combination of host factors and mechanical stimuli contribute to PCR.

  Host factors have been shown to include age, female sex and systemic disease. Mechanical stimuli could include orthodontic treatment, orthognathic surgery and prosthetic work [15]. The normal adaptive response of the temporomandibular joint (TMJ) seems to fail and a dysfunctional remodelling occurs. Historical PCR can present as an AOB and care must be taken to ensure that it is now static in nature.
- **Pathological:** trauma to the facial skeleton (e.g. condylar fracture, Le Fort I fractures) can also lead to a localized AOB and should not be overlooked.

Intra-orally the patient had a full dentition excluding third molars. The lower arch had mild crowding in the lower labial segment and premolar region. The upper arch had mild crowding, with proclination apparent in the premolar region. He had an overjet of 11 mm to 21 and an AOB. The molar and canine relationship was a full unit Class II on both sides. There was a crossbite on 16, and a centreline shift of the lower incisors 2 mm to the right. There was erosion noted on all first molars and poor oral hygiene throughout. No TMJ symptoms or problems were recorded.

According to the Orthodontic Index of Treatment Need scoring system this patient's malocclusion would need to be treated in secondary care. A decision about the need for a combined approach has recently led to attempts to produce an orthognathic treatment need scoring system. There are still shortfalls in scoring systems but they can provide some guidance in the assessment of patients (Box 14.1).

Box 14.1 Index of Orthognathic Functional Treatment Need [16].

This index applies to those malocclusions that are *not amenable to orthodontic treatment alone, due to skeletal deformity*, and will ordinarily apply to those patients who will have completed facial growth prior to surgery (commonly 18 years of age and older). It relates only to the *functional* need for treatment and should be used in combination with appropriate psychological and other clinical indicators.

5 **Very great need for treatment**
   5.1   Defects of cleft lip and palate and other craniofacial anomalies
   5.2   Increased overjet greater than 9 mm

(continued)

5.3 Reverse overjet ≥ 3 mm

5.4 Open bite ≥ 4 mm

5.5 Complete scissors bite affecting whole buccal segment(s) with signs of functional disturbance and/or occlusal trauma

5.6 Sleep apnoea not amenable to other treatments such as mandibular advancement device or continuous positive airway pressure (as determined by sleep studies)

5.7 Skeletal anomalies with occlusal disturbance as a result of trauma or pathology

4 **Great need for treatment**

4.2 Increased overjet ≥ 6 mm and ≤ 9 mm

4.3 Reverse overjet ≥ 0 mm and < 3 mm with functional difficulties

4.4 Open bite < 4 mm with functional difficulties

4.8 Increased overbite with evidence of dental or soft tissue trauma

4.9 Upper labial segment gingival exposure ≥ 3 mm at rest

4.10 Facial asymmetry associated with occlusal disturbance

3 **Moderate need for treatment**

3.3 Reverse overjet ≥ 0 mm and < 3 mm with no functional difficulties

3.4 Open bite < 4 mm with no functional difficulties

3.9 Upper labial segment gingival exposure < 3 mm at rest, but with evidence of gingival/ periodontal effects

3.10 Facial asymmetry associated no occlusal disturbance

2 **Mild need for treatment**

2.8 Increased overbite but no evidence of dental or soft tissue trauma

2.9 Upper labial segment gingival exposure < 3 mm at rest with no evidence of gingival/periodontal effects

2.11 marked occlusal cant with no effect on the occlusion

1 **No need for treatment**

1.12 Speech difficulties

1.13 Treatment purely for temporomandibular joint disease

1.14 Occlusal features not classified above

Reproduced with permission from Ireland A et al. An Index of Orthognathic Functional Treatment Need (IOFTN), *Journal of Orthodontics*, Volume 41, Issue 2, pp. 77-83, Copyright © 2014 British Orthodontic Society.

⊕ **Clinical tip** Assessment of anterior open bite

History, clinical assessment and cephalometric analysis aid in the assessment of AOB and help to ascertain the aetiology and hence plan further management.

As with all malocclusions, clinical examination should first include an assessment of any cranial base abnormality, ear position and ocular dystopia to help give an indication of any abnormality.

Extra-oral examination involves assessment of the patient in all planes: anterior, posterior, vertical and transverse. Clinical assessment of an AOB helps the clinician decide whether it is predominately skeletal or dental in origin. It is often a combination of both factors making classification difficult [10].

Assessment should include noting the severity of the AOB with regards to the posterior extension and the distance between the incisor teeth.

Mild AOBs that are confined to the incisor and canine teeth may be amenable to simple orthodontic camouflage treatment, or cessation of a digit sucking habit with or without the aid of an appliance. Deciduous or early mixed dentition AOBs are often a result of a digit sucking habit and upon cessation commonly resolve [12].

AOBs that extend to the molar region are more likely to be skeletal in origin, or a more complex combination of factors and require more complex treatment planning.

Clinical characteristics of a skeletal aetiology include an excess anterior face height (particularly the lower third), lip incompetence with the resting lip separation greater than 4 mm and a tendency for a

(continued)

Class II malocclusion and mandibular deficiency. However, there are some patients that may present with a hypoplastic maxilla and therefore have the facial appearance of a Class III malocclusion [17].

There is not uncommonly an associated high maxillary-mandibular planes angle with a vertical excess pattern. Proffit characterized this as 'long face' syndrome [9].

Intra-orally, the lower arch tends to be crowded with a narrow maxilla and posterior crossbite(s). Excessive eruption of the maxillary posterior teeth can lead to an AOB [14].

Attention must be given to any steps in the occlusion and the curves of Spee, as these will influence any pre-surgical orthodontics and surgical planning. Levelling the curve of Spee in the mandible in those with an increased lower face height will help to maintain the height and not increase it. A reverse curve of Spee in the mandible and reduced incisor eruption is indicative of a tongue posture habit [10].

Soft tissues will influence the AOB with note made to any tongue thrusting habits or mouth breathing.

Careful evaluation should be made as to whether the AOB is progressive or static in nature at presentation. Serial study models, historic photographs and clinical history will help to deduce this. Treatment should ideally be delayed until the AOB becomes static. PCR in high FMPA female patients can be a cause of a progressive AOB and needs careful treatment planning.

Standard investigations were done to include radiographs (orthopantomogram[OPG] and cephalometry), study models and clinical photographs. Clinical photographs included full right and left face in frontal, lateral and three-quarter views. Cephalometric analysis (Table 14.1) was performed and it was noted that the patient had a high FMPA and a very low sella–nasion–B point angle value. The A point–nasion–B point angle was large as was the OJ value; the OB value was negative (Figure 14.1).

❝ Expert comment Planning and imaging

Recent advances in medical imaging has led the field of orthognathic surgery into the realms of virtual three-dimensional planning and computer-aided surgery. The aim of three-dimensional virtual imaging for orthognathic surgery is to create one virtual anatomic model of the patient, including the triad of the facial soft mask, underlying bony structures and teeth [18].

Cone-beam computed tomography scanners (CBCT) have enabled good image acquisition at a low radiation dose and at a relatively lower cost than multi-slice CT as well as in-office imaging. At present the use of CBCT is limited as the scanned volume of CBCT is too small for all maxillofacial deformities and in some scanners the field of view is too short [18]. As technology progresses these problems will be overcome and CBCT will become the standard imaging modality in planning.

Three-dimensional virtual planning allows the clinician to have more information about the patient's anatomy in multiple planes. This becomes especially important for complex craniofacial deformities that might require complex orthognathic treatment planning. It allows three-dimensional facial harmonization rather than just focusing on facial profile [18]. It also allows the clinician to evaluate the postoperative outcome of surgery with soft tissue profiles.

At present the limitations of CBCT and the question of balance between radiation exposure of CBCT versus conventional radiography as well as cost makes virtual planning unjustified in many maxillofacial centres. However, as software packages develop, these differences will become negligible.

Further imaging may be needed for some AOB cases, especially if there is any doubt about the AOB being progressive in nature. If there is any suggestion that the AOB is progressive then SPECT (single-photon emission computed tomography) scanning may be needed. This shows areas of increased biological activity (i.e. high cellular turnover) and therefore may indicate if the AOB progression is due to PCR. If this was the case, then a delay in treatment would be prudent.

Table 14.1 Cephalometric values.

	Value	Norm
SNA	78.5°	82° ± 3°
SNB	68.0°	79° ± 3°
ANB	10.0°	3° ± 2°
MxP / MnP	40.5°	24° ± 3°
UAFH / LAFH	0.8	< 0.8 = > LAFH / > 0.8 = < LAFH
OJ	7.0 mm	2.0 mm ± 1.0 mm
OB	–5.5 mm	3.0 mm ± 1.0 mm
UI / MxP	116.5°	103° ± 6°
LI / MnP	93.5°	90° ± 5°
IIA	111.3°	135° ± 11°

SNA, sella–nasion–A point angle; SNB, sella–nasion–B point angle; ANB, A point–nasion–B point angle; MxP, maxillary plane; MnP, mandibular plane; UAFH, upper anterior face height; LAFH, lower anterior face height; OJ, overjet; OB, orbitale; UI, upper incisor; LI, labial inferior; IIA, inter-incisal angle.

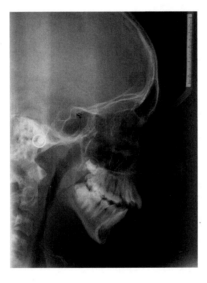

Figure 14.1 Lateral cephalogram demonstrating the extent of the anterior open bite.

Discussion with the patient at this time covered the planned orthodontic and future surgical treatment. Information was given verbally and a DVD made available during treatment.

The planned orthodontic treatment included maxillary arch expansion with a Quad Helix with non-extraction arch alignment and coordination. The proposed surgical approach consisted of a bimaxillary osteotomy and genioplasty. This was to include a differential Le Fort I maxillary impaction and advancement mandibular bilateral sagittal split osteotomy (BSSO) with advancement genioplasty.

> ⊕ **Learning point** Mandibular surgery alone
>
> Surgical treatment of AOB has traditionally involved the treatment of the maxilla alone or in combination with the mandible. The 'gold standard' has been maxillary procedures alone, in particular, superior repositioning and/or impaction, as they have been described as very stable and stable in Proffit's hierarchy (landmark paper) [19].
>
> However, appropriate case selected single mandibular jaw surgery is at least as stable as bimaxillary procedures, specifically BSSO with closing rotation and rigid internal fixation [20].
>
> (continued)

About one-third of patients have vertical maxillary excess (VME) and approximately 60% with VME also have an AOB or open bite tendency [21]. Therefore, the majority would require maxillary surgery, with or without mandibular surgery, and are regarded as stable procedures.

However, a proportion of patients may present with an acceptable vertical and anterior-posterior maxillary position and may be candidates for mandibular surgery alone. This avoids the undesirable effects of maxillary surgery on the upper lip position, alar base changes and alteration of dental display [22].

Patients that have short rami, normal condyles with no signs of resorption and a well-positioned maxilla should be considered for mandibular sagittal split osteotomy [21].

Class II patients with retrogenia and low FMPA may also be considered as the mandibular advancement and rotation may obviate the need for genioplasty [21].

Considerations for mandibular surgery alone:

1. Acceptable maxillary position.
2. Class II patients +/- retrogenia.
3. Small AOB.
4. Low FMPA patients.
5. Small anteroposterior discrepancy avoiding large mandibular advancements.
6. Short rami.
7. Normal condyles.

⊘ **Evidence base** Proffit's hierarchy of stability [21]

Prospective data on 2264 patients undergoing orthognathic surgery.

- Between 1975 and 2007.
- One-year follow-up for 1465 patients.
- Five-year or longer follow-up for 507 patients.
- Clinically significant relapse defined as > 2 mm.
- Figure 14.2 shows stability and predictability at one year postoperatively.

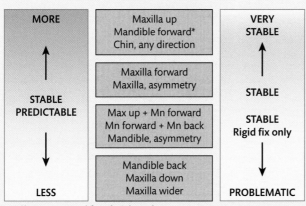

Figure 14.2 Surgical-orthodontic treatment: a hierarchy of stability.

A frank discussion was had with the patient about the need for strict oral hygiene and orthodontic treatment was commenced at age 16 years. The planned surgical intervention was in this case postponed until growth had finished.

At 18 years, the patient was seen for a final pre-surgical appointment in the orthognathic clinic. A detailed surgical plan was confirmed and discussed. This included a Le Fort I maxillary posterior impaction of 4 mm and 1 mm anteriorly and advancement of the mandible with rotation to the right by 1 mm to harmonize the centre lines with a BSSO, with 8 mm advancement genioplasty. This would leave the patient with a planned posterior open bite that would be closed post-surgically by orthodontics. This enabled positive OB correction creating a more stable occlusion and reducing relapse potential. Subsequent visits were to complete facebow registration, place hooks, metal ties and wafer try ins.

✪ Learning point Model surgery

Traditional planning of orthognathic cases involves formulating an integrated treatment plan based on the clinical, radiographic and model analysis. Success of surgery is by means of accurate model surgery that translates the planned clinical moves via a simulated postoperative model relationship to fabricate intermediate/final wafers [23]. Conventional model surgery and wafer fabrication are integral to the technical outcome of the surgical procedure as maxillary and bimaxillary surgery involve complex three-dimensional movements.

However, newer techniques advocate wafer fabrication from three-dimensional virtual planning and subsequent rapid prototyped wafers, but as yet they have not been shown to be superior in error elimination compared to conventional planning [24]. These are based on models scanned with CAD/CAM software. With time, virtual wafer planning and design will become as accurate and cost-effective as conventional model surgery.

Widely used model surgery techniques include the Lockwood key spacer and the Eastman anatomically orientated technique [25]. The Lockwood key spacer system incorporates thin plaster or plastic key spacers at the interface of the models and the articulator mounting assembly. These are held in place with elastics and casts can be moved accordingly and re-positioned as necessary.

The Eastman anatomically orientated technique uses multiple horizontal and vertical reference points on the mounting plaster to register the preoperative positions and the planned moves are in relation to these reference points [25].

Both techniques use a facebow registration in the supine centric occlusion mounted on a semi-adjustable articulator, as well as the Erickson measuring apparatus to provide reproducible model surgery. This apparatus allows recording of the maxilla in three dimensions to facilitate accurate model surgery. The Eastman technique has been shown to be significantly better in the vertical plane [25].

Errors in wafer fabrication, particularly the intermediate wafer, lead to inaccuracy in surgical technique. It has also been shown that errors were greater in cases where the planned movements were high (6–9 mm) and where differential maxillary impaction was planned [25].

This is important for severe AOB cases were relapse is common. Therefore, achieving the desired repositioning of the maxilla depends on accurate transfer of data using a reliable facial reference plane and reliable registration of the centric occlusion to obtain an accurate intermediate wafer [26].

---

❻ Expert comment Wafer checks

Preoperative wafer checks are important in the planning of all orthognathic cases. Adequate time should be given for any potential changes and re-check to be completed prior to surgery.

Checklist:

1. Intermediate and final wafer – separately. On models and on the patient.
2. Fit – stable, no interferences, no premature contacts, no rocking, positive seating of wafer.

(continued)

3. Occlusal surfaces.
4. Midline changes to planned move: co-incident or as accepted.
5. Correct direction.
6. Accurate replication of planned moves. Check each stage on the models in occlusion.

Successful bimaxillary osteotomy was performed with advancement genioplasty (Box 14.2). A Le Fort I impaction osteotomy with a standard advancement BSSO was completed. During the procedure, bony cuts were carried out with oscillating saws and non-locking plates were used for fixation. All maxillomandibular fixation and wafers were removed at the end of the procedure and elastics were placed post-operatively by the orthodontist on day one.

Box 14.2 Operative note

In order to reduce the potential for relapse in the vertical dimension, certain care should be taken during the technical procedure and certain areas of the osteotomy need special attention.

Whether one or two jaw surgery is completed, it has been shown that rigid internal fixation reduces the chances of relapse and it is now commonplace for plates or bicortical screws to be used for fixation.

Maxilla

If a Le Fort I osteotomy is performed, then ensuring that adequate bone removal occurs for posterior impaction is paramount. Care should be taken around the pterygoid plates and maxillary tuberosity and the maxilla should sit passively once the Le Fort I cuts and impaction have occurred. To enable this, special attention may be needed to the nasal septum as this can be an area of interference. To reduce alar base widening a non-resorbable cinch suture can be placed.

Advancements should consider the use of bone grafts or bone substitutes as these can act as a mechanical stop to prevent relapse [27].

Mandible

The BSSO is still the most commonly used technique, whether modified or conventional and attention should be paid to ensure that the medial pterygoid remains attached to the proximal segment and to strip the pterygomasseteric sling, medial pterygoid and stylomandibular ligament from the distal segment [21]. It is thought that adaptive changes occur in the muscle length and orientation that contribute to relapse therefore minimizing these effects is necessary [22].

The condyles should sit passively in the fossa without undue pressure as this can contribute to late condylar resorption and with high angle FMPA patients, this should be mandatory.

For large advancements, some studies have suggested that the technique of choice should be the inverted 'L' osteotomy with bicortical screws and bone grafts [27].

Establishment of a deep overbite surgically is essential to reduce the changes of relapse, with the post-surgical orthodontics aiming to maintain this overbite and hence potentially involving long-term retention.

A check OPG was performed post-operatively prior to discharge to assess condylar and plate position.

> **⊕ Learning point** Returns to theatre
>
> Regular follow-up postoperatively is essential to assess the success of the combined planned moves. As postoperative orthodontics continues, the opportunity to monitor potential relapse is possible.
>
> - **Immediate postoperative assessment:** Is there an AOB? How much positive OB and OJ is there? Is this similar to the planned move? Degree of relapse (in millimetres), is it progressive or static?
> - **Cause of the postoperative AOB:** Non-correction on the operating table? Poorly planned? Is the patient in pain and unable/unwilling to fully occlude? Have the muscles gone into spasm? Are there any soft tissue or dental interferences?
> - **Radiographic assessment:** Postoperative OPG ± lateral cephalogram. Are the condyles in the fossa? Is there a plating error? Was there adequate maxillary impaction?
>
> **How to approach?**
>
> 1. Review the original treatment plan with an orthodontist. Get a second opinion if necessary.
> 2. Fully assess the patient, to include postoperative radiography.
> 3. Review the operative procedure – difficulty of technical procedure, passive surgical correction of maxilla and mandibular condyles.
> 4. Discuss carefully with orthodontist if a trial of elastics is possible and if other operative factors have been explored and discounted. Could long-term retention cease the progression of the AOB without the need for surgical intervention?
> 5. What does the patient feel about the relapse and the potential for repeat surgery.
>
> **Return to theatre**
>
> Be clear with the patient about the planned procedure, re-plan the surgical moves and if necessary remake the intermediate/final wafers. Identify areas that need addressing during the operative procedure. Plan to return within one week of the original surgery.

Postoperative orthodontics were completed eight months after surgery and fixed retainers were placed after de-bonding. Review at one and two years demonstrated a stable occlusion with clinical photographs and radiographs to document this. The patient was pleased with this final outcome.

> **⊕ Learning point** Strategies to avoid relapse
>
> Avoidance of relapse of AOB can be difficult to achieve. A relapse may occur from just an incisal overlap but no contact, to complete lack of incisal contact and no overlap. Some strategies can be employed to reduce the potential for relapse and the degree that relapse could occur.
>
> - Accurate planning.
> - A clear assessment and management plan should be obtained for all patients. Subsequent planning needs to be realistic and achievable.
> - Intrusion versus extrusion of molars.
> - Overcorrection with posterior open bite.
> - Postoperative overeruption of the buccal segments.
> - Permanent retention.

Discussion

Management of the AOB is complex and this malocclusion depends on thorough assessment and precise planning. Correction is prone to relapse and figures range from 18% in surgical patients to 25% in non-surgical patients [28]. However, long-term outcome data on AOB patients is low and limited. Many studies fail to gain data on long-term results and often do not describe the degree of relapse in the vertical dimension, hence comparative analysis is difficult. Relapse has been attributed to tongue posture, growth pattern, treatment parameters and surgical instability [28]. The aetiology of relapse is difficult to attribute to one single cause and more likely to be multi-factorial in origin. Relapse factors related to tooth and bony movement are amenable to some clinician control and therefore careful planning of these factors can reduce relapse potential.

Rigid fixation has been shown to be more stable than wire fixation and although Le Fort I osteotomy remains the surgical treatment of choice, mandibular surgery has been shown to be at least as stable as bimaxillary osteotomy in selected cases. Creation of a positive overbite and stable occlusion are the aims of AOB correction. In many instances over correction allows for a degree of relapse, but this should not be at the expense of the functional and aesthetic outcomes of the patient.

A final word from the expert

AOB correction is one the most challenging malocclusions to correct and relapse can occur. Some relapse has little consequence functionally or aesthetically to some patients and the degree of relapse may also not pose any subsequent issues. Careful planning and assessment hopes to diminish any relapse potential and produce a stable outcome.

References

1. Miloro M.*Peterson's Principles of Oral and Maxillofacial Surgery.* New York: BC Decker, 2004.
2. Singer CP, Mamandras A, Hunter W. The depth of the mandibular antegonial notch as an indicator of mandibular growth potential. *Am J Orthod Dentofacial Orthop* 1987; 91(20): 117–24.
3. Lambrechts A, Harris A, Rossouw P, Stander I. Dimensional differences in the craniofacial morphologies of groups with deep and shallow mandibular antegonial notching. *Angle Ortho.* 1996; 66(4): 265–72.
4. Bjork A. Prediction of mandibular growth rotation. *Am J Orthod* 1969; 55: 585–99.
5. Nahom H, Horowitz S, Benedicto A. Varieties of anterior open-bite. *Am J Orthod* 1972; 61: 486–92.
6. Kim YH. Overbite depth indicator with particular reference to anterior open bite. *Am J Orthod* 1974; 65: 586–611.
7. Ng C, Wong W, Hagg U. Orthodontic treatment of anterior open bite. *Int J Paediatr Dent* 2008; 18(2): 78–83.
8. Reichert I, Figel P, Winchester L. Orthodontic treatment of anterior open bite: a review article-is surgery always necessary? *Oral Maxillofac Surg* 2014; 18(3): 271–7.
9. Proffit WR, Fields H, Sarver D.*Contemporary Orthodontics* fourth ed. St Louis: Mosby Inc, 2007.
10. Lin L, Huang G, Chen C. Etiology and treatment modalities of anterior open bite. *J Exp Med* 2013; 5(1): 1–4.
11. Beane R, Reimann G, Phillips C, Tulloch C. A cephalometric comparison of Black openbite subjects and Black norms. *Angle Orthod* 2003; 73: 294–300.
12. Olivieria J, Dutra A, Pereira C, De Toledo O. Etiology and treatment of anterior open bite. *J Health Sci Inst* 2011; 29(2): 92–5.

13. Burford D, Noar, J. The causes, diagnosis and treatment of Anterior Open bite. *Dent Update* 2003; 30: 235–41.
14. Ngan P, Fields W. Open bite: a review of etiology and management. *Pediatric Dentistry* 1997; 19(2): 91–8.
15. Arnett G, Milam S, Gottesman L. Progressive mandibular retrusion – idiopathic condylar resorption. Part II. *Am J Orthod and Dentofac Orthop* 1996; 110(2): 117–27.
16. Ireland A, Cunningham S, Petrie A, et al. An Index of Orthognathic Functional Treatment Need (IOFTN). *J Orthod* 2014; 41: 77–83.
17. Sassouni V. A classification of skeletal facial types. *Am J Orthod* 1969; 55(2): 109–23.
18. Swennen G, Mollemans W, Schutyser F. Three-dimensional treatment planning of orthognathic surgery in the era of virtual imaging. *J Oral Maxillofac Surg* 2009; 67: 2080–92.
19. Proffit W, Turvery T, Phillips C. The hierarchy of stability and predictability in orthognathic surgery with rigid fixation: a update and extension. *Head and Neck* 2007; 3: 21.
20. Oliveira J, Bloomquist D. The stability of the use of bilateral sagittal split osteotomy in the closure of anterior open bite. *Int J Adult Othodon Orthognath Surg* 1997; 12: 101.
21. Bisase B, Johnson P, Stacey M. Closure of the anterior open bite using mandibular sagittal split osteotomy. *Br J Oral Maxillofac Surg* 2010; 48: 352–5.
22. Stansbury C, Evans C, BeGole E. Stability of the open bite correction with sagittal split osteotomy and closing rotation of the mandible. *J Oral Maxillofac Surg* 2010; 68: 149–59.
23. Chowdhary R, Walker F, Mankani N. Model Surgery: a presurgical procedure for orthognathic surgeries – Revisited. *Int J Prosthodon and Restorative Dent* 2011; 1(1): 71–6.
24. Shqaidef A, Ayoub A, Khambay B. How accurate a rapid prototyped final orthognathic surgical wafers? A pilot study. *Br J Oral Maxillofac Surg* 2014; 52: 609–14.
25. Bamber M, Harris M, Nacher C. A validation of two orthognathic model surgery techniques. *J Orthod* 2001; 28: 135–42.
26. Park N, Posnick J. Accuracy of analytic model planning in bimaxillary surgery. *Int J Oral Maxillofac Surg* 2013; 42: 807–13.
27. Van Sickels J, Wallender A. Closure of anterior open bites with mandibular surgery: advantages and disadvantages of this approach. *Oral Maxillofac Surg* 2012; 16: 361–7.
28. Greenlee G, Huang G, Chen S, et al. Stability of treatment for anterior open-bite malocclusion: A meta-analysis. *Am J Orthod Dentofacial Orthop* 2011; 139(2): 159–69.

Severe Class II skeletal deformity

Lisa Greaney

Expert commentary Ken Sneddon and Jeremy Collyer

Case history

A 14-year-old Caucasian girl presented to clinic complaining of difficulty biting foods and a dislike of her diminutive chin. On examination she had a Class II division I incisor malocclusion on a severe Class II skeletal base with gross mandibular retrognathia. Her Frankfort-mandibular plane angle (FMPA) was increased with decreased lower posterior face height (LPFH) resulting in a 3 mm anterior open bite extending to the molar region and 8 mm overjet. Her permanent dentition had erupted with mild crowding of the upper arch and well-aligned lower arch, the latter facilitated by previous orthodontic extraction of four premolars. She had a bilateral crossbite with no mandibular deviation on closing. Medically she suffered with juvenile rheumatoid arthritis but was otherwise well.

Study models, a lateral cephalogram and a dental panoramic tomograph were taken for further assessment (Figure 15.1). Cephalometric analysis showed an A point–nasion–B point angle of 10° and FMPA of 42.5°. Both plain films confirmed the presence of diminutive condyles, narrow and posterior facing and short but wide rami with prominent antegonial notches.

✪ Learning point

The bird-face deformity of a severe Class II, high FMPA with significant retrogenia, often associated with diminutive condyles and reduced posterior face height poses many challenges to the orthognathic surgeon. Of greatest concern in these patients is the degree of mandibular advance required and the potential for relapse. Sagittal split osteotomy is the workhorse of mandibular surgery but has considerable limitations in this group of patients. Inverted 'L' osteotomy of the mandible is indicated in the management of this cohort but is a procedure that has largely fallen out of favour due to the need for an extra-oral approach and maxillomandibular fixation (MMF). The advent of distraction osteogenesis promised to be the answer for these cases, but now with close on 20 years of experience with these techniques it is clear that it does not represent the panacea that was hoped for. This case highlights the need to explore options that are not readily performed in most units today, in order to provide the best final outcome for the patient.

⊕ Expert comment

Management of the very severe Class II malocclusions, also known as the 'bird-face' deformity presents many challenges. The desired outcome is to provide a stable Class I occlusion in conjunction with correction of the aesthetic deformity.

This patient group presents anatomical features a number of standard deviations from the norm; there is reduced posterior face height secondary to underdevelopment of the mandibular condyles and ramus. The condyles themselves are generally diminutive and posteriorly angulated. Various syndromes or juvenile rheumatoid arthritis may be associated with their aetiology.

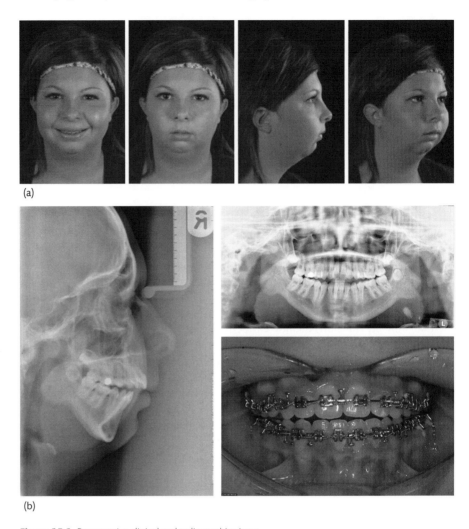

(a)

(b)

Figure 15.1 Preoperative clinical and radiographic views.

> ⭐ **Learning point** Frankfort-mandibular planes angle
>
> **Normal values**
>
> - High angle cases: growth is more vertical than horizontal with a posterior direction of rotational growth. The cranial base tends to be short (sella–nasion, S-N).
> - Low angle cases: growth is more horizontal than vertical with an anterior direction of rotational growth. The cranial base tends to be longer and flatter (S-N) (see Figure 15.2).
>
> (continued)

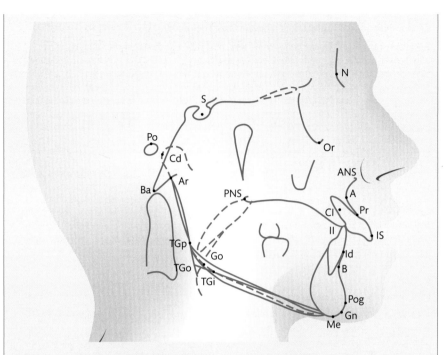

Figure 15.2 Normal cephalometric values. A, point A; ANS, anterior nasal spine; Ar, articulare; B, B point; Ba, basion; C↑, centroid of upper incisor; Cd, condylion; Gn, gnathion; Go, gonion; II, incision inferius; IS, incision superius; Id, infradentale; Me, menton; N, nasion; Or, orbitale; Po, porion; Pog, pogonion; PNS, posterior nasal spine; Pr, prosthion; S, sella; TG₁, inferior tangent point; TGp, posterior tangent point; TG₀, constructed gonion.

Reproduced with permission from WJB Houston, CD Stephens and WJ Tulley, *Textbook of Orthodontics*, Second Edition, Butterworth-Heineman, Elsevier, Oxford, UK, Copyright © Elsevier 1992.

Measurement	Mean ± normal range
SNA	82° ± 3°
SNB	79° ± 3°
ANB	3° ± 1°
A-B / FOP	90° ± 5°
MMPA	27° ± 5°
Face – height ratio	50–55%
FOP / Mx	10° ± 4°
UI / Mx	108° ± 5°
LI / Mn	92° ± 5°
UI / LI	133° ±10°
E↓ - APog	0–2 mm
E↓C↑	0–2 mm

SNA, sella–nasion–A point angle; SNB, sella–nasion–B point angle; ANB, A point–nasion–B point angle; A, point A; B, point B; FOP, functional occlusal plane; MMPA, maxillary-mandibular planes angle; Mx, maxillary plane; UI, upper incisor; Mn, mandibular plane; LI, lower incisor; E, E-point; APog, A-pogonion; C, centroid of upper incisor.

⭐ **Learning point** The treatment of severe Class 2 deformity

Treatment options included the conventional bilateral sagittal split osteotomy (BSSO), distraction osteogenesis and the inverted 'L' osteotomy. The advantages of the BSSO are numerous and include high operator familiarity and one-stage surgery; however, one must not overlook the risks to the inferior dental nerve, reported by Westermark [1] as 40 % of patients having some nerve dysfunction at two years post-surgery. Distraction osteogenesis promises to decrease early relapse by slowly increasing the pull on the pterygo-masseteric sling thus allowing compensatory adjustment. However, it requires surgery twice: to insert and then remove the distractor, leaving unavoidable extra-oral scars. It also requires high patient compliance both in follow-up attendance and daily perseverance turning the distractor. Complications such as pressure sores and infection have also been reported in the literature [2].

The inverted 'L' osteotomy first introduced by Caldwell [3] in 1968 has long fallen out of favour, mainly due to the use of an extra-oral approach to the rami and wired MMF. However, its primary indication according to Henderson [4] is 'mandibular hypoplasia where the deficiency is both horizontal (anteroposterior) and vertical'. The use of contemporary instrumentation obviates the need for extra-oral incisions and permits the use of semi-rigid fixation. This improves cosmesis as there is no visible scar. The procedure also greatly reduces risk to the inferior dental nerves as all cuts are made under direct vision superoposterior to the lingula.

➕ **Clinical tip** Technique for the inverted 'L' osteotomy

Access to the ramus is performed via standard intra-oral incision along the external oblique ridge and a mucoperiosteal flap is raised. Once a suitable subperiosteal envelope has been developed the Leverson-Merrell and Bauer retractors are inserted to provide good visualisation of the ramus and angle (Figure 15.3). A combination of Lindeman bur and right-angled saw are then used to perform the inverted 'L' osteotomy as previously described by Caldwell. The Lindemann bur is first used to make a horizontal cut through the bone extending to just beyond the lingula. A right-angled saw is then used to complete the vertical cut posterior to the lingula.

An acrylic wafer is used to hold the occlusion in its final position and secured with temporary MMF. The proximal and distal segments of the mandible are then plated into position and two blocks of harvested bone are slid into the defect, perpendicular to one another to form an 'L' shape. These are subsequently secured via the remaining holes in the plates (Figure 15.4). The wafer is then removed, occlusion checked, incisions closed with dissolvable suture material and maxillomandibular elastics applied in theatre.

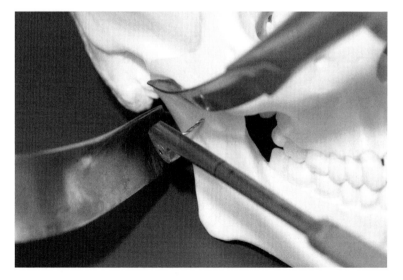

Figure 15.3 Retractors in position and right-angled drill.

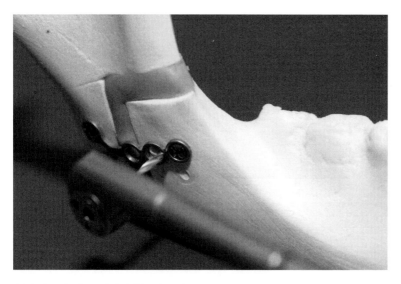

Figure 15.4 Use of right-angled drill for plate placement.

The advantages and disadvantages of both surgery and distraction techniques were discussed prior to embarking on a definitive treatment plan. A Le Fort I maxillary osteotomy, mandibular inverted 'L' osteotomy and advancement genioplasty were agreed. Pre-surgical orthodontics and surgically assisted rapid maxillary expansion were used to prepare for surgery.

The patient recovered uneventfully from surgery and was discharged home following a two-night hospital stay. She presented for follow-up and modification of elastics at one and two weeks post-surgery and was found to have a small dehiscence of her intra-oral mandibular wound, which subsequently healed with conservative management. Her occlusion remained stable throughout. Standard post-surgical orthodontic treatment was necessary (Figure 15.5).

Discussion

Severe Class II patients often present with highly distorted anatomy that account for their classic bird-face deformity. This treatment plan must not be thought of as a blanket prescription for all severe Class II individuals. Particular challenges included the necessary degree of advancement (12 mm) and the high potential for relapse with such unusual condylar anatomy.

Stability has always been a problem with larger movements in orthognathic surgery [5], but the dawn of semi-rigid fixation has minimized the need for wired MMF. Relapse has classically been divided into early and late relapse [6], with early being within six to eight weeks and attributed to movement at the osteotomy site itself [7]. Late relapse, seen radiographically between 6 and 17 months [7], is attributed to condylar resorption [8]. Due to her condylar anatomy, late resorption was of particular concern.

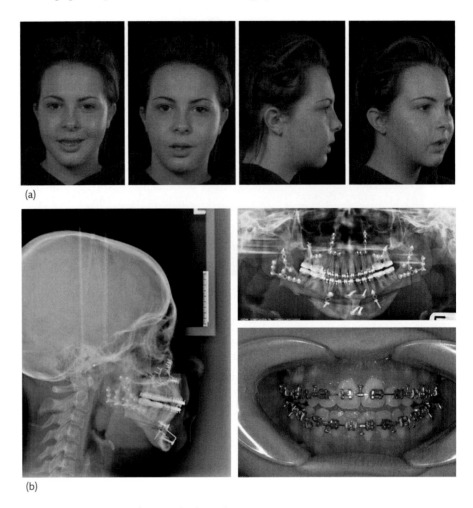

Figure 15.5 Postoperative clinical and radiographic views.

Early relapse at the osteotomy site is reportedly due to poor manipulation of the condyles intraoperatively and pull on the soft tissue envelope [7] in conjunction with little bony contact for rapid healing. During a BSSO the condylar head is subject to torque during fixation that forces the head into an abnormal position within the fossa. Maintaining the condyles in a passive position during the inverted 'L' osteotomy is easier since the proximal segment need only be manipulated to secure a plate rather than ensuring necessary overlap for adequate fixation. Stretching of the pterygo-masseteric sling is, however, unavoidable.

Distraction osteogenesis has also been considered as an alternative in all of our cases and would theoretically have less potential for early relapse due to controlled, slow pull on the pterygo-masseteric sling. However, this technique has its own disadvantages as referred to earlier.

Late relapse from progressive condylar resorption [9–15] will lead to eventual loss of posterior face height, which is especially relevant in this case. Change in condylar stresses due to intra-operative surgical positioning has been suggested as a cause [3]. Careful manipulation as with the BSSO is therefore imperative.

The inverted 'L', as with any surgical procedure, also has its own disadvantages. These include the need for a bone graft from the iliac crest in order to reconstruct the defect, creating a second surgical site with the potential for further complications. The duration of surgery is also longer than a conventional BSSO and the longer operating and anaesthetic time remains a disadvantage.

In this particular case, using the inverted 'L' osteotomy originally described in 1968 [3] with contemporary use of instruments and modified technique provided a cosmetically and functionally beneficial result for our patient with a severe Class II deformity, decreased LPFH and significant retrogenia (bird-face deformity). However, as described, there are several valid options for the treatment of patients with severe Class II skeletal bases, each with its own advantages and disadvantages. Each patient must be assessed individually and the merits of each option discussed in order to achieve the best final outcome.

A final word from the expert

The main issue in terms of the aesthetic outcome is the degree of retrogenia with which these patients present. This is often of sufficient degree that mandibular advance to achieve a Class I occlusion even when combined with a maximal genioplasty may still fail to fully correct the retrogenia.

Successful treatment requires a significant degree of mandibular advance and an increase in the posterior face height. These combined treatment goals raise concerns in terms of stability. It is widely accepted that the stability of any orthognathic procedure decreases with increasing magnitude of the move. Hence a large mandibular advance is inherently less stable than a smaller one. In addition it is conventional teaching that a bilateral sagittal osteotomy of the mandible cannot be used to increase posterior face height as this, in turn, leads to lengthening of the pterygo-masseteric sling and instability. One of the causes of late relapse following orthognathic surgery is idiopathic condylar resorption, this leading to a reduction in ramal height, clockwise rotation of the mandible and subsequent horizontal and vertical relapse with development of an anterior open bite. One of the identified risk factors for idiopathic condylar resorption is underdeveloped posteriorly angulated condyles, the very feature with which these patients present. It is apparent therefore that to treat these patients with BSSO is to court disaster and invite relapse.

The bilateral inverted 'L' osteotomy was described to manage patients where an increase in the posterior face height was indicated often associated with a large advance. The stability is provided by the interposition of blocks of cortico-cancellous bone graft into the osteotomy sites. The procedure as originally described was performed via bilateral neck incisions and required a protracted period of MMF. The introduction of semi-rigid fixation into orthognathic surgery largely removed the need for prolonged periods of MMF post-operatively and many tried to push the limits of the BSSO. The inverted 'L' fell somewhat out of fashion.

The decline in popularity was hastened by the introduction of distraction osteogenesis. This promised the ability to treat more significant defects than could be managed by conventional orthognathic means, to avoid the need for bone grafts and to offer greater stability. It was viewed by many as the panacea for the syndromic or extreme case. History will decide to what extent distraction osteogenesis has delivered upon its initial promise. There is no doubt that many cases that could not otherwise have been managed have produced some excellent results. It has found its place largely in craniofacial practice and syndromes such as hemi-facial microsomia. It also has a role in allowing early decannulation in patients with Pierre-Robin sequence. It is apparent, however, that distraction is not free of relapse. Neither is it an easy option for the patient. A distraction device suitable for a case such as this could be either an extra- or intra-oral device. The intra-oral devices have the benefit of being less obtrusive for the patient but are generally uni-vector, whereas the extra-oral devices can be multi-vector offering better control and distraction in three dimensions. The price to be paid for this greater flexibility is the requirement for trans-cutaneous pins and a much bulkier device. The drag of the pins can lead to unsightly scarring. In either case vector control can be difficult and achieving excellent occlusal results often requires considerable moulding of the regenerate with inter-maxillary elastics. The main drawback for the patient, however, is the high level of compliance required and the intensity of follow-up. The distraction phase may take up to three weeks followed by a prolonged period of consolidation.

Bearing in mind these limitations it is worth revisiting the inverted 'L' osteotomy in the light of developments in orthognathic surgery since it was first described. This procedure fell out of favour because of the need for extra-oral incisions, bone grafting and prolonged MMF. The requirement for bone grafting remains but with modern instrumentation, including specialized retractors and right-angle screwdrivers, this procedure can be carried out entirely intra-orally and internally fixed such that only guiding inter-maxillary elastics are required postoperatively.

The contemporary orthognathic surgeon must be aware that the BSSO is not the only mandibular procedure. While distraction osteogenesis has much to offer, in selected cases some of the older procedures when allied to modern techniques still have much to offer and may be an appropriate choice in patients such as that presented here.

References

1. Westermark A, Bystedt H, von Konow L. Inferior alveolar nerve function after sagittal split osteotomy of the mandible: correlation with degree of intraoperative nerve encounter and other variables in 496 operations. *Br J Oral Maxillofacial Surg* 1998; 36: 429–33.
2. Van Strijen PJ, Perdijk FBT, Becking AG, Breuning KH. Distraction osteogenesis for mandibular advancement. *Int J Oral Maxillofac Surg* 2000; 29: 81–5.
3. Caldwell JB, Hayward JR, Lister RL. Correction of mandibular retrognathia by vertical L osteotomy: a new technique. *J Oral Surg* 1968; 26: 259.
4. Henderson. A *Colour Atlas and Textbook of Orthognathic Surgery*. London: Wolfe Medical Publications, 1985.
5. Scheerlinck JPO, Stoelinga PJW, Blijdorp PA, et al. Sagittal split advancement osteotomies stabilized with miniplates. A 2-5 year follow-up. *Int J Oral Maxillofac Surg* 1994; 23: 127–31.
6. Van Sickels JE, Richardson DA. Stability of orthognathic surgery: a review of rigid fixation. *J Oral Maxillofac Surg* 1996; 34: 279–85.
7. Gassamann CJ, Van Sickels JE, Thrash WJ.Causes, location and timing of relapse following rigid fixation after mandibular advancement. *J Oral Maxillofac Surg* 1990; 48: 450–4.
8. Moore KE, Gooris PJJ, Stoelinga PJW. The contributing role of condylar resorption to skeletal relapse following mandibular advancement surgery. *J Oral Maxillofac Surg* 1991; 49: 448–60.

9. Kerstens HCJ, Tuinzing DB, Golding RP, van der Kwast WAM. Condylar atrophy and osteoarthritis after bimaxillary surgery. *Oral Surg Oral Med Oral Path* 1990; 69: 274–9.

10. Phillips RM, Bell WH. Atrophy of mandibular condyles after sagittal ramus split osteotomy: report of a case. *J Oral Surg* 1987; 36: 45–9.

11. Crawford JG, Stoelinga PJW, Blijdorp PA, Brouns JJA. Stability after reoperation for progressive condylar resorption after orthognathic surgery: report of seven cases. *J Oral Maxillofac Surg* 1994; 52: 460–6.

12. Merkx MAW, Van Damme PA. Condylar resorption after orthognathic surgery. *J Craniomaxillofac Surg* 1994; 22: 53–8.

13. Huang CS, Ross BR. Surgical advancement of the retrognathic mandible in growing children. *Am J Orthod* 1982; 82: 89–95.

14. Sesenna E, Raffaini M. Bilateral condylar atrophy after combined osteotomy for correction of mandibular retrusion. *J Maxillofac Surg* 1985; 13: 263–7.

15. Schendel SA, Epker BN. Results after mandibular advancement surgery: an analysis of 87 cases. *J Oral Surg* 1980; 38: 265–82.

16 The segmental maxillary osteotomy

Nabeela Ahmed

Expert commentary Dilip Srinivasan

Case history

A 16-year-old girl presented to the orthognathic joint clinic complaining of difficultly chewing and concern regarding the appearance of her anterior teeth (Figure 16.1 and 16.2). Clinical and cephalometric examination revealed an anterior open bite with posterior vertical maxillary excess. The maxillary central incisors were, however, in a satisfactory position. A step in the occlusal plane was noted between the maxillary canines and the first premolar. Based on these findings a bimaxillary procedure was considered with the potential option of a segmental maxillary osteotomy. Further to a discussion regarding the advantages and disadvantages of both surgical treatment options, she subsequently consented to a three-part maxillary osteotomy.

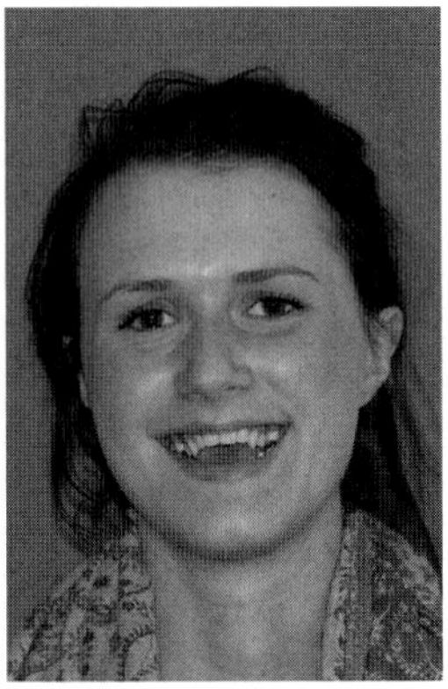

Figure 16.1 Preoperative facial view (smiling).

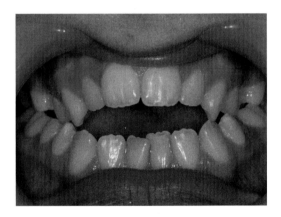

Figure 16.2 Preoperative occlusion. Note the position of the upper central incisors that are in the optimal position.

☼ Learning point First-line investigations

Base-line investigations for any patient presenting with a suspected or apparent facial deformity should include:

- an orthopantomogram (OPG)
- standardized lateral cephalogram
- upper and lower articulated study models
- clinical photographs (full face, lateral, closed and open mouth smile and occlusal views of the dental arches).

☼ Learning point History of anterior maxillary segmental osteotomies [1]

1921: Cohn-Stock gave the first account of this procedure.
1926: Wassmund reported a single-stage procedure that is undertaken via vestibular approach.
1962: Wunderer described a predominantly palatal technique.
1980: Bell described 'down-fracturing' of the maxilla and approached through a horizontal vestibular incision.

✚ Clinical tip

In order the achieve success with treating such a patient, a comprehensive history should be attained to conclude whether the issues the patient is concerned with are primarily aesthetic, functional or dental in nature.

The position of the maxillary central incisors is the key to achieving a good aesthetic outcome during the correction of dentofacial deformity using a segmental technique.

✪ Learning point Why undertake a segmental osteotomy?

Segmental maxillary osteotomy is a useful adjunct for the correction of vertical and transverse maxillary deformities. In some units, anterior segmental osteotomies are commonly used for the surgical correction of bimaxillary protrusion. However, the main indications are:

- Single-stage correction of transverse maxillary deficiency (which otherwise would be a two stage approach if undertaken with a surgically assisted rapid maxillary expansion followed by a traditional Le Fort I osteotomy).
- Correction of anterior open bite caused by posterior vertical maxillary excess.
- Need for differential movement of segments of the maxillary dentition.

Assessment of the patient for a segmental maxillary procedure

Consider the skeletal maxillary discrepancy in three dimensions:

- anteroposterior
- vertical
- transverse.

Assess the dentition and occlusion.
Evaluate the temporomandibular joint (TMJ).
Consider the facial soft tissues.

✪ Learning point

A multidisciplinary team meeting at which the patient is jointly assessed by the orthodontist and maxillofacial surgeon is mandatory. Embarking on an orthognathic treatment pathway involves commitment from the patient and prior to starting any orthodontic appliance therapy they should have a full understanding of the following:

- duration of treatment
- planned surgery (time frame)
- proposed surgical plan
- time required away from school / work
- frequency of appointments throughout treatment.

The end point following treatment is:

- improved function
- stability
- aesthetics
- minimal treatment time.

✪ Learning point Clinical assessment (as for all maxillary orthognathic procedures)

Are the facial midlines coincident? Are the facial and dental midlines coincident?

Assess the facial height:

- upper third
- middle third
- lower third.

Midface assessment

- Increased/decreased scleral show? Evidence of ocular dystopia.
- Frontonasal angle (ideally 30 to 40°).
- Paranasal hollowing.
- Nasaloabial angle: 85–105 degrees.
- Nasal projection 16–20 mm (measure from pronasale to subnasale).

(continued)

⊕ Clinical tip

The need for segmental surgery has reduced significantly with the wider availability of fixed orthodontic appliance therapy. Clearly there will be cases that are not amenable to treatment with orthodontics alone and cases with isolated discrepancies that are amenable to segmental osteotomy.

Consideration should be given to early identification of these patients. Thus combined orthodontic and surgical treatment planning can ensue, in order to optimize the tooth movement required to achieve the outcome required surgically.

❝ Expert comment

Correct identification of the exact site of skeletal and dental abnormality is the key to success.

❝ Expert comment

We know that transverse maxillary discrepancy has the highest risk of relapse when just orthodontic correction is performed [2].

- Alar width (increased / decreased).
- Lip competence.
- Incisal show:
  - at rest (2 – 4 mm)
  - smiling (full tooth crown to 2 mm of the gingiva).
- Upper lip length (22 mm in males, 20 mm in females +/- 2 mm).

Mandibular assessment

- Skeletal pattern.
- Chin throat length (normal approximately 42 mm ± 6 mm).
- Chin throat angle (normally 110°).
- TMJ – assess range of movement and evidence of temporomandibular joint dysfunction syndrome.
- Labial-mental angle (should be at least 130°).
- Lower lip length (44 mm for males and 40 mm for females ± 2 mm).

Dental midlines

- Maxillary midline to facial midline.
- Maxillary to mandibular midline.
- Mandibular midline to chin relationship.
- Is there an occlusal cant?

Intra-oral examination

- Presence of third molars.
- Angles relationship:
  - molar
  - canine
  - incisor.
- Overjet (+3.5 mm ± 2.5 mm).
- Overbite (3–5 mm).
- Presence of any crossbites (and document which teeth, if not symmetrical).
- Gingival health (including thick / thin gingival biotype).

Radiological evaluation

As a basic evaluation, OPG, lateral cephalogram and periapical views of the planned osteotomy sites should be considered mandatory.

The pre-surgical orthodontic phase of her treatment lasted for two years. During this period she underwent arch alignment, decompensation and creation of space between the maxillary canines and premolars to allow the osteotomies to be performed safely. She subsequently underwent operative intervention (Box 16.1).

Box 16.1 Operative note

We elected to perform a Y-shaped osteotomy in this case with concurrent advancement of the maxilla.

After infiltration with local anaesthetic, the mucoperiosteal incision was made in the premolar region, ensuring that at least 1 cm cuff was maintained from the attached gingivae. The approach is as for a Le Fort I osteotomy and then the segmental osteotomy is performed after the down fracture has occurred. The midline osteotomy was performed using a fissure bur and the interdental bone cuts were made and joined, after which these segments are mobilized. A fissure bur is used for these bone cuts, which are completed with a fine osteotome.

(continued)

In the case of the U-shaped osteotomy, a U-shaped channel is created to preserve the central portion of the maxilla and the radial segmental osteotomy bone cuts allowed to join up.

The palatal mucosa is not divided in these situations and care is ensured to keep in intact to preserve the viability of these segments post surgically. A Mitchell's trimmer is often used to mobilize the mucosa over the osteotomized segments.

The intraoperative splint was then positioned and maxillomandibular fixation (MMF) placed to allow the segments to be immobilized prior to fixation. Any interferences between segments can be reduced with a fine fissure bur. At this point 1.5 mm titanium osteosynthesis miniplates were utilized. If bone grafting is required, then this too can be placed and stabilized as usual. Soft tissue closure after hard tissue fixation has occurred needs to be meticulous and is completed after the MMF has been removed.

> ✪ **Learning point** Complications of maxillary procedures
>
> **Immediate**
>
> - Malocclusion (immediate).
> - Haemorrhage [4].
> - Vascular compromise and necrosis.
> - Neurosensory deficit transient.
>
> **Late**
>
> - Malocclusion.
> - Permanent neurosensory deficit. The most common neurosensory deficit in maxillary procedures is that of the infra-orbital nerve that recovers rapidly and is experienced in approximately 25% of patients [5]. Impairment of the greater and lesser palatine nerves and nasopalatine and superior alveolar nerves, is less frequently reported by patients and tends to be better tolerated.
> - Damage to the dentition. Given the nature of the Le Fort I osteotomy and sectioning of the maxilla for segmental procedures, damage to the roots is a concern, as is damage to the gingival tissue. However, periodontal concerns following surgery are no higher in this group of patients [6].
> - Nasal deformity can be caused by buckling of the nasal septal cartilage in cases with maxillary impaction or setback. This can be avoided by careful trimming of the nasal septum, spines and cartilage. Some clinicians might also consider fixation of the nasal septum to prevent displacement in the immediate postoperative period. The literature also refers to airway changes following Le Fort I osteotomy [3].

Following recovery, light anterior elastic traction was placed. She remained as an inpatient overnight and was discharged home with elastics in situ. She was subsequently reviewed on a weekly basis and the guiding elastics were used for the first two weeks post surgery only. Otherwise she made an uncomplicated recovery with total healing of the surgical wounds and no evidence of compromise of the segments or a palatal fistula. The occlusion was noted to be even and bilateral at this stage and coincident with the pre-surgical model surgery.

Close follow-up via the orthognathic joint clinic was maintained and she underwent five months of post-surgical orthodontic treatment to fine-tune the arch alignment. She has now been reviewed for one year following cessation of treatment and there has been no evidence of relapse of the anterior open bite (Figure 16.3 and 16.4).

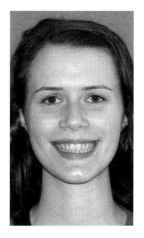

Figure 16.3 Facial view following segmental osteotomy and orthodontic debond (smiling).

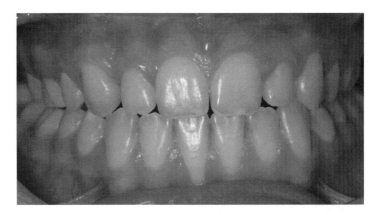

Figure 16.4 Occlusion following segmental osteotomy and orthodontic debond.

> **❝ Expert comment**
>
> Isolated segmental maxillary osteotomy can be performed without a Le Fort I osteotomy. These include:
>
> - anterior maxillary osteotomy:
>   - ○ Wassmund technique (requires removal of the first premolar)
>   - ○ Wunderer technique (removal of the second premolar [7])
> - posterior maxillary osteotomy:
>   - ○ Schuchardt procedure
>   - ○ Bell and Perko technique [8].
>
> Other techniques include the bird wing osteotomy [9]. Segmental osteotomies can also be undertaken in the mandible. The most commonly undertaken is the Kole osteotomy, which alongside the Wassmund technique, can close an anterior open bite associated with bimaxillary proclination [10]. Posterior segmentalization of the maxilla is known as the Schuchardt procedure, which is unstable due to incomplete mobilization of the maxilla [11].

Discussion

Complications specific to segmental maxillary procedures

One of the biggest reported complications of segmental osteotomies is loss of tooth vitality [12]. However, with careful planning and meticulous surgery, the incidence of complications is low [3,6]. A systematic review of segmental osteotomies concluded that soft tissue response is difficult to predict in this style of surgery [13]. There are case reports that detail the use of maxillary segmental osteotomies to correct malocclusion and improve aesthetics after trauma, with successful results [14]. The literature is in agreement that this is a safe method of treating discrepancies of the maxilla in either dimension, as long as the orthodontic preparation is complementary to the surgical planning [15].

> **✅ Evidence base** Facial soft tissue response to anterior segment osteotomies [13]
>
> - Systematic review, level 4 retrospective evidence.
> - Eleven centres.
> - Studies between 1983 and 2008.
>
> (continued)

- Lateral cephalometry in all studies.
- Preponderance of Asians and females.
- Anterior segment osteotomy leads to reduction in labial prominence and increase in nasolabial angle.
- Soft tissue changes confined to oro-labial region.

Source: data from Jayaratne Y et al. Facial soft tissue response to anterior segmental osteotomies: A systematic review, *International Journal of Oral and Maxillofacial Surgery*, Volume 39, Issue 11, pp.1050-1058, Copyright © 2010 International Association of Oral and Maxillofacial Surgeons; published by Elsevier Inc. All rights reserved.

In addition to the techniques discussed thus far, it has been proposed that anterior maxillary segmental distraction can be used in cleft patients [16]. Despite limited numbers the suggestion was that distraction in this format would increase the sella – nasion - point A angle and improve midface convexity. This procedure would also allow lengthening of the arch and allow correction of crowding associated with a hypoplastic maxilla.

Overall the need for segmental surgery has reduced with advances in orthodontics and particularly the use of temporary anchorage devices. However, segmental procedures are a vital part of the armamentarium of the orthognathic surgeon and should be considered in appropriate cases at the joint assessment phase.

A final word from the expert

The decision to do a segmental osteotomy needs to be made at the start of the treatment. This allows the orthodontist to move the teeth to a position that facilitates the osteotomy and also position the maxillary anterior teeth to give optimal lip support at the end of the procedure.

References

1. Stoelinga JWP. Segmental surgery of the jaws. In:Langdon JD, Patel MF, Ord RA, Brennan PA (eds) *Operative Oral and Maxillofacial Surgery* second edition. London: Hodder and Stoughton Limited; 2011: pp 635–7.
2. Proffit W, Turvey T, Phillips C. Orthognathic surgery: a hierarchy of stability. *Int J Adult Orthodon Orthognath Surg* 1995; 11(3): 191–204.
3. Chen Y-R, Yeow VK. Multiple-segment osteotomy in maxillofacial surgery. *Plast Reconstr Surg* 1999; 104(2): 381–8.
4. Ho M, Boyle M, Cooper J, et al. Surgical complications of segmental Le Fort I osteotomy. *Br J Oral Maxillofac Surg* 2011; 49(7): 562–6.
5. Karas ND, Boyd SB, Sinn DP. Recovery of neurosensory function following orthognathic surgery. *J Oral Maxillofac Surg* 1990; 48(2): 124–34.
6. Carroll WJ, Haug RH, Bissada NF, et al. The effects of the Le Fort I osteotomy on the periodontium. *J Oral Maxillofac Surg* 1992; 50(2): 128–32.
7. Wassmund M. *Lehrbuch der Praktischen Chirurgie des Mundes und der Kiefer*. Leipzig: H Meusser, 1935.
8. Sanghai S, Chatterjee P. *A Concise Textbook of Oral and Maxillofacial Surgery*. London: Jaypee Brothers Publishers; 2008.
9. Kannan V, Ahamed A, Sathyanarayanan G, et al. Anterior maxillary osteotomy: A technical note for superior repositioning: A bird wing segment. *J Pharm Bioallied Sci* 2014; 6(5): 107.

10. Lachard J, Blanc J, Lagier J, et al. [Kole's operation]. *Revue Stomatol Chir Maxillo-Faciale*. 1986; 88(5): 306–10.

11. Schuchardt K. Experiences with the surgical treatment of some deformities of the jaws: prognathia, micrognathia, and open bite in Wallace. Transactions of Second Congress, International Society of Plastic Surgeons, London; 1959.

12. Pepersack WJ. Tooth vitality after alveolar segmental osteotomy. *J Oral Maxillofac Surg* 1973; 1: 85–91.

13. Jayaratne Y, Zwahlen R, Lo J, Cheung L. Facial soft tissue response to anterior segmental osteotomies: A systematic review. *Int J Oral Maxillofac Surg* 2010; 39(11): 1050–8.

14. You K-H, Min Y-S., Baik H-S Treatment of ankylosed maxillary central incisors by segmental osteotomy with autogenous bone graft. *Am J Orthod Dentofacial Orthop* 2012; 141(4): 495–503.

15. Rosen H. Segmental osteotomies of the maxilla. *Clin Plast Surg* 1989; 16(4): 785–94.

16. Wang XX, Wang X, Li ZL, et al. Anterior maxillary segmental distraction for correction of maxillary hypoplasia and dental crowding in cleft palate patients: a preliminary report. *Int J Oral Maxillofac Surg* 2009; 38(12): 1237–43.

SECTION 6

Temporomandibular joint disease

17 Temporomandibular joint replacement

Nabeela Ahmed

Expert Commentary Andrew Sidebottom

Case history

A 17-year-old male was referred from a district general hospital for consideration of bilateral joint replacement for progressive condylar resorption. His presenting complaint was of a changing facial profile and difficulty with eating certain foods.

Clinical examination showed a classic bird-face deformity, with an overjet of 9 mm, a complete overbite and maximal incisal opening of 38 mm. He denied any jaw pain. Given his age and the limitations and restrictions on consideration for joint replacement, options for initial management included:

1. Watch and wait.
2. Standard bimaxillary osteotomy with counter-clockwise rotation and significant advancement of the mandible.
3. Distraction osteogenesis.
4. Inverted 'L' shaped osteotomy and bone graft interposition.
5. Bilateral temporomandibular joint replacement.

Due to his age at initial presentation, following a lengthy discussion it was elected to watch this patient and review him clinically over time. At a subsequent review four years later, his overjet was still 9 mm, the overbite was now 1 mm and the maximal incisal opening 38 mm. He again denied pain. Repeat orthopantomogram (OPG) and lateral cephalogram at this stage showed progressive condylar resorption with subsequent displacement of the condyle anteriorly out of the fossa region (see Figures 17.1 and 17.2).

Following a further discussion of surgical options, he elected to proceed with bilateral temporomandibular joint (TMJ) replacement as he felt that other options were less definitive and reliable [1].

His clinical features of functional occlusal derangement and condylar collapse complied with National Institute of Health and Care Excellence (NICE) guidelines and funding was applied for from his local Primary Care Trust. He was sent for patch testing via his general practitioner to nickel, cobalt, chromium and molybdenum. A computed tomogram (CT) scan was also arranged that showed destruction of the condylar head on the right (see Figure 17.3).

In order to confirm the joint pathology diagnosis a CT or magnetic resonance scan as a minimum is required (not just plain radiographs). A CT scan is preferable as it can subsequently be used for construction of the custom made prosthesis. He then proceeded to total replacement of the TMJ (Boxes 17.1 and 17.2).

> **Clinical tip**
>
> As in any clinical scenario, a thorough history and examination are imperative. As a baseline, details regarding occlusal relationship, overbite and overjet are mandatory. Recording maximal incisal opening, protrusive and lateral excursive movements are also useful in cases where joint ankylosis and restriction are reported. A visual analogue scale is used to record pain and dietary scores (and are a useful repeatable, reproducible measure).

⊕ **Clinical tip**

In cases where progression of joint disease is expected or suspected, serial OPGs may be more useful than initial investigation with a CT scan as subsequent TMJ replacement planning will require a repeat scan to be performed. Initial investigations can include an OPG and lateral cephalogram.

Study models and an occlusal bite record may be of clinical use in monitoring progression of disease. In patients where a joint replacement will take place, patch testing is recommended [2,3].

Preoperative OPG and lateral cephalogram

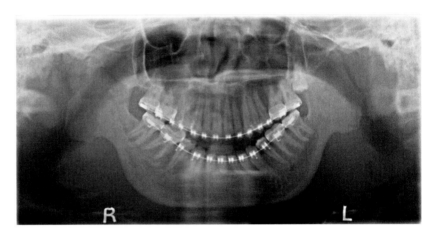

Figure 17.1 Note the absence of the condyles bilaterally and classic antegonial notching of a long-standing process with attempted muscle functional growth. There was no pre-existing history of trauma.

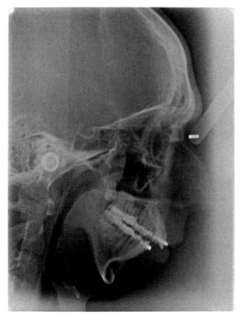

Figure 17.2 Lateral cephalogram again showing absence of condyles and retrognathic mandibular appearance as a result.

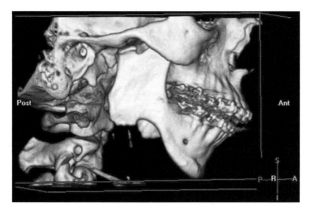

Figure 17.3 Three-dimensional reconstruction from CT scan images showing absence of right condyle. This level of scanning and image quality is required for construction of the 3-dimensional model and surgical planning stents (if they are used). They also allow the generation of a screw guide to be created to show the length of screw to use for securing the condylar and fossa components.

> ✚ **Clinical tip**
>
> Approximately 21% of patients have pneumatization of the zygomatic arch and complex that needs to be appreciated in order to prevent postoperative infective sequelae. This is an extension of the pneumatization of the temporal and mastoid bone [4]. This can be factored in by the company manufacturing the TMJ prosthesis, or if not requires review by the attending surgeon if using stock prosthesis.

> ⭐ **Learning point** Guidelines for temporomandibular joint replacement
>
> In order to comply with NICE guidance, there is a prerequisite for failed conservative management (including arthroscopy if possible). The UK guidelines also suggest the following clinical indications for joint replacement [5]:
>
> - diseases involving condylar bone loss
> - degenerative joint disease (osteoarthrosis)
> - inflammatory joint disease such as rheumatoid, ankylosing spondylitis, psoriatic arthritis [6]
> - ankylosis
> - post-traumatic condylar loss or damage
> - postoperative condylar loss (including neoplastic ablation)
> - previous prosthetic reconstruction
> - previous costochondral graft
> - serious congenital deformity
> - multiple previous procedures.
>
> Clinical indications under which a TMJ replacement should be considered are usually a combination of the following:
>
> - dietary score of < 5/10 (liquid scores 0, full diet scores 10)
> - restriction of mouth opening (< 35 mm)
> - occlusal collapse (anterior open bite or retrusion)
> - excessive condylar resorption and loss of height of vertical ramus
> - pain score > 5 out of 10 on visual analogue scale (combined with any of the others)
> - reduced quality of life score (these give an idea of pain and functional disability and permit some assessment of outcome).
>
> Overall long-term success rate for TMJ replacement is quoted as 90% [7].
>
> Contraindications to temporomandibular joint replacement:
>
> - any local infective process (consider dental, otological and skin sources)
> - severe immunocompromise (systemic and acquired)
> - severe coexistent diseases (American Society of Anaesthesiologists Grade III).
>
> Reprinted from *British Journal of Oral and Maxillofacial Surgery*, Volume 46, Issue 2, Sidebottom AJ, Guidelines for the replacement of temporomandibular joints in the United Kingdom, pp.146–147, Copyright © 2007 The British Association of Oral and Maxillofacial Surgeons, with permission from Elsevier, http://www.sciencedirect.com/science/journal/02664356.

❝ Expert comment

It is important to consider the anaesthetic difficulties that may be encountered when considering TMJ replacement. These are both general medical problems and local airway problems. From the general health point of view rheumatoid patients may be on steroids or immunosuppressant therapy and one should consider stopping this to facilitate healing. In addition, involvement of the cervical spine may make flexion of the neck either dangerous due to compromise of the spinal cord, or difficult due to restricted movement either from ankylosis of the spine or surgical fusion.

The local anatomy of a retrusive chin, fixed flexion of the cervical spine, or restricted mouth opening may make intubation difficult and therefore an experienced airway anaesthetist is often required who is capable of performing fibre-optic aided awake intubation. Likewise the models and scans may prove a useful guide to the anaesthetist with respect to the gauge of the nasal airway on each side [8].

Box 17.1 Operative note

The procedure is performed under general anaesthetic, with care given to maintaining sterility of the joint space, as intra-oral access is required at the time of securing the prosthetic condylar component.

Some surgeons will use a urology drape for this purpose to separate the oral cavity from the skin (and position the patient so that contamination with oral secretions is not possible). Maxillomandibular fixation (MMF) screws / Leonard buttons can also be applied before the joint space is accessed to minimize the potential contamination intraoperatively. Alternatively the use of adhesive sterile drapes with the mouth free to be covered can be used [9].

The hair is shaved to the level of the pinna superiorly. The drapes can then be secured to the patient, which also helps to exclude hair from the surgical field. The ear canal should be cleansed and then excluded. A Jelonet (Smith & Nephew, UK) plug can be inserted into the external auditory meatus to plug this point (and should be documented as placed so that it can be removed at the end of the operation).

Using a pre-auricular approach with temporal extension the incision line is marked (Figure 17.4) and infiltrated with anaesthesia, which can also be introduced deep into the joint space itself and onto the zygomatic arch. Other access approaches have been described in the literature, but this is the preferred choice of the senior author.

The incision is made to the depth of the temporal fascia. Once this has been suitably exposed along the line of the skin incision, this is incised vertically at the root of the zygomatic arch with 45-degree superoanterior release of the superficial envelope of the fascia to protect the temporal branch of the facial nerve. Subperiosteal dissection is continued along the arch with blunt stripping inferiorly to expose the joint capsule. The position of the joint is confirmed by manipulation of the mandible and the joint is then opened. Throughout meticulous haemostasis should be observed. Once the anterior and posterior margins of the condylar neck are exposed subperiosteally the condylar neck can be safely divided with care being taken to preserve the medial periosteum and deeper maxillary vessels. The use of a piezoelectric saw can also help to preserve the soft tissues around the joint, but is often slower.

✪ Learning point Retromandibular approach

An incision line is marked 0.5 cm posterior to the ascending ramus of the mandible and 2–3 cm in length. Infiltration with local anaesthetic containing adrenaline is advised to aid with haemostasis. This incision is extended down to the level of the parotid fascia, with haemostasis throughout.

The parotid fascia is then divided with blunt dissection through the parotid looking for the branches of the facial nerve, which are often found lying in the masseteric fascia. Once the branches are isolated the masseter is released from the pterygoid along the posterior and inferior border of the ramus. Release of the pterygomasseteric sling permits subperiosteal dissection up to the sigmoid notch and also allows exposure of the coronoid if this requires removal at the time of surgery. As an approximate guide, you need to be able to visualize the angle fully and sigmoid notch (through both the upper and lower incision).

Box 17.2 Operative note (continued)

Condylectomy and eminectomy

A Dautreys retractor can be used behind the condylar neck and into the sigmoid notch to protect the underlying soft tissues and vessels whilst the residual condylectomy is performed, usually with a fissure bur.

The eminence can also be reduced using a fissure bur to 'postage stamp' the eminence that can then be fractured off or removed using a chisel. A large burr can then be used to smooth the resultant surface. The alternative is to use an oscillating rasp [10].

Insertion and securing the prosthesis

The prosthetic components should be pre-soaked in antibiotic-containing solution and the site irrigated with a similar solution to help prevent local infection. The fossa component is fixed first and three screws as a minimum are used to secure it.

The mandibular component is introduced and secured after the patient has been placed into MMF. At this stage a change of gloves will be necessary as intra-oral access has been made. The condylar component is secured, again with three screws and the resulting occlusion checked. There should be a minimum gap of 5 mm between the fossa and the distal mandibular segment. If dislocation or malocclusion occurs, repositioning of the mandibular component may be required, hence it is important initially not to use all the screw holes. Once the occlusion is secure then attempt dislocation of the prosthesis, particularly where a coronoidectomy has been performed. Should this occur then a week of light elastic traction should be maintained to prevent dislocation occurring in the postoperative period (11).

Once the fit is deemed suitable, the remaining fixation screws can be applied, with care taken to change gloves each time the oral cavity is accessed to check the occlusion. Throughout the surgical procedure, irrigation is performed with copious amounts of gentamicin solution.

Wound closure

Drainage from the wound should be achieved with a small suction drain to both the retromandibular and pre-auricular site with one drain traversing the two sites. This should be removed the following day to prevent risk of infection. Care must be taken to prevent it being sutured into place during wound closure. Closure of both wounds needs to occur in layers. A 3/0 Vicryl/PDS (Ethicon Inc. US) can be used to close parotid and temporal fascia. Failure to close the parotid fascia meticulously can increase the risk of a sialocoele developing. Subcuticular closure may be performed with 3/0 Vicryl. Skin closure is attained with 6/0 Ethilon or Prolene (Ethicon Inc. US) and a continuous suture can be used on the pre-auricular and retromandibular incisions.

Postoperative care

Patients will normally need 24 hours of admission and intravenous antibiotics. Individual surgeon preference should then be sought as to the duration of inpatient care.

However, all patients need to be instructed on the use of a Therabite (Atos Medical, USA) and this needs to be started on the first postoperative day. The average length of stay in the UK is 3.2 days.

Instructions on how to use this device are based on the 7 × 7 × 7 approach: seven times a day, they use the appliance and stretch their opening as wide as is comfortable, seven times and hold for seven seconds each time. There is a diary within the Therabite appliance packaging (which are single use only) that allows the patient to document their progress. It should be increased as much as possible each day, but will tend to fall back a little overnight. Progress can be monitored at a similar time daily.

Skin sutures can be removed after five to seven days (by their practice nurse) and the patient is usually seen six weeks later.

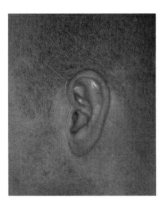

Figure 17.4 Diagram of pre-auricular incision.

✪ **Learning point** Complications

Immediate

- Bleeding (may necessitate access to the neck to tie off the branch of the external carotid). In cases of ankylosis, a preoperative magnetic resonance angiogram may be of use here, with a stent cutting guide and consideration of using a piezoelectric knife to complete the condylectomy).
- Dislocation of the TMJ, of which the highest incidence is in the first week [11] and more common in cases where there is a pre-existing anterior open bite. Use of MMF or elastics should be considered immediately post-operatively to minimize this risk. These can be discontinued after one week.
- Neuropraxia of facial nerve branches; temporary or permanent.
- Infection (consider prophylaxis pre- and postoperatively and early removal of drains).
- Deafness (this may occur as the ear pledget may not have been removed postoperatively, or they have a clot which requires removal from postoperative bleeding).

Delayed

- Pre-auricular scar.
- Malocclusion (perceived and real).
- Neuropraxia of facial nerve branches; temporary or permanent. Most are transient, and resolved by time of the 6-week follow up appointment.
- Temporal hollowing particularly if the temporalis is fully divided.
- Limited movement of the mandible (no lateral excursions possible due to detachment of lateral pterygoid).
- Allergy to the prosthesis (reduced with preoperative testing).
- Frey's syndrome.

Discussion

TMJ surgery has evolved significantly over the last ten years and is increasingly performed by designated surgeons. Early referral is advisable in cases where such treatment is indicated, as currently funding permission is a rate-limiting step in management. Where possible, referral to surgeons with a specialist TMJ practice is also advisable for holding/diagnostic measures such as arthroscopy and arthrocentesis given the better outcomes achieved in such units.

The procedure itself arguably has significant aesthetic, anatomical, and functional benefits and increasingly is being offered to more patients as confidence in the procedure and correct patient selection has improved.

A final word from the expert

Alternatives to joint replacement

- Accept limitation of movement (but accept lifelong risks to patient with restricted intra-oral access requiring intubation for any other purpose).
- Changing facial profile cannot be corrected any other way.
- Difficulty with function/eating.
- Pain and quality of life issues are known to improve with TMJ replacement [7,13].
- Consider alternative joint salvage procedures such as costochondral grafting.

In young patients, give consideration to delaying the joint replacement as long as possible given the life expectancy of a prosthetic joint and limitations of access to replacement (and

(continued)

revision surgery being more complicated) in the patient's lifetime. Costochondral grafting is still considered to be the first option of management in children [14], although simple gap arthroplasty and temporalis interposition will give the desired improvement in function with less morbidity, but will necessitate later reconstruction once growth is complete.

There are also reported cases of patients who have developed idiopathic condylar resorption whilst undergoing orthodontic treatment who may benefit from a combined TMJ/orthognathic surgical approach, or who have previously had failed joint surgery [15].

References

1. Hoppenreijs TJ, Freihofer HPM, Stoelinga PJ, et al. Condylar remodelling and resorption after Le Fort I and bimaxillary osteotomies in patients with anterior open bite: A clinical and radiological study aesthetic and reconstructive surgery. *Int J Oral Maxillofac Surg* 1998; 27(2): 81–91.
2. Sidebottom A, Speculand B, Hensher R. Foreign body response around total prosthetic metal-on-metal replacements of the temporomandibular joint in the UK. *Br J Oral Maxillofac Surg* 2008; 46(4): 288–92.
3. Sidebottom A, Mistry K. Prospective analysis of the incidence of metal allergy in patients listed for total replacement of the temporomandibular joint. *Br J Oral Maxillofac Surg* 2014; 52(1): 85–6.
4. Ladeira D, Barbosa G, Nascimento M, et al. Prevalence and characteristics of pneumatization of the temporal bone evaluated by cone beam computed tomography. *Int J Oral Maxillofac Surg* 2013; 42(6): 771–5.
5. Sidebottom AJ. Guidelines for the replacement of temporomandibular joints in the United Kingdom. *Br J Oral Maxillofac Surg* 2008; 46(2): 146–7.
6. Sidebottom A, Salha R. Management of the temporomandibular joint in rheumatoid disorders. *Br J Oral Maxillofac Surg* 2013; 51(3): 191–8.
7. Mercuri LG, Edibam NR, Giobbie-Hurder A. Fourteen-year follow-up of a patient-fitted total temporomandibular joint reconstruction system. *J Oral Maxillofac Surg* 2007; 65(6): 1140–8.
8. O'Connor M, Sidebottom A. Is the 3-D CT model useful to our anaesthetists? *Br J Oral Maxillofac Surg* 2013; 51(3): 262–3.
9. Sidebottom AJ. Total prosthetic replacement of the temporomandibular joint. In:Langdon J, Ord R, Brennan P (eds) *Operative Maxillofacial Surgery* second edition. Oxford: CRC Press; 2010. p. 573.
10. Sainuddin S, Currie A, Saeed NR. Use of reciprocating rasp in articular eminectomy. *Br J Oral Maxillofac Surg* 492011. p.e42–e43.
11. Mustafa EM, Sidebottom A. Risk factors for intraoperative dislocation of the total temporomandibular joint replacement and its management. *Br J Oral Maxillofac Surg* 2014; 52(2): 190–2.
12. Idle MR, Lowe D, Rogers SN, Sidebottom AJ, Speculand B, Worrall SF. UK temporomandibular joint replacement database: report on baseline data. *Br J Oral Maxillofac Surg* 2014; 52(3): 203–7.
13. Burgess M, Bowler M, Jones R, Hase M, Murdoch B. Improved outcomes after alloplastic tmj replacement: Analysis of a multicenter study from Australia and New Zealand. *J Oral Maxillofac Surg* 2014: 72(7): 1251–7.
14. Sidebottom AJ. Current thinking in temporomandibular joint management. *Br J Oral Maxillofac Surg* 2009; 47(2): 91–4.
15. Hills AJ, Ahmed N, Matthews NS. Concurrent bilateral total temporomandibular joint replacement surgery and conventional maxillary osteotomy utilizing virtual surgical planning web-based technology. *J Craniofac Surg* 2014; 25(3): 954–6.

18 Osteochondroma of the mandibular condyle / temporomandibular joint

Alan Attard

⊕ Expert commentary Jason Green

Case history

A 37-year-old woman was referred for assessment and management of a facial deformity. She presented with a five-year history of progressive deviation of her lower jaw to the right hand side, associated with pain in the left pre-auricular area and decreasing mouth opening. She denied any history of trauma, had no generalized joint symptoms and her past medical history was clear. Extra-oral examination showed bowing of the left lower border of mandible and the chin point deviated to the right of the facial midline. On palpation tenderness of the left temporomandibular region was noted. Examination of the external auditory meata was unremarkable. Her interincisal distance on maximum mouth opening was limited to 18 mm. Intra-oral examination showed good oral hygiene with a healthy periodontal status and well-restored dentition. In addition, a maxillary cant with a left-sided tilt and a left lateral open bite was noted. An orthopantomogram (OPG) (Figure 18.1) showed an exophytic mass of the left mandibular condyle with mixed density and a sclerotic appearance.

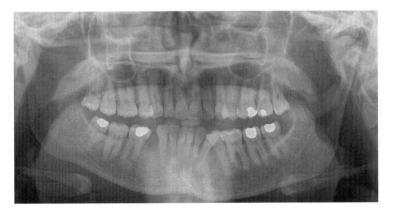

Figure 18.1 Orthopantomogram demonstrating enlargement of the left mandibular condyle.

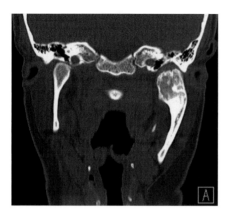

Figure 18.2 Coronal slice of a computed tomogram demonstrating the left-sided anomaly.

Cross-sectional imaging offered further diagnostic and three-dimensional information on this lesion. A computed tomogram (CT) scan showed a large exostosis of the left mandibular condyle with intact cortices and no bony ankylosis (Figure 18.2).

In order to assess whether this lesion was actively growing and thus predict whether the deformity was progressive, a nuclear medicine bone single-photon emission computerized tomogram (SPECT) was requested. This showed a marked area of increased uptake in the region of the left mandibular condyle corresponding to the condylar lesion seen on the CT scan (Figure 18.3).

> ✅ **Evidence base** SPECT scintigraphy for condylar hyperplasia [1]
> - Hodder et al. in 2000.
> - Eighteen patients with suspected unilateral condylar hyperplasia.
> - Twenty-three SPECT scans for this cohort.
> - Patients reviewed at six-monthly intervals.
> - A difference in uptake of 55: 45% between the condyles was regarded as indicative of condylar hyperplasia.
> - Compared with a group of 11 age-matched controls.
> - Concluded that SPECT is useful to assess bone activity that may lead to the development of an asymmetry.
>
> *Source:* data from Hodder SC et al., SPECT bone scintigraphy in the diagnosis and management of mandibular condylar hyperplasia, British Journal of Oral and Maxillofacial Surgery, Volume 38, Issue 2, pp.87–93, Copyright © 2000 The British Association of Oral and Maxillofacial Surgeons, Published by Elsevier Ltd.

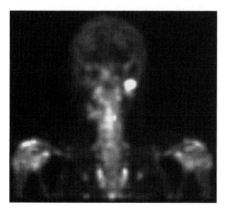

Figure 18.3 Single-photon emission computerized tomogram scan showing marked uptake in left condyle.

Based on the history, clinical examination and medical imaging findings, the diagnosis of osteochondroma of the left temporomandibular joint (TMJ) was made.

The following issues were identified:

1. Neoplasia of the left TMJ.
2. Progressive lower facial deformity.
3. Chin point deviated to the right.
4. Painful left TMJ.
5. Limited mouth opening.
6. Maxillary cant.
7. Malocclusion.
8. Left-sided lateral open bite.

The patient's desired management outcomes were:

1. Relief of left-sided pre-auricular pain.
2. Improved mouth opening.
3. Improved masticatory function.
4. Alignment of the chin point.
5. Correction of the malocclusion.

⨁ Expert comment

Several conditions may present with progressive symptoms as seen in this case. Limitation of mouth opening in patients may be attributed to both intra- and extra-articular pathology. In this case the patient has reported a slow but noticeable change in facial appearance with movement of the chin point and bowing of the mandible. Whilst these features are seen in other conditions such as condylar hyperplasia and hemimandibular hyperplasia, they are not generally associated with trismus.

The patient provided old photographic evidence to show the progressive nature of the facial deformity, which can be invaluable in both diagnosis and treatment planning. This case also demonstrates the value of plain radiography in diagnosis. The OPG clearly shows a mixed radio-opacity mass at the left condyle. I find that plain radiography is essential in managing all TMJ conditions.

The difficulty in this type of case is to decide whether or not a biopsy is warranted prior to definitive surgery. Whilst malignant conditions of the TMJ are rare, they should be borne in mind in any condition where there is a gross change in condylar morphology. In this case, the slow progressive nature and subsequent cross-sectional and nuclear medicine images were strongly suggestive of an osteochondroma. Where there is a question as to the underlying pathology, I would advocate open biopsy to confirm the diagnosis prior to definitive surgery.

Following discussion a treatment plan that addressed the patient's desired management outcomes was proposed to achieve optimum function, aesthetics and stability. This consisted of the following steps:

1. Excision of the neoplastic lesion to arrest further growth of the lower jaw.
2. Le Fort I maxillary osteotomy to correct maxillary cant and malocclusion.
3. Bilateral sagittal split mandibular osteotomy to correct left mandibular bowing and malocclusion.
4. Sliding genioplasty to centralize the chin point.

The treatment plan was discussed with the patient. After careful consideration and taking into account the patient's concerns the plan was revised. The finalized treatment accepted by the patient consisted of:

1. Excision of the neoplastic lesion to arrest further growth of the lower jaw and correct mandibular asymmetry.
2. Le Fort I maxillary osteotomy to correct maxillary cant and malocclusion (Box 18.1).

Box 18.1 Operative note

Under general anaesthesia, a partial condylectomy of the left mandibular condyle to include the entire lesion was performed through an extended temporal pre-auricular approach. The condylar stump was contoured to the shape of a condylar head, allowing it to seat passively in the glenoid fossa over the well-preserved articular disc. A standard Le Fort I differential impaction osteotomy was performed to level the maxillary cant and obtain a satisfactory occlusion (Figure 18.4). The patient was placed in light elastic maxillomandibular fixation for four weeks. The surgery achieved optimal functional and aesthetic results with good stability noted three years post procedure. The patient remains under yearly outpatient follow up.

> ⊕ **Clinical tip**
>
> Preparation and work-up for this case is identical to that seen with conventional orthognathic surgery. Accurate clinical assessment, cephalometrics and photographic records are essential. Standard articulated study models allow both the surgeon and technician to accurately plan surgery, prepare surgical wafers and allow manufacture of custom made arch bars - the latter invaluable for intra- and postoperative inter-maxillary fixation or traction.
>
> In addition, we used a three-dimensional stereolithograhic model to help with the planning and positioning the surgical cuts for the maxilla. The increasing ease of access to this type of model means their use in surgical planning has become increasingly common. The model helps the surgeon visualize and plan three-dimensional movements and even allow a 'dry run' of the planned surgical procedure.

> ⊕ **Expert comment**
>
> In most cases, the osteochondroma can be resected through a conventional pre-auricular incision. Additional surgical access from a submandibular or retromandibular approach may be required with larger lesions or as a second access point for reconstruction. Where I have needed to access the ramus, I prefer to use a high submandibular, transmasseteric (upper Risdon) approach. This gives a very broad access to the mandibular ramus with minimal preoperative morbidity.

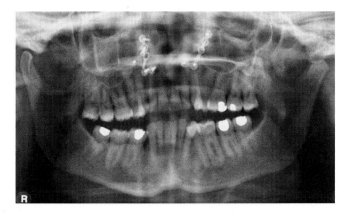

Figure 18.4 Postoperative orthopantomogram.

Discussion

The neoplasms and pseudo-tumours of the TMJ are relatively uncommon. Their early identification is essential in order to establish a diagnosis and if required provide early treatment. This may minimize potential associated secondary facial deformity developing.

TMJ lesions include osteochondroma, osteoma, osteoblastoma, synovial chondromatosis, ganglion, synovial cyst, simple bone cyst, aneurysmal bone cyst, epidermal inclusion cyst, haemangioma, non-ossifying fibroma, Langerhan's cell histiocystosis, plasma cell myeloma and sarcoma. The bone or cartilage-forming tumours are the most common lesions of the mandibular condyle. They are readily identified as they lead to facial asymmetry and malocclusion. Conversely, the intraosseous condylar lesions are difficult to diagnose as their symptoms – painful or painless swelling, dull pain in the pre-auricular region, clicking sound and discomfort during mastication – are similar to the symptoms of temporomandibular disorders (TMDs). Therefore, these pathologies are often initially overlooked, as patients are treated conventionally for TMDs [2].

✪ Learning point   Definition of osteochondroma

The World Health Organization defines osteochondroma (also known as osteocartilagenous exostosis) as a 'cartilage-capped bony protrusion on the external surface of bone' [3]. It is one of the most common benign bone tumours and occurs in any bone that develops by endochondral ossification [4]. The craniofacial regions are not common sites of osteochondromas. Reported regions of occurrence in the craniofacial skeleton include the skull base, maxillary sinus, zygomatic arch and mandible. Mandibular osteochondromas have been reported to occur in the coronoid process, condyle, ramus, body, angle and symphyseal regions [5]. The embryonic development of the mandibular condyle by endochondral ossification makes this area the most frequent facial site for this type of tumour, followed by the coronoid process of the mandible [6]. Review of the literature indicates that patients with these tumours present mainly in the fourth decade of life with a mean age of 39.7 years and a male to female ratio of 1:1.5 [7]. Malignant transformation has been reported but has been very rare (<1%) in cases of solitary lesions. Although a recurrence rate of 2% has been reported for osteochondromas that occur all over the body, no case of either recurrence or malignant transformation has been reported in the mandible [8].

The aetiology for osteochondromas is uncertain, with proposed aetiological factors being traumatic, inflammatory, developmental, reparative and genetic mutations.

Condylar osteochondromas are typically situated on the anteromedial surface of the condylar head at the insertion of the lateral pterygoid muscle. Similarly, osteochondromas of the mandibular coronoid process arise at the insertion of the temporalis muscle. The tumours are thought to develop from the tendinous attachment of these muscles, similar to the tendency of long bone osteochondromas to arise at the tendinous attachments [7]. It has been suggested that these lesions arise from hyperplasia of chondrocyte nests in the periosteum that are stimulated by mechanical stress from the tendinous insertions [9].

ⓕ Expert comment

The benign nature of osteochondromas mean that are unlikely to recur. At the time of surgery there is often a delineation between normal condyle and the benign growth. In these cases it is possible

(continued)

to 'remove' the osteochondroma and preserve as much as the anatomical condyle as possible. The articular surface of the condyle is surgically remodelled to give as smooth a surface as possible. In this case, it was expected that there would be little if no useful portion of the meniscus remaining. In actual fact, the meniscus was completely preserved and could be left in situ. If meniscectomy is performed, the surgeon needs to decide on what, if any, interpositional graft is required.

In some cases, the condyle is completely replaced with the osteochondroma that necessitates a decision as to how to reconstruct the condyle. There are many options of restoring function to the damaged condyle. These vary from the very simple gap arthroplasty (which can be very well tolerated by some patients), all the way through to total alloplastic replacement. The possible surgical options are discussed below. Total joint replacement can be carried out at the same time as surgical resection.

> ✪ **Learning point** Presentation
>
> Osteochondromas of the mandibular condyle often cause symptoms similar to those of temporomandibular dysfunction syndrome. Clinical findings associated with osteochondroma of the condyle may include a palpable, painless temporomandibular mass with lower facial asymmetry and prognathic deviation. Other features include malocclusion with open bite on the affected side and cross-bite on the contralateral side [10]. In some cases severe pain, hypomobility and clicking and locking of the TMJ, as well as headaches and cervical pain may be present [11].

> ✪ **Learning point** Imaging
>
> The radiographic presentation of osteochondroma in the mandibular condyle region is that of a sclerotic mass. Osteochondromas are found most often on the medial aspect of the mandibular condyle (52%), followed by an anterior location (20%) and rarely in the lateral or superior positions (< 1%) [12].
>
> CT is useful for both diagnostic and treatment planning purposes. A feature considered diagnostic of osteochondromas on CT is the continuation of the cortex and medulla of the parent bone with that of the tumour [13]. CT scans may be used to generate three-dimensional reconstructed images and in the production of printed models, both useful to the surgeon in preoperative planning.
>
> Osteochondroma of the mandibular condyle must be distinguished from unilateral condylar hyperplasia. Radiographically an osteochondroma usually shows a globular projection extending from the margins of the condylar head with the normal outline of the condylar head being maintained, whereas unilateral condylar hyperplasia shows an enlarged condylar process. CT plays a decisive role in differentiating the two entities. On CT an osteochondroma is seen as a growth arising from the morphologically normal condyle, whereas condylar hyperplasia is seen as enlargement of the condylar process [14].

> ✪ **Learning point** Histology
>
> Histologically an osteochondroma shows a thickened cellular periosteum, deep to which lies a sheet of proliferating chondrocytes. Beneath this cartilaginous cap is a zone of ossification resulting in the formation of cancellous bone [7,10].

Treatment objectives
1) Establish diagnosis.
2) Complete excision of lesion.
3) Relieve symptoms.
4) Restore function.
5) Correct maxillary and occlusal plane.
6) Correct malocclusion.
7) Restore facial symmetry.

> ✪ **Learning point** Management
>
> There are no large studies available for review because most of the existing literature consists of single case reports. In consideration of the benign nature of the lesion and its extremely low likelihood of recurrence, immediate reconstruction after extirpation of condylar lesions is usually advocated [5].

Surgical options
1. Partial condylectomy (vertical ramus height preserved).
2. Condylectomy (vertical ramus height compromised) + reconstruction (reconstitute vertical ramus height) with or without articular disc preservation and repositioning.

    a. Ipsilateral ramus lengthening osteotomy; sagittal split osteotomy / sliding vertical; subsigmoid osteotomy / distraction.

    b. Autogenous reconstruction: rib graft / sternoclavicular grafts / bone graft.

    c. Prosthetic TMJ replacement: stock joint; custom joint.

3. With or without con**ventional orthognathic surgery.**

A final word from the expert

This is a very interesting case that links together several maxillofacial disciplines to achieve a desirable surgical outcome. The patient presented with a progressive facial deformity in conjunction with common temperomandibular joint symptoms. Despite the size of the osteochondroma, surgery was performed without the need for complex and expensive reconstruction and the patient now has no temperomandibular joint symptoms and functions normally. Her interincisal clearance is over 30 mm and she is pain free. She is able to eat a normal diet and as yet has shown no sign of recurrence of the osteochondroma, four years after surgery.

Whilst uncommon, osteochondromas represent a challenge for the surgeon in terms of planning and surgical reconstruction. Each individual case is different in terms of symptomatology and presentation, surgical planning and reconstructive surgery.

References

1. Hodder SC, Rees JIS, Oliver TB, et al. SPECT bone scintigraphy in the diagnosis and management of mandibular condylar hyperplasia. *Br J Oral Maxillofac Surg* 2000; 38: 87–93.
2. More CB, Gupta S. Osteochondroma of mandibular condyle. *J Nat Sci Biol Med* 2013; 4(2): 465–8.
3. Schajowicz, F, Ackerman, LV, Sissons, HA. *International Histological Classification of Tumors*. No. 6. Histological Typing of Bone Tumors. Geneva: World Health Organization, 1972.
4. Forssell H, Happonen RP, Forssell K, Virolainen E. Osteochondroma of the mandibular condyle report of a case and review of the literature. *Br J Oral Maxillofac Surg* 1985; 23: 183–9.
5. Wolford LM, Mehra P, Franco P. Use of conservative condylectomy for treatment of osteochondroma of the mandibular condyle. *J Oral Maxillofac Surg* 2002; 60(3): 262–8.
6. Utumi ER, Pedron IG, Perrella A, et al. Osteochondroma of the temporomandibular joint: a case report. *Braz Dent J* 2010; 21(3): 253–8.
7. Avinash KR, Rajagopal KV, Ramakrishnaiah RH, et al. Computed tomographic features of mandibular osteochondroma. *Dentomaxillofac Radiol* 2007; 36: 434–6.
8. Wolford LM, Movahed R, Dhameja A.Allen WR. Low Condylectomy and Orthognathic Surgery to Treat Mandibular Condylar Osteochondroma: A Retrospective Review of 37 Cases.*J Oral Maxillofac Surg* 2014; 72(9): 1704–28.
9. Gonzalez-Otero S, Navarro-Cuellar C, Escrig-de Teigeiro M, et al. Osteochondroma of the mandibular condyle: Resection and reconstruction using vertical sliding osteotomy of the mandibular ramus. *Med Oral Patol Oral Cir Bucal* 2009; 14(4): E194–7.
10. Marks RB, Carlton DM, Carr RF. Osteochondroma of the mandibular condyle: report of a case with 10 year follow up. *Oral Surg Oral Med Oral Pathol* 1984; 58: 30–2.
11. Sanders B, McKelvy B. Osteochondromatous exostosis of the condyle. *J Am Dent Assoc* 1977; 95: 1151–3.

12. Peroz I, Scholman HJ, Hell B. Osteochondromas of the mandibular condyle: a case report. *Int J Oral Maxillofac* Surg 2002; 31: 455–6.
13. Murphey MD, Choi JJ, Kransdorf MJ, et al. Imaging of osteochondroma: variants and complications with radiologic - pathologic correlation. *Radiographics* 2000; 20: 1407–34.
14. Saito T, Utsunomiya T, Furutani M, Yamamoto H. Osteochondroma of the mandibular condyle: a case report and review of literature. *J Oral Sci* 2001; 43: 293–7.

19 Management of the Wilkes Grade III temporomandibular joint

Grigore Mihalache

Expert commentary Ahmed Messahel

Case history

A 28-year-old female presented to her general medical practitioner with a history of a loud click, frequent locking and pain from her right temporomandibular joint (TMJ). She was subsequently referred to the local oral and maxillofacial surgery unit for treatment.

On presentation the patient complained of a 12-month history of pain and ongoing discomfort from her right TMJ with a persistent audible click during function. This was sometimes so distressing to her that she often avoided dining in public. She denied bruxism or clenching and there were no associated ear, nose and throat problems. No bad habits (such as nail biting) were identified and no previous trauma to the facial area reported.

Her past medical history was unremarkable.

Clinical examination revealed that her mouth opening was 31 mm with an audible click from the right TMJ. The muscles of mastication were unaffected. The contra-lateral TMJ demonstrated no abnormalities. There was obvious tenderness over the right TM joint line.

On intra-oral examination the patient had a Class III incisal relationship in conjunction with congenitally absent lower central incisors with retained deciduous incisors. There was a very slight left lateral open bite.

The orthopantomogram (Figure 19.1) demonstrated no bony pathology, adequate condylar length, and no dental pathology. The working diagnosis of right TMJ anterior disc displacement with reduction (ADDWR) was made.

In order to establish a definitive diagnosis a TMJ protocol magnetic resonance imaging (MRI) scan was organized and the patient considered for early surgical intervention due to her frequent troublesome painful locking following an adequate period of non-surgical management (bite splint/analgesia/jaw rest).

> **Expert comment**
>
> TMJ dysfunction is a common complaint with a recent increase in numbers referred to secondary care for advice and management. The condition occurs in up to 30% of the population and is commonly seen in young female patients.
>
> Management tends to vary between centres; however, all patients should initially undergo a period of evidence-based conservative treatment that consists of jaw rest, non-steroidal anti-inflammatory drugs (NSAIDs) and a bite splint for at least six weeks. Patients who fail to respond to these routine conservative measures for pain, restricted opening and locking should be considered for therapeutic
>
> (continued)

arthrocentesis or arthroscopy, both of which are associated with symptomatic improvement in 70% of patients. For acute closed lock you should consider proceeding directly to arthrocentesis / arthroscopy.

In addition, arthroscopy had the added advantage of providing diagnosis that is far superior to MRI imaging alone.

The MRI scan demonstrated anterior displacement of both menisci, with reduction in anterior translation of the condyles, but there was evidence of capture bilaterally (Figures 19.2 and 19.3). This places her into the Wilkes III classification of dysfunction (see 'Learning point: Staging of internal derangement').

On review, the right TMJ continued to be symptomatic, demonstrating a painful opening click with continued associated locking during function. Her symptoms were having a marked effect on her quality of life at this stage and conservative measures had limited success. We proceeded with an arthrocentesis of the right TMJ under day case general anaesthesia (Box 19.1).

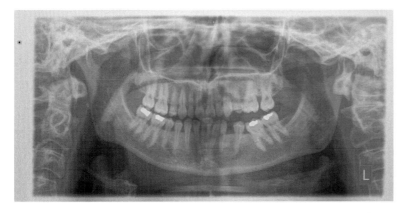

Figure 19.1 Orthopantomogram with no evidence of bony pathology of the temporomandibular joints.

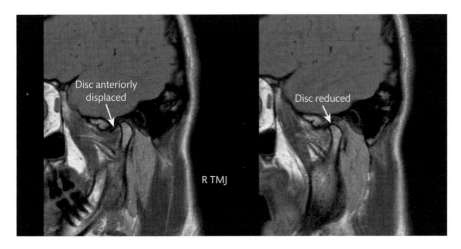

Figure 19.2 Right temporomandibular joint with mouth closed and mouth opened (ADDWR).

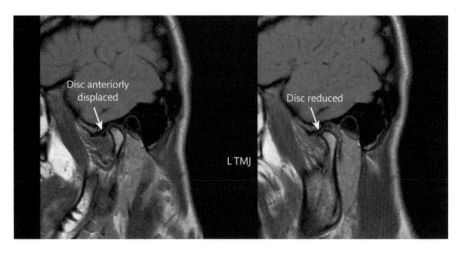

Figure 19.3 Left temporomandibular joint with mouth closed and opened (ADDWR).

Expert comment

During the process of arthrocentesis/arthroscopy, lysis of adhesions by hydro-dissection occurs as a result of the joint space being distended by fluid under pressure. In addition, during arthroscopy adhesiolysis also occurs by passage of the arthroscope through the adhesions under direct vision. The advantage of using an arthroscope to directly visualize the joint includes future planning for further surgical intervention should failure to improve occur.

Clinical tip

Place a small amount of Jelonet (Smith & Nephew, UK) (or equivalent) into the external ear canal. This prevents fluid entering the ear and patients complaining of temporary hearing loss after the procedure. Be sure to include this piece of material in your swab counts.

Clinical tip

Start off with a 5 ml syringe and 21G (green) needle loaded with sterile normal saline 0.9%. This is easy to handle and allows you to target the joint accurately. It also prevents you distending the superior joint space too much during the initial access phase. You should only inject 2–3 ml initially to distend the joint. Ensure you angle the needle forwards away from the external ear canal to prevent inadvertent injury to the external/middle ear structures.

Clinical tip

Look carefully for the following: movement of the chin to the opposite side; needle/syringe flick on gentle movement of the mandible; and back pressure on the syringe during initial injection of 2–3 ml of sterile 0.9% saline to confirm correct positioning within the superior joint space.

Clinical tip The Nitzan surgical technique [1,2]

A straight line is drawn from the lateral canthus to the tragus. The first point is made 10 mm anterior to the tragus on this line and the needle is inserted 2 mm caudal to this line. The second point is marked 20 mm anterior to the tragus on the straight line and needle is inserted 10 mm inferior to this. This should give excellent access to the upper joint space and the two needles can be triangulated appropriately (Figure 19.4).

Box 19.1 Operative note

The surgical field is prepared with an appropriate antiseptic solution such as povidone-iodine, and a single dose of intravenous broad-spectrum antibiotics is administered on induction. The upper joint space was accessed using the Nitzan technique. A 21-guage (40 mm green) needle was inserted at each of the landmark points with lavage of a least 200 ml of normal saline (0.9%) under continuous pressure. Excellent backflow was achieved. Manipulation under anaesthesia demonstrated a maximum incisal distance of 54 mm without dislocating the mandible. After the procedure was completed, an injection of 1.5 ml solution containing 1.0 ml bupivacaine 0.5% with 1:200,000 epinephrine and 0.5 ml triamcinolone was placed in the upper joint space.

Postoperative recovery was unremarkable and routine follow-up demonstrated complete resolution of painful symptoms with no further locking and mouth opening improving to 48 mm with excellent pain free lateral excursions.

Clinical tip

In difficult access joints where you have attempted more than one initial pass, be aware that upon injection of lavage fluid you may be at risk of extravasation into the surrounding tissues. This is particularly important if you are using local anaesthetic injection into the joint after the procedure as the patient may experience temporary facial nerve palsy.

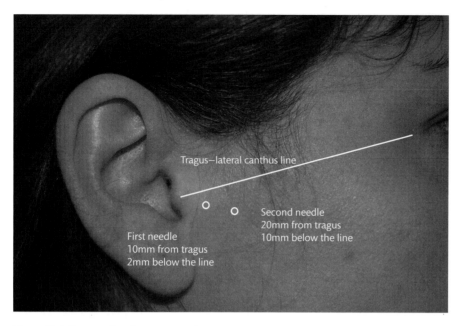

Figure 19.4 Two-needle arthrocentesis technique.

> ✪ **Learning point** TMJ lavage [3]
>
> Ohnishi: Arthroscopy with trochar in joint space
>
> Nitzan: Two-needle arthrocentesis: needle one 10 mm from the tragus on tragus-lateral canthus line and 2 mm inferior to the line; needle two 20 mm from the tragus-lateral canthus line and 10 mm inferior to the line.
>
> Laskin: Two needle arthrocentesis: needle one 10 mm from the tragus on tragus-lateral canthus line and 2 mm inferior to the line; needle two 2-3 mm in front of first needle.
>
> Alkan: Double needle cannula arthrocentesis: 10 mm from the tragus on tragus-lateral canthus line and 2 mm inferior to the line.
>
> Guarda-Nardini: Single needle arthrocentesis: 10 mm from the tragus on tragus-lateral canthus line and 2 mm inferior to the line.
>
> Reham: Single Shepard cannula with two lumens: 10 mm from the tragus on tragus-lateral canthus line and 2 mm inferior to the line.
>
> Rahal: Single-puncture arthrocentesis: 10 mm from the tragus on tragus-lateral canthus line and 2 mm inferior to the line.
>
> Alkan: Two needle arthrocentesis: needle one 7 mm from the tragus on tragus-lateral canthus line and 2 mm inferior to the line; needle two 10 mm from the tragus on tragus-lateral canthus line and 2 mm inferior to the line
>
> Reprinted from *British Journal of Oral and Maxillofacial Surgery*, Volume 49, Issue 4, Tozoglu S, et al., A review of techniques of lysis and lavage of the TMJ, pp.302–309, Copyright © 2011 The British Association of Oral and Maxillofacial Surgeons, with permission from Elsevier, http://www.sciencedirect.com/science/journal/02664356

Discussion

Temporomandibular joint dysfunction (TMD) is a complex term that covers all the structures involved in pathologic aspects concerning the TMJ. This relates to bony structures, musculature with ligaments, cartilaginous and neural structures [4].

⊕ Learning point Temporomandibular joint and related musculoskeletal disorders [4]

I. Intra-articular
(intracapsular pathology)
A. Articular disc
- Displacement
- Deformity
- Adhesions
- Degeneration
- Injury
- Perforation
- Anomalous

B. Disc attachments
- Inflammation
- Injury (laceration, haematoma, contusion)
- Perforation
- Fibrosis
- Adhesions

C. Synovium
- Inflammation/effusion
- Injury
- Adhesions
- Synovial hypertrophy/hyperplasia
- Granulomatous inflammation
- Infection
- Arthritides (rheumatoid, degenerative)
- Synovial chondromatosis
- Neoplasia

D. Articular fibro cartilage
- Hypertrophy/hyperplasia
- Degeneration (chondromalacia)
  - Fissuring
  - Fibrillation
  - Blistering
  - Erosion

E. Mandibular condyle and glenoid fossa (see also musculoskeletal)
- Osteoarthritis (osteoarthrosis, degenerative joint disease)
- Avascular necrosis (osteonecrosis)
- Resorption
- Hypertrophy
- Fibrous and bony ankylosis
- Implant arthropathy
- Fracture / dislocations

II. Extra-articular (extracapsular pathology)
A. Musculoskeletal
- Bone (temporal, mandible, styloid)
  - Anomalous developmental (hypoplasia, hypertrophy, malformation, ankylosis)
  - Fracture
  - Metabolic disease
  - Systemic inflammatory disease (connective tissue/arthritides)
  - Infection
  - Dysplasias
  - Neoplasia
- Masticatory muscles and tendons
  - Anomalous development
  - Injury
  - Hypertrophy
  - Atrophy
  - Fibrosis, contracture
  - Metabolic disease
  - Infection
  - Dysplasias
  - Neoplasia
  - Fibromyalgia

B. Central nervous system / peripheral nervous system
  - Reflex sympathetic dystrophy

The aetiology of TMD can be very broad and multifactorial and can include causes such as injury to the jaws, TMJ, neck, masticatory muscles, stress that sequentially produces muscle fatigue, bruxism or clenching of teeth, dislocation of the disc, osteoarthritis and rheumatoid arthritis [5].

The prevalence of TMD is more common in women than in men. The average age of presentation is around 30 years old [4].

Diagnosis is based on a detailed history of the disorder, past and current medical history, along with a thorough physical examination including intra-oral and extra-oral structures. Initial imaging joint imaging should include an orthopantomogram, at the very least to exclude a bony or dental cause. Specialist imaging can include CT scans for suspected bony pathology and anky-losis, MRI scans for suspected internal derangement and other specialist imag-ing such as radio nucleotide bone scans that might be considered for increased cellular activity [6].

✪ Learning point Staging of internal derangement (Wilkes) [7–9]

Stage	Clinical	Imaging	Surgical
I. Early	Painless clicking No restricted motion	Slightly forward disc, reducing[a] Normal osseous contours	Normal disc form Slight anterior displacement Passive in coordination (clicking)
II. Early/intermediate	Occasional painful clicking Intermittent locking Headaches	Slightly forward disc, reducing Early disc deformity Normal osseous contours	Anterior disc displacement Thickened disc
III. Intermediate	Frequent pain Joint tenderness, headaches Locking Restricted motion Painful chewing	Anterior disc displacement, reducing early progressing to non-reducing[a] late Moderate to marked disc thickening Normal osseous contours	Disc deformed and displaced Variable adhesions No bone changes
IV. Intermediate/late	Chronic pain, headache Restricted motion	Anterior disc displacement, non-reducing Marked disc thickening Abnormal bone contours	Degenerative remodelling of bony surfaces Osteophytes Adhesions, deformed disc without perforation
V. Late	Variable pain Joint credits Painful function	Anterior disc displacement, non-reducing with perforation and gross disc deformity Degenerative osseous changes	Gross degenerative changes of disc and hard tissues; Perforation Multiple adhesions

[a] Refers to disc position in relation to the condyle when the mouth is open
Reproduced with permission from American Society of Temporomandibular Joint Surgeons: Guidelines for diagnosis and management of disorders involving the temporomandibular joint and related musculoskeletal structures revised April 2001 and approved by ASTMJS 2001, *CRANIO® The Journal of Craniomandibular & Sleep Practice*, Volume 21, Issue 1, pp.68–76, Copyright © 2003 W. S. Maney & Son Ltd; permission conveyed through Copyright Clearance Center, Inc.

Disc movement and displacement may be usefully visualized on MRI. A normal TMJ demonstrates anterior movement of the disc on mouth opening. In the early stages of TMD, when the mouth is closed, the disc is displaced anteriorly and is reduced when the mouth is opened, along with a clicking thus constituting ADDWR. In the late stages of TMD, the anteriorly displaced disc is not reduced when the mouth is opened thus constituting anterior disc displacement without reduction (ADDWOR) (Figure 19.5) [4].

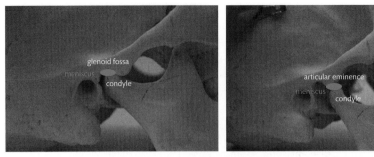

Normal Disc Placement

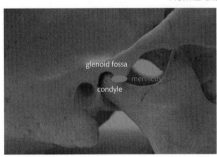
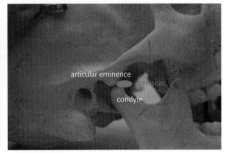

ADDWR

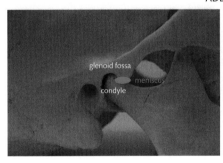
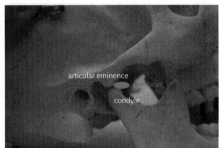

ADDWOR

Figure 19.5 Representation of various stages of internal derangement.

⭐ **Learning point** Treatment algorithm for temporomandibular dysfunction

Non-surgical	Surgical
• Soft diet	• Manipulation under anaesthesia
• Medication	• Arthrocentesis
○ NSAID's (ibuprofen)	• Arthroscopy
○ Analgesics (paracetamol)	• Condylotomy (indirect arthroplasty)
○ Antidepressants (amitriptyline, nortriptyline)	• Arthrotomy
○ Neuropathic pain drugs (gabapentin)	• Discectomy
○ Local anaesthetic injections	• Coronoidotomy or coronoidectomy
○ Steroid injections	• Styloidectomy (Eagle's syndrome)
○ Botulinum toxin	• Joint replacement
• Splints (hard / soft, upper / lower)	
• Physical therapy	
• Cognitive behavioural therapy	
• Psychological therapy	

Temporomandibular joint dysfunction is complex and modalities of treatment include surgical or non-surgical approaches. The clinician should be focused towards the reduction of pain, improvement of TMJ function and reducing the progression of any internal disc derangement.

Non-surgical treatment is based on soft diet, analgesia, maxillomandibular appliances, physiotherapy and possibly behaviour changes (e.g. nail biting). The patient should employ either a liquidized or soft diet for a period of about a week before returning to a normal diet. Drug therapy consists of simple analgesia such as paracetamol and consideration should be given to the use of NSAIDs such as ibuprofen if the patient can tolerate these. The use of tricyclic antidepressants such as nortriptyline and centrally acting pain-modifying drugs such as gabapentin should be reserved for those who do not respond to initial simple measures and use of simple analgesics. Injections into the joint space with steroids (kenalog) has also shown to be beneficial but must be used with caution and reserved for those individuals when there is a strong suspicion of an inflammatory nature to their joint pain (e.g. arthritis/capsulitis). The introduction of botulinum toxin into the affected muscle groups can provide benefit to these patients for periods of three to six months and often needs to be repeated. There is evidence that maxillomandibular appliances in any form (upper/lower, hard/soft) can be of benefit in treating TMD. In some cases they may exacerbate symptoms and their use may need to be discontinued. Behaviour recognition is very important in the treatment of TMD and avoidance bad habits like clenching the teeth, bruxism and chewing gum should be avoided. Psychological therapy could be very helpful in coping with stress that is strongly associated with TMD.

The most commonly used surgical treatment for Wilkes Stages III and IV is arthrocentesis [10]. There are eight different methods of performing the procedure [3,7,11] and we routinely employ the Nitzan technique (see Figure 19.4).

A Wilkes Stage I requires reassurance and usually discharge from the clinic at the first visit. Stage II is also non-surgical with use of the conservative measures discussed earlier. Wilkes Stages III and IV have been shown to benefit from therapeutic treatment such as arthrocentesis/arthroscopy in collaboration with non-surgical treatment and for late stage V more invasive surgical treatment should be considered.

A final word from the expert

Arthrocentesis/arthroscopy of the upper joint space reduces pain by removing inflammatory mediators from the joint, increasing mandibular mobility by removing intra-articular adhesions, eliminating the negative pressure within the joint, recovering the articular disc and fossa space and improving disc mobility, which reduces the mechanical obstruction caused by the anterior position of the disc.

Arthrocentesis/arthroscopy has an intermediate place between the medical and the surgical forms of treatment. The ease, lower costs and excellent published results so far, include this technique in the international protocol for the treatment of TMJ dysfunction.

References

1. Nitzan DW, Samson B, Better H. Long term outcome of arthrocentesis for sudden-onset, persistent, severe closed lock in the TMJ. *J Oral Maxillofac Surg* 1997; 55: 151.

2. Nitzan DW, Price A: The use of arthrocentesis for the treatment of osteoarthritic TMJ. *J Oral Maxillofac Surg* 2001; 59: 1154–9.

3. Tozoglu S, Al-Belasy FA, Dolwick MF. A review of techniques of lysis and lavage of the TMJ. *Br J Oral Maxillofac Surg* 2011 Jun; 49(4): 302–9.

4. American Society of Temporomandibular Joint Surgeons: Guidelines for diagnosis and management of disorders involving the temporomandibular joint and related musculo-skeletal structures revised April 2001 and approved by ASTMJ S2001. *Cranio* 2003; 21(1): 68–76.

5. Ingwale S, Goswami T: Temporomandibular joint: disorders, treatments, and biomechanics. *Ann Biomed Eng* 2009; 37(5): 976–96.

6. De Riu G, Stimolo M, Meloni SM, et al. Arthrocentesis and Temporomandibular Joint Disorders: Clinical and Radiological Results of a Prospective Study. *Int J Dent* 2013; 2013: 790648.

7. Guarda-Nardini L, Manfredini D, Ferronato G. Arthrocentesis of the temporomandibular joint: a proposal for a single-needle technique. *Oral Surg Oral Med Oral Pathol Oral Radiol Endod* 2008; 06: 483–6.

8. Wilkes CH: Internal derangements of the temporomandibular joint: Pathological variation. *Arch Otolaryngol Head Neck Surg* 1989; 115: 469.

9. Wilkes CH: Surgical treatment of internal derangements of temporomandibular joint. *Arch Otolarngol Head Neck Surg* 1991; 117: 64.

10. Neeli AS, Umarani M, Kotrashetti SM, Baliga S. Arthrocentesis for the treatment of internal derangement of the temporomandibular joint. *J Maxillofac Oral Surg* 2010; 9(4): 350–4.

11. Shinohara EH, Pardo-Kaba SC, Martini MZ, Horikawa FK. Single puncture for TMJ arthrocentesis: An effective technique for hydraulic distention of the superior joint space. *Natl J Maxillofac Surg* 2012; 3(1): 96–7.

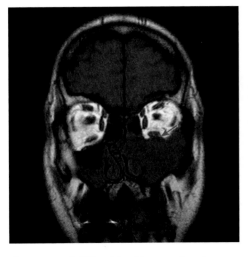

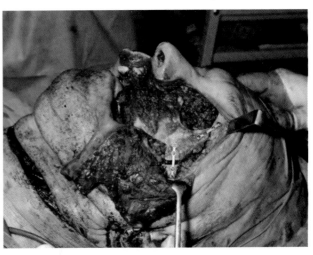

Figure 1.1 MRI (T2-weighted) in coronal section demonstrating the tumour in the left maxillary antrum and invading the left orbital floor (arrow).

Figure 1.3 Deep circumflex iliac artery inset.

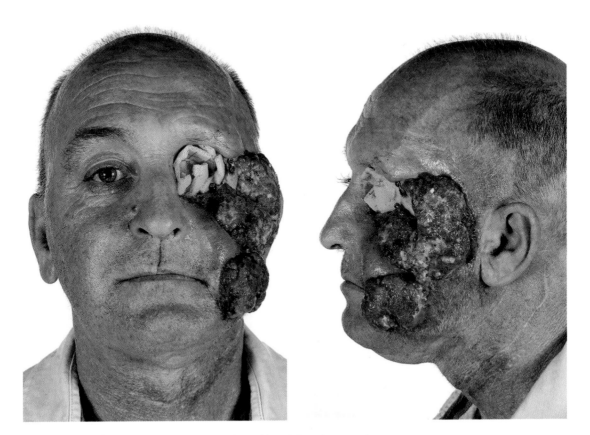

Figure 1.4 Immediate pre-operative anteroposterior and lateral views demonstrating recurrence.

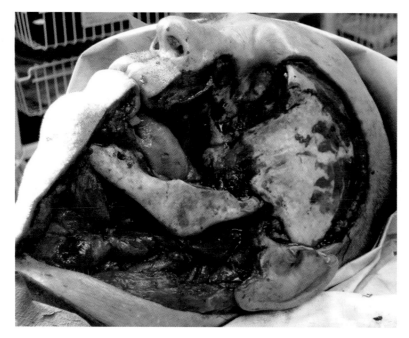

Figure 1.6 Following resection of recurrence.

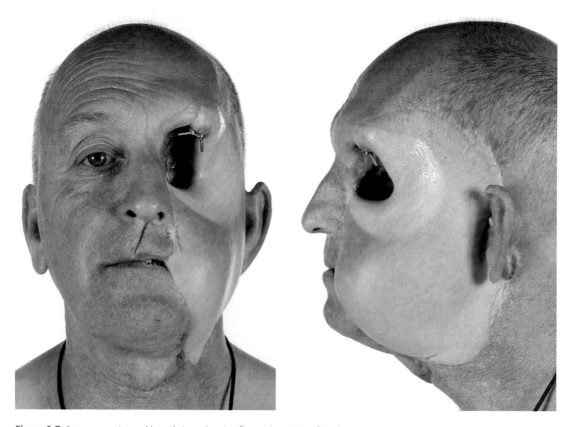

Figure 1.7 Anteroposterior and lateral views showing flap and position of implants.

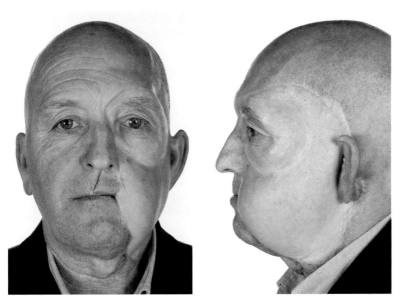

Figure 1.8 Anteroposterior and lateral views with prosthesis in position.

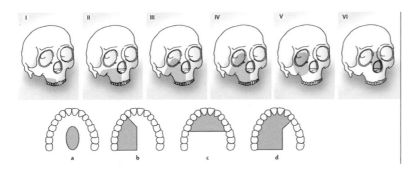

Figure 1.9 Brown classification.

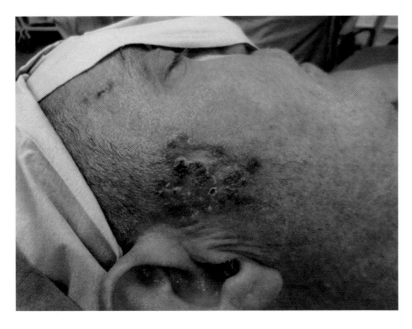

Figure 2.1 Right pre-auricular morphoeic basal cell carcinoma.

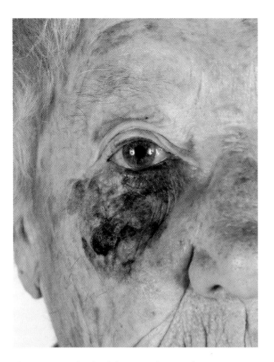

Figure 2.2 Right cheek lentigo maligna melanoma.

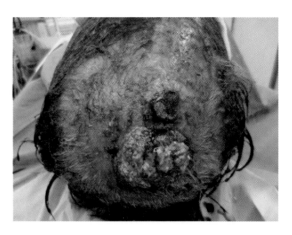

Figure 2.3 Pre-operative image of scalp squamous cell carcinoma.

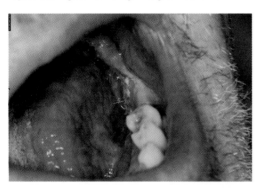

Figure 3.1 Exposed bone with surrounding erythematous oral mucosa.

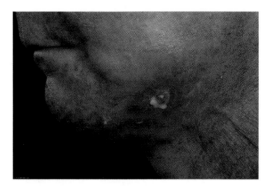

Figure 3.5 Extra-oral breach of the skin with discharge of pus and subsequent fistulation.

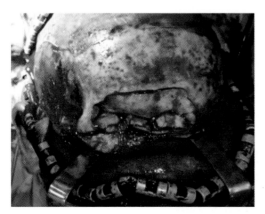

Figure 4.2 Comminuted fracture of the anterior wall of the frontal sinus and anterior orbital roof.

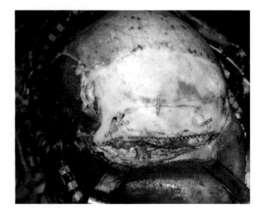

Figure 4.3 Fixation of right frontal sinus fracture with miniplates.

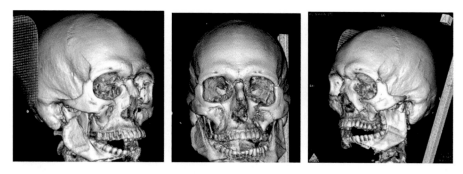

Figure 5.1 Three-dimensional reconstruction of computed tomogram demonstrating panfacial fractures.

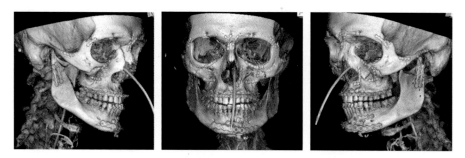

Figure 5.2 Three-dimensional reconstruction of CT illustrating the post-operative appearance.

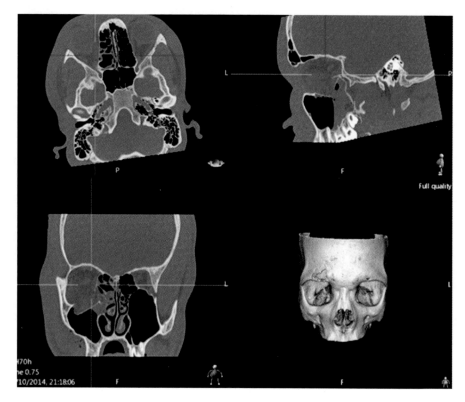

Figure 6.1 Axial, sagittal, coronal and three-dimensional reformatting of CT showing a right orbital floor fracture.

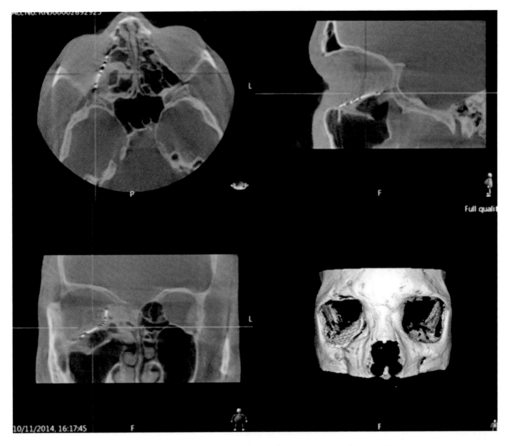

Figure 6.2 Post-operative CT demonstrating appropriate orbital reconstruction plate position

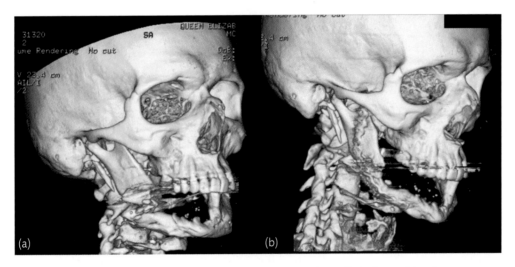

Figure 10.1 Three-dimensional CT reformats of the original comminuted mandibular fracture (a) and following application of a custom-made pre-bent reconstruction plate (b).

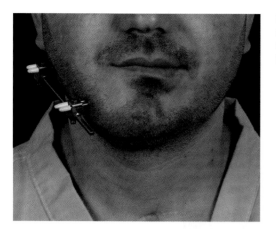

Figure 12.2 Postoperative view (following commencement of distraction) with the distraction device in place demonstrating the Synthes transcutaneous single-vector device.

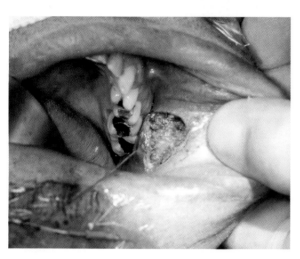

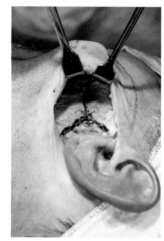

Figure 20.3 Raising of skin flap with marking of the parotid duct.

Figure 20.2 Intra-oral exposure of the duct.

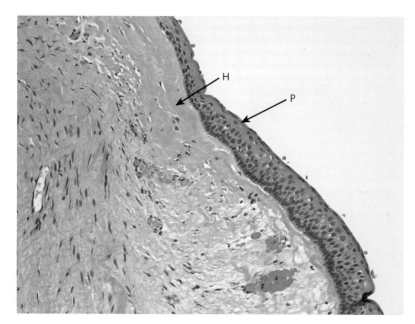

Figure 23.3 Haematoxylin & eosin stain of keratocystic odontogenic tumour removed by enucleation at first presentation showing epithelial parakeratosis (P) and subepithelial hyalinization (H) – both now known to be predictors of high risk of recurrence [1,2].

Reproduced courtesy of Dr Jenish Patel, Consultant Cellular Pathologist

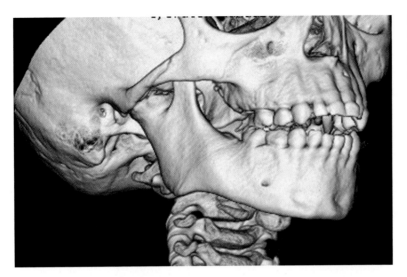

Figure 24.1 Computed tomogram (three-dimensional, coronal, and axial formats) demonstrating ankylosis of the right temporomandibular joint.

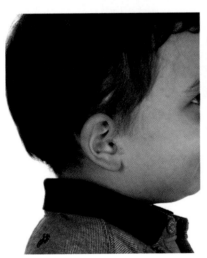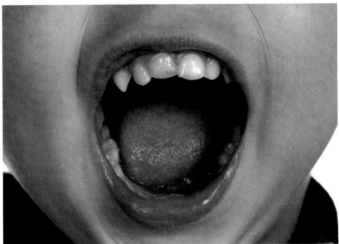

Figure 24.2 (a) Post-operative photographs demonstrating the pre-auricular and retromandibular scars. **(b)** Intra-oral view with mouth opening of 32 mm.

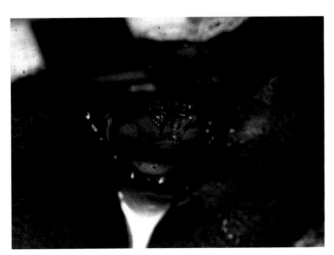

Figure 26.3 Image of orbital floor through a transconjunctival approach. Fat herniation into the fracture can be clearly identified and must be released.

SECTION 7

Salivary gland

Case 20   Salivary calculi

20 Salivary calculi

Jahrad Haq

ⓘ Expert commentary Mark McGurk

Case history

A 50-year-old man was referred by a secondary unit with a three-month history of intermittent swelling to the left parotid region. He was seen in the multidisciplinary one-stop salivary gland clinic. This clinic consists of an oral and maxillofacial surgeon, oral medicine consultant and a consultant dental radiologist.

Associated with the swelling was a foul taste, despite which he had not suffered from any overt infective episodes requiring antibiotics. The swelling was also not strictly related to mealtimes and resolved spontaneously after a period of minutes.

He was conscious of a lump within the left cheek that was stable in form and position. There was no other relevant medical or drug history and this was the first such episode that the patient had experienced.

On examination, there was no swelling on inspection. However, a firm lump was palpable in the mid-third of the left parotid duct. This was consistent with a large salivary calculus and it was not possible to milk saliva through the affected duct. The contralateral parotid examination was normal and there was no lymphadenopathy or facial nerve deficit.

He underwent ultrasound imaging, which demonstrated a 9 mm × 5 mm stone in the left parotid duct (Figure 20.1). The gland showed signs of atrophy consistent with previous inflammation and obstruction.

The treatment options were discussed with the patient. As the stone was considered too large for primary basket retrieval, consideration was given to either

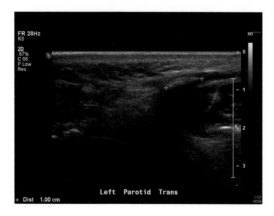

Figure 20.1 Ultrasound scan showing a calculus in the parotid duct.

> **✪ Learning point**
>
> First line investigations for salivary gland obstructive pathology:
>
> 1. Ultrasound (US).
> 2. Plain film radiograph if a small stone is lodged near the punctum.
> 3. Sialography is becoming redundant because of improvements in US imaging, but still has application when strictures or abnormalities of the duct are being investigated.

extra-corporeal shockwave lithotripsy (ECSL) or surgical removal of the stone by a gland-preserving technique using endoscopic guidance. The patient was keen to avoid surgical intervention and opted for a course of ECSL. It was explained that the chance of success would be around one in three for a stone of 10 mm maximum dimension.

The patient underwent three sessions of ECSL over a ten-week period using 4/3000 initially then 4/3500 for the final two sessions. This was tolerated well and arrangements were made for a review in three months.

At outpatient review, it was noted that the patient had been asymptomatic since the ECSL; however, the stone was still palpable. Repeat ultrasound demonstrated the large stone (10 mm × 5 mm) in the distal third of the duct with two smaller fragments lying proximally.

In light of the failure of the ECSL to sufficiently fragment the stone to permit spontaneous discharge or basket retrieval, the option of surgery was offered to and accepted by, the patient. It was decided to perform gland-preserving endoscopic assisted stone removal under general anaesthesia.

This combined approach relies upon the traditional pre-auricular approach to the parotid (extra-oral modified Blair access with a sub-superficial musculoaponeurotic system [SMAS] flap), but with a smaller access incision. The duct is identified and skeletonized, guided by the light on the end of the endoscope. The stone is then found and released by a simple longitudinal incision in the duct wall.

The patient was consented for this and counselled regarding the general and possible specific complications including scarring, facial nerve weakness (uncommon), duct stenosis (uncommon), salivary fistula (rare), Frey's syndrome (rare) and sialocele (common if there is a distal stricture in the duct).

At the time of surgery the stone was palpable distally in the parotid duct, at the anterior edge of masseter. The duct orifice was dilated with Nettleships and the sialendoscope was passed. It was apparent that several smaller stones were present as well as the larger 10 mm stone.

> **❝ Expert comment**
>
> One of the disadvantages of failed lithotripsy is there is no longer a single large stone to retrieve but multiple fragments. This presents a practical problem at surgery and fragments can lodge near the ostium or back in the hilum. It is also easy to miss fragments and occasionally the shockwaves push fragments outside the duct system into the connective tissue.
>
> If fragments are left in the duct the risk is that they will gradually enlarge requiring a further operative procedure. As is normally the case, a second surgical procedure is much more difficult to undertake and the risk of complications increases. As a precaution, if a patient has previously had lithotripsy then the surgeon should have an ultrasound machine at hand during surgery to make sure all stone fragments are identified and retrieved.

Due to the distal position of one of the stones (2 cm from the ostium) it was decided to attempt trans-ductal basket retrieval using a non-releasing five-wire helical basket under endoscopic visualization. Once the stone had been grasped by the basket it was drawn towards the ostium, but became impacted in the duct about 1cm from the ostium.

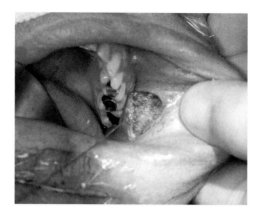

Figure 20.2 Intra-oral exposure of the duct.
See colour plate section.

> **ⓒ Expert comment**
>
> The size of a stone cannot be assessed through an endoscope so it is easy to try and retrieve a stone that is too big to pass down the duct lumen. The parotid ostium is functionally very delicate and every attempt should be made to leave it intact. Only stones visible or protruding through the ostium should be released by incising the ostium. Stones lying within ~ 1 cm or adjacent to the lumen should be approached via a semi-lunar incision that identifies the duct within the cheek (using the endoscope). The stone is then released by a vertical incision through the duct wall.

An intra-oral semi-lunar incision was made and the duct was dissected out (Figure 20.2). Great care is taken to prevent trauma to the duct orifice, which would likely lead to stenosis. A ductotomy was performed directly onto the palpable stone, which was then extracted using a dental caries excavator. In this instance the stone was firmly attached to the duct wall and required release from the soft tissue. The net result was that the duct wall fragmented into layers and the lumen was lost. This meant the endoscope could not be reintroduced due to the presence of false passages.

This presented a significant disadvantage because the endoscope could not be used to guide the surgeon onto the duct system when the gland was approached by the traditional pre-auricular approach. Additional stones were present in the remaining proximal duct system, the dissection on to the duct had to be blind.

With continuous nerve monitoring in place, a sub-SMAS flap was raised from a modified Blair incision. The surface landmarks of the parotid duct were marked on the parotid capsule and the flaps were raised and reflected to a point 2 cm beyond that of the anticipated stone position (Figure 20.3). The buccal branch of the facial nerve was identified and isolated. The duct was then located and skeletonized with careful dissection in an antegrade manner. Once the duct was isolated, the position of the remaining stones became apparent and they were released through a longitudinal ductotomy.

A thorough washout of the gland was then performed and both ductotomy sites were closed with 6/0 Vicryl Rapide (Ethicon Inc. US). The skin flap and intra-oral incisions were closed and a pressure dressing was placed.

At review appointment in one month, the scar was healing well, there was no evidence of facial nerve deficit or salivary fistula and the patient was asymptomatic.

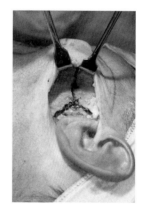

Figure 20.3 Raising of skin flap with marking of the parotid duct. See colour plate section.

Discussion

Aetiology

The prevalence of symptomatic salivary gland stones in the UK is 5.9:100,000 and represents the majority of salivary gland pathology in middle-aged patients [1].

The submandibular gland is the most common site for calculi, some 80–90% are found here, compared with 5–10% in the parotid gland and approximately 5% in the sublingual and other minor salivary glands [2].

✪ Learning point

The aetiology of sialothiasis is not completely understood, but the best explanation has been provided by Harrison [3]. The salivary glands contain micro-vesicles full of destructive enzymes. If these enzymes are released prematurely they would destroy the cell and so are neutralized by calcium ions to make a micro-calculus. These are being shed all the time into the duct lumen and if these micro-calculi are held up in the duct system they act as a nidus to initiate stone formation (saliva is supersaturated with calcium). Why the micro-calculi should be trapped is unclear, but as most stones develop at the bends in the duct pure anatomical reasons probably play an important role in the genesis of salivary stones.

Salivary stones are generally round or ovoid in form and consist of an inorganic portion of carbonated calcium phosphates as well as organic components of proteins, glycoproteins, mucopolysaccharides and lipids. These form around a central core of precipitated calcium salts aggregated on an organic nidus of desquamated epithelial cells, bacteria and salivary mucins. The makeup of submandibular stones differs from parotid stones with the ratio of inorganic to organic material being 18:82 compared to 51:9, respectively [4,5]. As well as varying degrees of mineralization, the stones also demonstrate either concentric or globular growth and fractal patterns. This is thought to have an effect on the vulnerability of a stone to lithotripsy [6].

Presentation

The presentation of a patient with salivary stones is classically described as the 'mealtime syndrome'. Pain and/or swelling of the affected gland associated with the eating or thought of food is typical. Massage of the gland may lead to a temporary relief of the obstruction around the stone, or cause the stone to move to a position whereby the duct is rendered patent.

Ongoing or intermittent sialadenitis usually follows a year or two after the first episode of obstruction and results in chronic enlargement or tenderness of the gland, with purulent discharge from the duct orifice when a subacute infection converts to an acute one. It may also be possible to palpate the stone by bimanual examination. This is certainly the case with stones lying in the mid and distal thirds of the submandibular duct. It may not be possible to milk saliva from the affected gland. A single duct obstruction is not the cause of a dry mouth.

It is important to note that salivary calculi are not the sole cause of obstructive sialadenitis. The duct may become stenosed secondary to trauma or may be prone to mucous plugging, both of which can lead to a similar presentation. The differential diagnoses can be narrowed by further investigations, either in the form of imaging, or direct visualization of the duct lumen using sialoendoscopy.

⚙ **Learning point** Imaging

Ultrasound

Ultrasonography is now the initial imaging modality of choice for salivary gland disease. It has been reported to have a sensitivity of 94% and a specificity of 100% and is therefore regarded by some to be the method of choice in salivary stone imaging [7]. The stones, if present, produce a characteristic acoustic shadow from an echogenic round or oval structure. The duct anatomy can be discerned as well, with proximal duct dilatation being a key feature of an obstructive pathology [8].

Ultrasonography can be performed by radiologist or a trained surgeon in the setting of a one-stop clinic and is also readily available, cheap, non-irradiating and acceptable to patients due to its non-invasive nature.

Plain radiography

The radiopacity of salivary calculi varies depending on the proportion of inorganic matter they contain. As a result of this, 50% of parotid and 20% of submandibular stones are radiolucent [5]. Plain film radiographs are most useful for identifying small stones lodged at the orifice of the glands that are difficult to identify by other imaging modalities.

Sialography

Sialography describes the retrograde administration of radiopaque water-soluble contrast into the ductal system of the gland under investigation. The duct is first dilated and cannulated, the dye is then instilled under positive pressure (maximum 75 mmHg) whilst the region is imaged by plain film radiography [9]. A series of exposures can demonstrate the progressive filling of the ductal system as well as the rate of drainage.

Sialography is useful for illustrating changes in the anatomy of the duct and any strictures or filling defects typical of the presence of salivary calculi. The technique can be combined with digital subtraction, which uses post-processing subtraction of the bony background and contrast enhancement of the salivary ducts [10,11].

It is advised to wait for approximately six weeks from any acute infective or inflammatory episode prior to sialography.

Computed tomography

Unenhanced computed tomography (CT) is useful in cases of painful saliva glands where ultrasound or sialography may be technically difficult. Fine-cut CT has the ability to differentiate between clusters of small stones and one larger stone, which is helpful in deciding on treatment modality [12]. However, the duct is poorly visualized and the patient will be exposed to ionizing radiation.

Cone-beam (CB) CT may permit a lower exposure if the field of interest is limited just to the gland and ductal system in question. CBCT machines are becoming more commonplace now and may therefore play more of a part in the investigation of salivary calculi in the near future.

Magnetic resonance imaging

Magnetic resonance (MR) sialography does not require any invasive ductal cannulation and allows for precise evaluation of the ductal system up to the level of the third order branches [13]. In order to diagnose the presence of a stone, indirect features of ductal dilatation and signal loss are identified. For this reason, smaller stones that do not affect the ductal anatomy may be missed. MR sialography has the advantage of being appropriate in the presence of acute inflammation unlike conventional sialography [7].

Modes of management

The decision on how to proceed following the diagnosis of a salivary calculus relies on a number of variables. These include: which gland is affected, the location of the stone, the presence of multiple stones, the size of the stone and anatomy of the duct, as well as whether the stone is mobile within the duct.

✪ **Learning point**

Criteria for basket retrieval

- Small stone 3–5 mm (or stone up to 30% larger than the duct – occasionally get a dilated duct- that ideally are mobile).
- No stricture in front of the stone.

Criteria for extra-corporeal shockwave lithotripsy

- Stone ~ 5–8 mm in length.
- Minimally invasive approach with low morbidity consequently good for children and patients with a complex medical history who are unfit for general anaesthetic.
- Drawback is the cost of equipment (~ £100,000), protracted course of treatment with a minimum of three attendances of one hour each and unreliable results (60% stone clearance) at six months.
- Difficult to treat patients who live at a distance from the centre.
- Intra-corporeal lithotripsy can be performed using LASER but this is time consuming and not efficient. Also temperature changes in the duct lead to strictures. Pneumatic lithotripter is a new entity that is deployed in renal calculi but is largely unproven in the management of salivary stones.

Criteria for surgical removal of calculi

- Stones ideally ~ 8 mm or larger.
- Patient medically fit for a 90-minute operation.
- Drawback is that an open parotid procedure is required.
- Advantages are that the procedure reliably retrieves the stone, it is quick (overnight stay) and morbidity is low. Over time the author has moved away from lithotripsy to surgery for large stones for reasons of efficiency.

Sialoendoscopy

With the advent of endoscopes small enough to make passage through the salivary ductal system, the diagnostic gap has been filled by the ability to directly visualize the causative pathology.

The diameter of endoscopes available are from 0.6 mm to 1.6 mm and contain an irrigating channel and in some instances a working channel in order to pass baskets, drills, endoluminal lithotripters, or optical fibres for laser.

Such procedures can be performed under local anaesthesia and are generally well tolerated by patients. The overriding advantage of sialendoscopy is the benefit of combining diagnostic with possible therapeutic events simultaneously. Should it not be possible to retrieve the stone directly with a basket due to large size or immobility, the endoscope light can also serve as an excellent guide as to the position of the stone in order to direct a combined surgical approach [14–16].

> ⊕ **Clinical tip**
>
> - The parotid duct orifice is dilated by means of a Nettleship dilator (much easier in the parotid) and in the submandibular gland a papillotomy has been superseded by the introduction of a disposable dilator introduced by Cook Medical Ltd based on the Seldinger technique.
> - The optimal size is the 6000 pixel 0.9 mm scope and the 10,000 1.1 mm scope. The 1.6 mm version is too big for practical application.

> ❝ **Expert comment**
>
> The risk is that with dormia-type baskets once a stone is captured in the basket it cannot be released. If the stone is badly selected and will not pass down the duct the embarrassed operator is left with a patient firmly attached to a long wire basket! Cook Medical Ltd have helped overcome this problem by introducing a special basket that can grasp and then drop a stone if required.

Radiologically guided basket retrieval

In a similar fashion to endoscopic basket retrieval, dormia baskets can be introduced and advanced into the ductal system but using fluoroscopic or ultrasound guidance instead [17]. The small, mobile stone must first be visualized on the screen, then the basket can be monitored and advanced until it lies proximal to the stone. Capture of the stone should occur on withdrawal of the open basket.

Lithotripsy

ECSL describes a repetitive pressure wave generated by an electromagnetic source applied to the patient's body surface by means of a water-filled cushion. A frequency of around 120 Hz is adopted, with sessions of up 5000 shockwaves. A course of treatment may consist of up to five sessions [18].

Following this, repeat imaging will demonstrate the effect of the ECSL on the salivary calculi. If fragmented suitably, the particles may now be spontaneously washed out of the duct orifice, or indeed be amenable for basket retrieval.

> ✔ **Evidence base** Extra-corporeal shock wave lithotripsy [18]
>
> - In a series by Escudier et al 2003, 33% of patients were cured of submandibular calculi and another 35% were rendered symptom free although some stone fragments persisted in the duct.
> - Treatment was slightly more effective in the parotid gland, with 30 of 38 patients symptom free compared with 53 of 84 after treatment of submandibular stones.
> - The cut-off point is 7 mm diameter, above which lithotripsy is seen to be less effective.
>
> *Source:* data from Escudier MP et al., Extracorporeal shockwave lithotripsy in the management of salivary calculi, *British Journal of Surgery*, Volume 90, Issue 4, pp.482–485, Copyright © 2003 British Journal of Surgery Society Ltd. Published by John Wiley & Sons, Ltd.

Minimally invasive surgery

Intra-oral surgical release of stones can be guided by manual palpation in the case of larger submandibular stones, as well as endoscopic-assisted combined approaches for proximal duct small submandibular stones and parotid duct stones.

The surgical approaches for parotid stones have been described in the case report. With regard to submandibular stones the operative technique can be under general or local anaesthesia [19]. A floor of mouth incision and dissection medial to the sublingual gland is continued, permitting full skeletalization of the submandibular duct. The lingual nerve is kept under direct vision at all times and is therefore unlikely to be damaged. A ductotomy directly onto the underlying stone is performed and the stone is delivered into the oral cavity using a dental excavator. The ductotomy site is closed with 6/0 Vicryl Rapide (Ethicon Inc. US) and the floor of mouth incision with 4/0 Vicryl Rapide.

Gland removal

The minimally invasive surgery techniques outlined in this case study almost entirely obviate the need for gland removal. With appropriate examination, imaging and treatment stratification 97% of patients can be rendered symptom free, whilst the glands integrity is preserved [20].

Gland removal should be a last resort, for example, for intra-parenchymal stones causing ongoing symptoms refractory to the management as described above.

⊘ Evidence base [20]

- An observational study of 4691 consecutive patients (parotid n = 1165; submandibular n = 3526) treated by lithotripsy, endoscopy, basket retrieval and/or surgery in five centres from 1990 to 2004 inclusive.
- Results: salivary calculi were eliminated in 3775 out of 4691 (80.5%) cases and partly cleared in 782 out of 4691 (16.7%) patients. Salivary glands were removed in 134 out of 4691 (2.9%) of patients with symptoms in whom treatment failed.

Source: data from Iro H et al., Outcome of minimally invasive management of salivary calculi in 4,691 patients, *The Laryngoscope*, Volume 119, Issue 2, pp.263–268, Copyright © 2009 The American Laryngological, Rhinological, and Otological Society, Inc.

A final word from the expert

Salivary calculi are the most common of salivary gland pathologies in middle age and such patients are frequently seen in maxillofacial and ear, nose and throat clinics with the typical mealtime syndrome presentation. This case has described a complex patient who has progressed along the treatment algorithm and is now rendered symptom free and still in possession of their gland.

The salivary gland surgeon should possess a repertoire of skills: clinical, surgical and ideally radiological in order to provide the full remit of options to their patient. Minimally invasive options have now consigned the vast majority of salivary stone interventions as clinic based or as day surgery.

References

1. Escudier MPM, McGurk MM. Symptomatic sialoadenitis and sialolithiasis in the English population, an estimate of the cost of hospital treatment. *Br Dent J* 1999; 186(9): 463–6.
2. Combes J, Karavidas K, McGurk M. Intraoral removal of proximal submandibular stones - an alternative to sialadenectomy? *Int J Oral Maxillofac Surg* 2009; 38(8): 813–6.
3. Harrison JD.Causes, natural history, and incidence of salivary stones and obstructions. *Otolaryngol Clin North Am* 2009; 42(6): 927–47.
4. Bodner L. Parotid sialolithiasis. *J Laryngol Otol* 1999; 113: 266–7.

5. Moghe S, Pillai A, Thomas S, Nair PP. Parotid sialolithiasis. *BMJ Case Rep* 2012; 2012, pii: bcr 2012007480.

6. Nolasco P, Anjos AJ, Marques JMA, et al. Structure and Growth of Sialoliths: Computed Microtomography and Electron Microscopy Investigation of 30 Specimens. *Microsc Microanal* 2013; 19(05): 1190–203.

7. Rzymska-Grala I, Stopa Z, Grala B, et al. Salivary gland calculi - contemporary methods of imaging *Pol J Radiol* 2010; 75(3): 25–37.

8. Joshi AS, Lohia S. Ultrasound Indicators of Persistent Obstruction after Submandibular Sialolithotomy. *Otolaryngol Head Neck Surg* 2013; 149(6): 873–7.

9. Som PM, Shugar JMA, Train JS, et al: Manifestations of parotid gland enlargement: radiographic, pathologic, and clinical correlations. Part I: The autoimmune pseudosialectasias. *Radiology* 1981; 141(2): 415–9.

10. Forman WH: Subtraction sialography. *Radiology* 1977; 122(2): 533.

11. Buckenham TM, George CD, McVicar D, et al: Digital sialography: imaging and intervention. *Br J Radiol* 1994; 67(798): 524–9.

12. Yousem DM, Kraut MA, Chalian AA. Major salivary gland imaging. *Radiology* 2000; 216(1): 19–29.

13. Capaccio P, Cuccarini V, Ottaviani F, et al: Comperative ultrasonographic, magnetic resonance sialographic, and videoendoscopic assessment of salivary duct disorders. *Ann Otol Rhinol Laryngol* 2008; 117(4): 245–52.

14. Nahlieli O, London D, Zagury A, Eliav E. Combined approach to impacted parotid stones. *J Oral Maxillofac Surg* 2002; 60(12): 1418–23.

15. Marchal F. A combined endoscopic and external approach for extraction of large stones with preservation of parotid and submandibular glands. *Laryngoscope* 2007; 117: 373–7.

16. McGurk M, MacBean AD, Fan KF, et al. Endoscopically assisted operative retrieval of parotid stones. *Br J Oral Maxillofac Surg* 2006; 44: 157–60.

17. Drage NA, McAuliffe NJ. Ultrasound-guided basket retrieval of salivary stones: a new technique. *Br J Oral Maxillofac Surg* 2005; 43(3): 246–8.

18. Escudier MP, Brown JE, Drage NA, McGurk M. Extracorporeal shockwave lithotripsy in the management of salivary calculi. *Br J Surg* 2003; 90(4): 482–5.

19. Combes J, Karavidas K, McGurk M. Intraoral removal of proximal submandibular stones - an alternative to sialadenectomy? *Int J Oral Maxillofac Surg* 2009; 38(8): 813–6.

20. Iro H, Zenk J, Escudier, MP, et al. Outcome of minimally invasive management of salivary calculi in 4, 691 patients. *The Laryngoscope* 2009; 119(2): 263–8.

SECTION 8

Dentoalveolar surgery

21

Sagittal split osteotomy for the removal of a lower third molar

Matthew Idle

ⓘ **Expert commentary** Stephen Dover

Case history

A 48-year-old male was referred to the regional Oral and Maxillofacial Surgery Department by his general dental practitioner (GDP) with a five-year history of recurrent pain and swelling from around the right angle of the mandible. The signs and symptoms were, however, complex and he was initially diagnosed by his GDP, incorrectly, with temporomandibular joint dysfunction syndrome. During the year prior to his referral he had experienced two episodes of right-sided facial swelling and trismus that were attributed to pericoronitis surrounding an unerupted lower right third molar. Each presentation required treatment with a seven-day course of oral antibiotics and subsequent resolution of the infection was achieved without hospitalization. The GDP decided at this juncture that the patient met the National Institute for Health and Care Excellence (NICE) guidance [1] for surgical intervention (see 'Learning point: NICE Guidance for wisdom tooth removal').

⭐ **Learning point** NICE Guidance for wisdom tooth removal [1]

Prophylactic removal of pathology-free third molars should be discouraged.

Surgical removal should be limited to patients with evidence of pathology, namely:

- unrestorable caries
- non-treatable pulpal and/or periapical pathology
- cellulitis
- abscess
- osteomyelitis
- internal/external resorption of the tooth or adjacent teeth
- fracture of tooth
- disease of the follicle including cyst/tumour
- tooth/teeth impeding surgery or reconstructive jaw surgery
- tooth involved in the field of tumour resection
- one severe episode of pericoronitis
- second or subsequent episode of pericoronitis.

From National Institute for Clinical Excellence (2000) *TA 1 Guidance on the Extraction of Wisdom Teeth*. London: NICE. Available from www.nice.org.uk/TA1. Reproduced with permission. Material accurate at the time of publication.

Lopes et al. demonstrated that of 300 prospectively collected referrals from GDPs for third molar extraction(s), 82% were compliant with NICE guidance [2].

Source: data from Kim DS et al., Influence of NICE guidelines on removal of third molars in a region of the UK, *British Journal of Oral and Maxillofacial Surgery*, Volume 44, Issue 6, pp.504–506, Copyright © 2005 The British Association of Oral and Maxillofacial Surgeons, Published by Elsevier Inc.

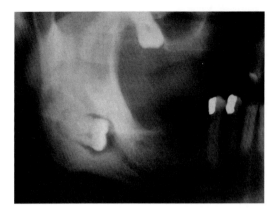

Figure 21.1 Orthopantomogram indicating the horizontally impacted lower right third molar with loss of the white lines of the inferior alveolar canal

He was noted to have a medical history including ulcerative colitis and hypertension. There were no known allergies and his repeat prescription included prednisolone and lisinopril.

Clinical examination revealed an unerupted lower right third molar (48) and a chronic sinus in the buccal sulcus over the angle of the right mandible. An orthopantomogram (OPG) demonstrated that the lower right third molar was horizontally impacted and in very close proximity to the inferior alveolar nerve (IAN) (Figure 21.1). These radiographic findings prompted a computed tomogram (CT) of the mandible (Figure 21.2) and this demonstrated that the inferior alveolar neurovascular bundle was immediately adjacent to the follicle in a medial (lingual) orientation and that there was evidence of buccal perforation of the mandibular cortex. The follicle surrounding the tooth was not noted to be pathologically enlarged. In view of high risk of injury to the IAN and of fracture of the mandible during extraction, the patient elected to leave the tooth in situ and was discharged back into the care of his GDP.

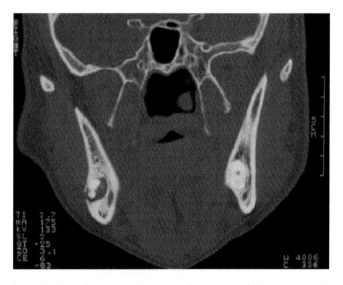

Figure 21.2 Coronal section of a computed tomogram (bone window) demonstrating a buccal perforation of the mandible. The IAN is positioned medially (lingually) to the lower right third molar.

🕐 **Evidence base** Radiological predictors of inferior alveolar nerve injury [3]

- Retrospective and prospective surveys.
- 1560 impacted third molars requiring surgical extraction.
- Radiological signs of close relationship between third molar and IAN:
  a. Darkening of the root.
  b. Deflection of the root.
  c. Narrowing of the root.
  d. Dark and bifid root.
  e. Interruption of the white line(s) of the inferior alveolar canal.
  f. Diversion of the inferior alveolar canal.
  g. Narrowing of the inferior alveolar canal.
- Retrospective:
  ○ Randomized 553 patients (800 third molars), impairment of labial sensation-2.4%.
  ○ Radiological signs 73 out of 800 (9.1%).
- Prospective:
  ○ 552 patients (760 third molars), impairment of labial sensation - 3.08%.
  ○ Radiological signs 157/760 (20.66%).
- Signs most commonly associated with nerve injury (in order):
  a. Diversion of the inferior alveolar canal ($p < 0.001$).
  b. Darkening of the root ($p < 0.001$).
  c. Interruption of the white line ($p < 0.001$).
- Signs unrelated to nerve injury
  a. Narrowing of the root.
  b. Dark or bifid root.
  c. Narrowing of the inferior alveolar canal.
  d. Deflected root.
- 104 patients with 'positive' x-ray findings did not sustain nerve injury.

Source: data from Rood JP, Nooraldeen Shebab BAA, The radiological prediction of inferior alveolar nerve injury during third molar surgery, *British Journal of Oral and Maxillofacial Surgery*, Volume 28, Issue 1, pp.20–25, Copyright © 1990 Elsevier Inc.

❝ Expert comment

Recurrent pain and swelling are not usually associated with temporomandibular dysfunction; they are more likely to be due to infection. The referral to hospital for assessment of 48 was appropriate given the episodes of infection. Given the history, chronic intra-oral sinus and CT findings there was a high likelihood of recurrent infection. Not withstanding the risks to the inferior dental nerve, the risks of continuing symptoms and a severe infection were significant. Surgical removal should have been recommended and if declined, the patient reviewed with a repeat CT to assess progression of the radiolucent area around the wisdom tooth.

However, four years later he presented to the Emergency Department with a significant right-sided facial swelling and a short history of a pyrexial illness. On this occasion there was a discharging sinus on the skin overlying the right angle of the mandible and trismus of 8 mm (interincisal) was noted. As there was no upper airway compromise the patient was deemed suitable for an urgent head and neck CT. This demonstrated that the lower right third molar was the nidus of infection and an associated abscess cavity measuring 12 × 6 × 3 cm was present (Figure 21.3).

The patient was transferred immediately to the operating theatre and underwent exploration of the perioral and parapharyngeal tissue spaces via an intra-oral buccal sulcus incision and an extra-oral submandibular incision. Corrugated surgical drains were placed into the abscess cavity to allow further drainage postoperatively. Culture

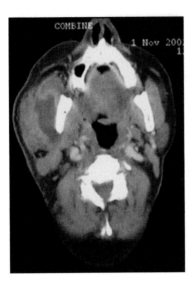

Figure 21.3 Axial slice of a computed tomogram (soft tissue window) demonstrating an abscess cavity surrounding the right angle of the mandible.

of a swab from the cavity indicated a heavy growth of *Staphylococcus aureus*, but no anaerobes. The patient made a significant improvement and the drains were removed at day 2 postoperatively with subsequent discharge home on a course of oral antibiotics.

Once the acute infection had settled over a period of weeks, arrangements were made to remove the tooth. A standard intra-oral approach would result in the need for significant bone removal (with increased risk of intra-/postoperative fracture) and place the IAN at unnecessary risk of injury. Thus the decision was made to perform a unilateral (right) sagittal split osteotomy (SSO) to remove the tooth [4].

A right sagittal split ramus osteotomy with a Hunsuck modification [5] was performed under general anaesthesia and the lower right third molar was removed with the neurovascular bundle seen intact. It was noted that a potential communication existed between the follicle and the skin of the right cheek and this was curetted simultaneously. Temporary intraoperative maxillomandibular (MMF) fixation was achieved with Leonard buttons and an upper Gunning splint. The buccal osteotomy site was fixed with a Leibinger 2.0 mm, four-hole (4 mm space) osteosynthesis minipate (Stryker, US) using 6 mm monocortical screws. This was augmented with a bicortical screw proximally to further stabilize the fragments (Figures 21.4 and 21.5). The osteotomy site was pre-plated to ensure correct anatomical position of the proximal and distal fragments postoperatively.

✚ Clinical tip History of the sagittal split osteotomy [6]

1957: First described by Obwegeser and Trauner.

1961: Dal Pont modified to create a vertical osteotomy between the first and second molars allowing greater contact surfaces between the cut bone.

1968: Hunsuck modified to create a shorter horizontal medial cut just past the lingula to minimize the soft tissue dissection. Anterior vertical cut similar to Dal Pont.

1976: Spiessel introduced internal fixation rather than six weeks of MMF.

1977: Epker proposed less stripping of the masseter to preserve the vascular pedicle and reduce bone resorption at the gonial angle. Also limited medial dissection which reduced postoperative swelling, haemorrhage and manipulation of the IAN.

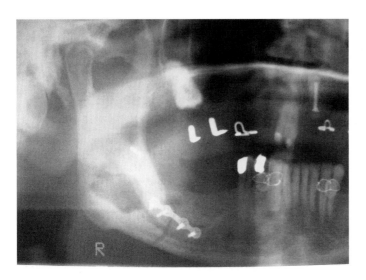

Figure 21.4 Orthopantomogram demonstrating miniplate and bicortical positional screw fixation and the Gunning splint in the upper jaw

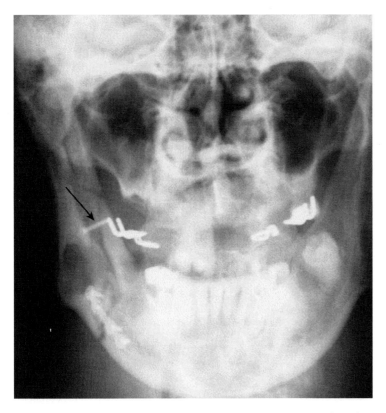

Figure 21.5 Postoperative posteroanterior view of the jaws showing bicortical screw (arrow).

He was subsequently discharged home on postoperative day 1 with paraesthesia reported in the distribution of the right mental nerve. No lingual nerve deficit was noted. At subsequent review, the cutaneous sinus on the right cheek had resolved and the paraesthesia was improving.

Discussion

The extraction of third molars is one of the ten most common procedures performed within the National Health Service. In England according to the Hospital Episode Statistics between 2012 and 2013 there were 69,366 independent episodes of third molar extraction [7].

The acknowledged risks associated with lower third molar extraction are: discomfort, swelling, trismus, bleeding, infection, alveolar osteitis and temporary or permanent deficit to the IAN or lingual nerve. Many differing figures are quoted for injury to these branches of the trigeminal nerve. Bataineh reported an incidence of IAN injury of between 0.4% and 8.4% based on 28 papers. Lingual nerve injury was reported in the range of 0% to 23% again based on 28 publications [8]. Renton et al. [9] report temporary deficit in the IAN of up to 8% and permanent injury in 3.6%. Robinson et al. [10] report deficit to the lingual nerve in about 4% of cases, but this is rarely permanent. In a case such as this the concern is that the risk of IAN injury is greatly increased in view of the findings on the OPG and subsequent CT.

In a clinical scenario as described above it is worth considering adjunctive imaging. The use of CT of the mandible still has a place, but cone-beam CT (CBCT), where available, has largely replaced this as the imaging of choice in view of the reduction in the effective radiation dose (see the Learning point).

✪ Learning point Cone-beam computed tomography [11].

CBCT uses a cone-shaped x-ray beam and an amorphous silicon flat panel as the detector. The image creation process is divided into three stages:

- data acquisition
- primary reconstruction
- secondary or multiplanar reconstruction.

CBCT is defined by the field of view:

- small, limited or dento-alveolar (approximately 4 cm^2)
- medium or maxillofacial (approximately 8 cm^2)
- large or craniofacial (+/- the skull vault).

Effective radiation doses of varying imaging modalities:

- OPG: 0.002–0.003 mSv
- dentoalveolar CBCT: 0.01–0.67 mSv
- craniofacial CBCT: 0.03–1.1 mSv
- CT mandible: 0.25–1.4 mSv.

A study by Matzen et al. [12] showed that CBCT influenced the treatment plan in 12% of cases of lower third molar extraction. Umar et al. [13] state that CBCT should be employed in the assessment of third molars to reduce risk to the IAN during extraction [13].

Inherent to this case is an elevated risk of intra- or postoperative mandibular fracture. Ethunandian et al. [14] state an incidence of 0.0033% to 0.0049% in their report on 130 mandibular fractures following lower third molar extraction. The literature demonstrates a 2.4:1 M:F ratio, but mentions that intraoperative fractures are more common in females (1:1.3 M:F). The decision to undertake a unilateral SSO was based on the increased risk of IAN injury and mandibular fracture, especially taking into consideration the perforation of the buccal cortex on CT.

Speculand and Ahmed [15] reported on 23 cases of ectopic third molars and the mode of extraction. An intra-oral approach was employed in 11 cases, including one endoscopic removal and one SSO. Extra-oral access to the ectopic third molar included: three preauricular, one submandibular, one retromandibular, one endaural and two cases where the access route was not described. The remaining four cases were managed conservatively. They also report three 'in-house' cases of markedly ectopic third molars of which two were approached extra-orally and one intra-orally. An extra-oral approach should be considered, but will also place branches of the facial nerve at risk and this should be discussed as part of the treatment planning phase.

Coronectomy has been discussed as an alternative to extraction in appropriate cases to reduce the risk of IAN injury. This was disregarded as a treatment option in this case in view of the significant amount of bone removal that would have been required. It was also noted on CT that significant pericronal and periradicular infection was present around lower right third molar that was in addition, horizontally impacted. According to Gady and Fletcher [16] these two findings represent a contraindication to coronectomy. Renton [17] concurs with these authors that immunomodulating drugs are a further contraindication and this patient was on long-term prednisolone for ulcerative colitis.

The landmark paper by Renton et al. (as discussed in the Evidence base box) does advocate the use of coronectomy in appropriate clinical cases. Certainly from a medico-legal standpoint it is imperative that the patient has been counselled regarding this surgical option if indicated.

🕑 **Evidence base** Coronectomy versus extraction [9]

- Randomized selection of 128 patients undergoing removal of 196 third molars.
- Selection criteria; patients at high risk of injury to the IAN based on radiographic findings.
- Features as described in Landmark paper by Rood et al. [3].
- New feature described; juxta-apical area.
- IAN injury: higher with removal (18.6%) versus coronectomy (0%).
- Radiographic features associated with injury to the nerve:
  o Juxta-apical area ($p = 0.04$).
  o Deviation of the canal ($p = 0.007$).
- Radiographic features associated with failed coronectomy:
  o Conical root formation ($p < 0.001$).
  o Narrowing of the roots within the canal ($p = 0.017$).
- In patients at high risk of IAN injury coronectomy reduces the chance of injury with no adverse effects on morbidity.

Source: data from Renton T et al., A randomised controlled clinical trial to compare the incidence of injury to the inferior alveolar nerve as a result of coronectomy and removal of mandibular third molars, *British Journal of Oral and Maxillofacial Surgery*, Volume 43, Issue 1, pp.7-12, Copyright © 2004 The British Association of Oral and Maxillofacial Surgeons. Published by Elsevier Inc.

The need for intervention for ectopic lower third molars is rare. They will usually remain asymptomatic and unknown to both the patient and the GDP. However, when they do present a problem to the patient and fulfil the NICE guidance [1] for extraction then appropriate investigations, careful planning and detailed consent should be undertaken with the aim of reducing risk to the patient.

A final word from the expert

Appropriate access and exposure of an operative site is a basic tenet of any surgical procedure. The sagittal split used in this case achieved both and gave every opportunity to minimize bone removal and protect the inferior alveolar bundle. It was wise to pre-plate the osteotomy site to achieve correct anatomical re-positioning of the fragments and to use a positional rather than lag screw. This avoids compression of the fragments, squeezing of the inferior dental bundle and potential malrotation of the mandibular condyle.

Buried wisdom teeth communicating via a sinus into the mouth or on to the skin of the face should be removed. They are a continuing source of infection with the potential for serious and potentially life-threatening sequelae.

References

1. National Institute of Health and Care Excellence. Guidance on the extraction of wisdom teeth, TA1 London: National Institute for Health and Care Excellence, 2000. https://www.nice.org.uk/guidance/ta1 (accessed 6 June 2014).
2. Kim DS, Lopes J, Higgins A, Lopes V. Influence of NICE guidelines on removal of third molars in a region of the UK. *Br J Oral Maxillofac Surg* 2006; 44: 504–6.
3. Rood JP, Nooraldeen Shebab BAA, The radiological prediction of inferior alveolar nerve injury during third molar surgery. *Br J Oral Maxillofac Surg* 1990; 28: 20–5.
4. Jones T, Monaghan A, Garg T. Removal of a deeply impacted mandibular third molar through a sagittal split ramus osteotomy approach. *Br J Oral Maxillofac Surg* 2004; 42: 365–8.
5. Hunsuck EE. A modified intraoral sagittal splitting technique for correction of mandibular prognathism. *J Oral Surg* 1968; 26: 250–3.
6. Monson LA. Bilateral sagittal split osteotomy. *Semin Plast Surg* 2013; 27(3): 145–8.
7. Hospital Episode Statistics, Admitted Patient Care, England- 2012- 13. Leeds: Health and Social Care Information Centre. Pub. November 5, 2013. http://www.hscic.gov.uk/hes (accessed 7 June 2014).
8. Batanineh AB. Sensory nerve impairment following mandibular third molar surgery. *J Oral Maxillofac Surg* 2001; 59: 1012–7.
9. Renton T, Hankins M, Sproate C, McGurk M. A randomised controlled clinical trial to compare the incidence of injury to the inferior alveolar nerve as a result of coronectomy and removal of mandibular third molars. *Br J Oral Maxillofac Surg* 2005; 43: 7–12.
10. Robinson PP, Loescher AR, Yates JM, Smith KG. Current management of damage to the inferior alveolar and lingual nerves as a result of removal of third molars. *Br J Oral Maxillofac Surg* 2004; 42: 285–92.
11. Whaites E, Drage N.*Essentials of Dental Radiography and Radiology* fifth edition. Edinburgh: Churchill Livingstone; 2013.
12. Matzen LH, Christensen J, Hintze H, et al. Influence of cone beam CT on treatment plan before surgical intervention of mandibular third molars and impact of radiographic factors on deciding on coronectomy vs surgical removal. *Dentomaxillofac Radiol* 2013; 42(1): 98870341.
13. Umar G, Obisesan O, Bryant C, Rood JP. Elimination of permanent injuries to the inferior alveolar nerve following surgical intervention of the "high risk" third molar. *Br J Oral Maxillofac Surg* 2013; 51: 353–7.

14. Ethunandan M, Shanahan D, Patel M. Iatrogenic mandibular fractures following removal of impacted third molars: an analysis of 130 cases. *Br Dent J* 2012; 212(4): 179–84.

15. Ahmed NM, Speculand B. Removal of ectopic mandibular third molar teeth: literature reviewand a report of three cases. *Oral Surgery* 2012; 5: 39–44.

16. Gady J, Fletcher MC. Coronectomy: indications, outcomes, and description of technique. *Atlas Oral Maxillofac Surg Clin North Am* 2013; 21(2): 221–6.

17. Renton T. Notes on coronectomy. *Br Dent J* 2012; 212(7): 323–6.

22

Implant restoration of the atrophic maxilla with concurrent mandibular rehabilitation

Elizabeth Gruber

✪ **Expert commentary** Graham James

Case history

A 29-year-old woman was referred by her general dental practitioner to the oral and maxillofacial surgery department with a diagnosis of aggressive periodontal disease. Her failing dentition had already been scheduled for extraction. She was fit and well, not taking any regular medications and had no relevant family history of periodontal disease. She did not smoke, had been under periodontal supervision for many years and was well motivated to comply with oral hygiene requirements.

Clinical examination revealed mobility of all residual teeth, in both the upper and lower arches. Initial investigation involved an orthopantomogram (OPG) radiograph that revealed severe bone loss (Figure 22.1). Due to periodontally migrated teeth and loss of occlusal support, the vertical dimension of occlusion was dramatically reduced.

A full dental clearance was undertaken and the patient was provided with immediate complete upper and lower dentures. Four months later the patient was reassessed and was not tolerating the dentures well, as they were poorly retained. A further OPG was obtained (Figure 22.2) and a cone-beam computed tomogram scan (Figure 22.3) for preoperative planning for bone augmentation and implant surgery (Box 22.1).

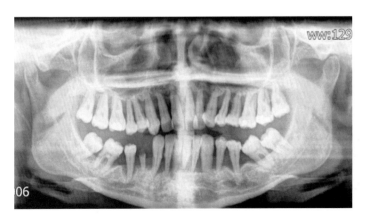

Figure 22.1 Orthopantomogram demonstrating aggressive generalized periodontal disease.

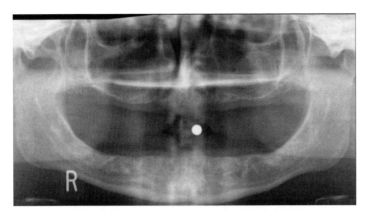

Figure 22.2 Postoperative orthopantomogram for implant planning.

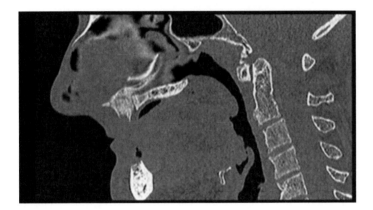

Figure 22.3 Cone-beam computed tomogram for implant planning.

Box 22.1 Operative note

A Le Fort I osteotomy was undertaken with 7 mm anterior and 7 mm downward displacement. An interpositional, corticocancellous bone graft, harvested from the iliac crest, was positioned with screws. OPG and lateral cephalogram radiographs show the immediate postoperative appearance (Figure 22.4 and 22.5).

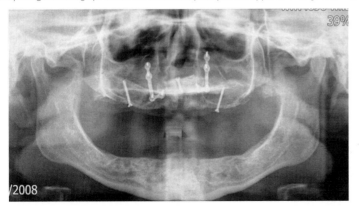

Figure 22.4 Orthopantomogram immediately following Le Fort I downward displacement and bone graft.

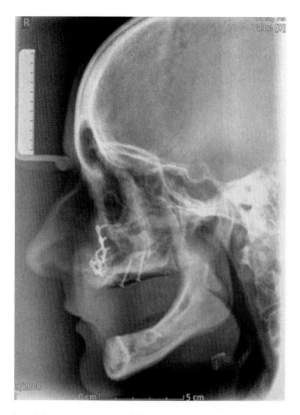

Figure 22.5 Lateral cephalogram immediately following surgery.

After four months, bone levels were deemed to be satisfactory on OPG radiograph (Figure 22.6) and six standard dental implants were surgically placed into the maxilla (Figure 22.7). Two dental implants were placed into the mandible five months later (Figure 22.8). Implant loading was delayed. Implant-retained dentures were constructed by a restorative dental specialist and these continue to be well tolerated by the patient. Follow-up at five years with OPG revealed stable peri-implant bone levels and no loss of vertically augmented bone volume.

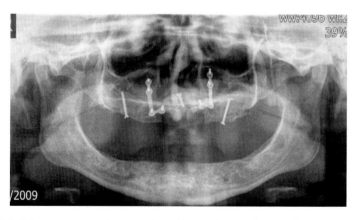

Figure 22.6 Orthopantomogram demonstrating stable bone levels at four months.

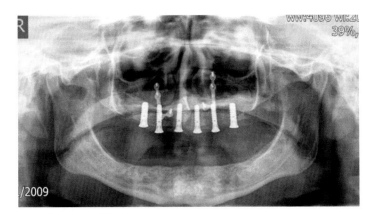

Figure 22.7 Six maxillary implants placed at four months.

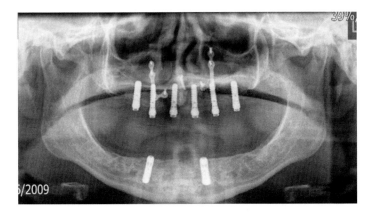

Figure 22.8 Two mandibular implants placed nine months following the initial bone graft.

Discussion

Approach to management of the atrophic maxilla

Any tooth loss may be followed by extensive resorption of the alveolar ridge. Due to the resulting bone loss, the alveolar anatomy and morphology will undergo various changes over time. The normal process leads to buccal / labial bone loss followed by reduction in height. This bone loss may be localized or generalized.

> ✓ **Evidence base** Cawood and Howell Classification [1]
>
> There are several alveolar bone morphologic classifications. The most frequently used system was proposed by Cawood and Howell in 1988 and describes the residual alveolar ridge form [1]. A classification of the edentulous jaws was developed based on a randomized cross-sectional study from a sample of 300 dried skulls. It was noted that whilst the shape of the basal process of the mandible and maxilla remains relatively stable, changes in shape of the alveolar process are highly significant in both the vertical and horizontal axes. In general, the changes of shape of the alveolar process follow a predictable pattern.
>
> - Class I: dentate.
> - Class II: immediately post-extraction.
>
> (continued)

> ⊗ **Learning point**
>
> It is important to undertake a thorough history and examination in patients with periodontal disease. Local risk factors include poor oral hygiene and removable and fixed appliances. Systemic risk factors include diabetes, smoking, immunosuppression and a positive family history for periodontal disease.

> ✚ **Clinical tip**
>
> Assessment of bone levels on OPG to grade severity of bone loss, which can be categorized as localized or generalized and as mild, moderate, or severe.

> ❝ **Expert comment**
>
> When assessing the atrophic maxilla, the defect can be localized or generalized. Causes include periodontal disease (inflammation), trauma, tumour, congenital, iatrogenic, or a natural process following tooth loss.

- Class III: well-rounded ridge form that has adequate height and width.
- Class IV: knife-edge ridge form, adequate in height but inadequate in width.
- Class V: flat ridge form with inadequate height and width.
- Class VI: depressed ridge form with evident basal bone loss.

⊘ Evidence base Lekholm and Zarb Classification [2]

Bone quality was classified into four categories by Lekholm and Zarb in 1985 based on its radiographic appearance and the resistance to drilling.

- Type 1: bone in which almost the entirety is composed of homogenous compact bone.
- Type 2: bone in which a thick layer of compact bone surrounds a core of dense trabecular bone.
- Type 3: bone in which a thin layer of cortical bone surrounds a core of dense trabecular bone.
- Type 4: bone characterized as a thin layer of cortical bone surrounding a core of low-density trabecular bone of poor strength.

Type 1 bone is more commonly found in the mandible and Type 4 in the posterior maxilla. Lower density bone is more prone to resorption following tooth loss. Types 2 and 3 are the most favourable for the osseointegration of implants and they provide a balance between adequate density for implant primary stability and blood supply for healing.

Pneumatization is enlargement of the maxillary sinus by resorption of alveolar bone that formerly served to support a missing tooth or teeth. This then occupies the edentulous space, sometimes leaving only a thin cortex of bone. This phenomenon was demonstrated radiographically, after the extraction of maxillary posterior teeth, by Sharan and Madjar in 2008 [3]. If a dental implant is planned in these cases, immediate implantation and/or immediate bone grafting should be considered to assist in preserving the three-dimensional bony architecture of the sinus floor at the extraction site.

A full facial and oral examination with radiographic imaging are essential in the appropriate assessment of maxillary resorption and morphology aiding in planning of bone augmentation and implant placement. OPG radiograph is important in assessing the vertical bone height, sinus floor and the presence of pathology; lateral cephalogram for occlusal vertical dimension and cone-beam computed tomography scan for accurate three-dimensional surgical implant planning and assessment of the local antomy, including the maxillary sinus and nasal floor.

Planning with full involvement by the restorative dental specialist from the outset is essential to achieve the best outcome.

Key parameters to be assessed in patients with completely edentulous jaws:

- any opposing dentition
- vertical inter-arch relationship (reduced or increased space)
- horizontal or transverse inter-arch relationship
- status of maxillary sinus (presence or absence of pathology or septa)
- presence or absence of keratinized mucosa.

> ✪ **Learning point** Ridge augmentation
>
> Augmentation procedures to increase the volume of deficient or atrophic alveolar bone have been extensively described in the literature. Various surgical techniques have been developed to treat bone defects of different shapes and sizes, regardless of whether they result from ridge atrophy, trauma, inflammation, tumours or malformation.
>
> Ridge augmentation has three main objectives:
>
> 1. **Function:** create sufficient volume of vital bone to accommodate a dental implant that is long and wide enough for its ideal restorative and functional position.
> 2. **Aesthetics:** provide bony support for the associated soft tissues, for good aesthetics of gingival / mucosal and facial structures.
> 3. **Prognosis:** sufficient bone volume must be created around the neck of the implant. This covers the endosseous implant segment and ensures a tight soft tissue seal, giving a predictable long-term prognosis of the implant.

The considerations in selecting a specific approach relate to complexity of surgical technique, morbidity of the procedure, healing time, predictability and cost. Limitations and complications may be due to general medical issues, dental status, extent and location of the bone defect, patient preference and budget restrictions.

There may be one or several restorative options to meet the functional and aesthetic requirements of an individual patient. It is the responsibility of the clinician to select the best option(s) and present these to the patient with the expected outcome, either in the form of a provisional set-up and try-in or using appropriate software. Treatment planning has become 'restoration-driven' and this allows the bone to be reconstructed to meet the restorative needs, rather than accepting a restorative compromise. It is therefore essential to be aware of all possible techniques and refer to a specialist if necessary.

Treatment may be carried out via a 'staged' approach where procedures of ridge augmentation are performed in healed sites in preparation for delayed implant placement. This differs from simultaneous procedures of bone augmentation and implant placement. Staged procedures of augmenting the alveolar process are usually indicated in the presence of advanced bone resorption. The purpose of augmentation may be to enable implant insertion of adequate dimensions or to create suitable conditions for an aesthetic and functional implant-supported restoration. This requires a correct inter-arch relationship, ideal soft tissue support and a reasonable height of the crowns involved in the planned prosthesis.

It should be remembered that there are conventional options of non-implant prosthetic treatment. Alternatives to staged augmentation include complete removable dentures, short implants and bone augmentation with simultaneous implant placement.

> ✪ **Learning point** Techniques of ridge augmentation
>
> There are a variety of defect situations of varying complexity and different bone augmentation techniques may be more suitable depending on the defect.
>
> ● **Onlay bone grafting:** autologous onlay bone grafting procedures are effective and predictable for severely resorbed edentulous ridges to allow implant placement. Implant survival rates are slightly lower than those placed in native bone.
>
> ● **Horizontal ridge augmentation:** autologous bone blocks, with or without the use of barrier membranes, result in higher gains in ridge width and lower complication rates than using particulate materials with or without a membrane. The survival rates of implants is high.
>
> (continued)

- **Vertical ridge augmentation:** predictability is lower and the complication rate is higher than with techniques for horizontal ridge augmentation. Autologous bone blocks are the 'gold standard' (as in this case). Survival rates of implants high.

- **Le Fort I osteotomy with interpositional autologous bone grafts:** this can be used successfully to treat atrophy of the maxilla, including cases associated with severe intermaxillary discrepancy. It may be suitable for management of Cawood and Howell Class IV, V, or VI atrophy. Interpositional or 'sandwich' grafting is an interesting alternative to traditional techniques of vertical bone augmentation such as onlay grafting or guided bone regeneration (GBR). This technique was first described in 1976 by Schettler [4] and 1977 by Bell et al. [5]. Excellent long-term results have been reported by Nyström et al. 2009 [6] and by Chiapasco et al. 2009 [7] with an implant survival rate of 86.6%.

- **Maxillary sinus floor elevation (transalveolar approach):** this technique is predictable for augmenting bone in the posterior maxilla, however, this is essentially a blind, uncontrolled procedure. A height of 3 mm is the maximum achievable with this technique. A variety of materials may be safely and predictably used, alone or in combination. These include autografts, allografts, xenografts and alloplastic materials. It is not currently clear whether the use of a grafting material improves the prognosis.

- **Maxillary sinus floor elevation (lateral approach):** this can be simultaneous or delayed using a xenograft spacer. The use of autografts with this technique does not influence survival rates of rough surface implants, but may reduce healing times. The quality and quantity of bone in the residual maxilla influence implant survival rates, independent of the type of grafting procedure. For rough surface implants placed in augmented maxillary sinuses the survival rates are similar to those of implants inserted in native bone.

- **Split-ridge techniques:** split-ridge and expansion techniques are effective for the correction of moderately resorbed edentulous ridges, in selected cases. Survival rates of implants are similar to those in native bone.

- **Vertical distraction osteogenesis:** useful in selected cases, however, there is a high complication rate. These include change of distraction vector, incomplete distraction, fracture of distracting device and partial relapse of initial bone gain. Survival rates of implants are similar to those in native bone.

★ **Learning point** Augmentation materials

Autografts

- Bone may be harvested from several intraoral sites, most commonly in the mandible from the buccal cortical plate of the horizontal ramus or the symphyseal (chin) region. Only a limited volume of bone can be harvested. Patients may experience less discomfort from intraoral than extra-oral donor sites [8].
- Extra-orally preferred sites are the iliac crest and calvarium and large amounts of cortical and cancellous bone can be harvested. These may offer better resistance to resorption and faster healing than at intraoral sites.
- Advantages: osteogenesis.
- Disadvantages: donor site morbidity, resorption.

Alloplastic (biomaterials)

- Bone substitute (e.g. Geistlich Bio-Oss, Bio-Gide collagen membrane – prevents soft tissue ingrowth).
- Can be combined with autograft techniques.
- Advantages: no donor site, stable scaffold for bone formation and low resorption rate

Guided bone regeneration

- GBR is a surgical procedure that utilises grafting materials and barrier membranes to stimulate and direct the growth of new bone into defect sites.
- Osteoconduction is the process of guiding the reparative growth of natural bone.
- Osteoinduction is the process of encouraging undifferentiated cells to become active osteoblasts.
- Osteogenesis occurs when living bone cells in graft material contribute to bone remodelling – this only occurs with autografts.

Implant options

Dental implants function through the process of osseointegration. This is the direct structural and functional connection between living bone and the surface of a load-bearing artificial implant. The majority of implants are made of titanium, although other materials such as ceramics can be used. The intraosseous surface of the implant is rough to increase the surface area for integration, which improves biomechanical and functional stability. The majority of dental implants will integrate within two to six months. They are then used to support either fixed or removable prostheses.

- **Conventional osseointegrated implants:** these can be placed as a one-stage procedure with a sinus floor elevation or as a delayed procedure. It is not possible to demonstrate the superiority of one augmentation technique over another based on implant survival rates. The material, surface, thread design and dimensions of an implant are all important biomechanical factors that can influence the quality and strength of osseointegration, the bone-implant interface and the long-term success.
- **Short implants:** implants as short as 4 mm (e.g. Bicon and Straumann) are now available and are particularly useful in the posterior maxilla where limited vertical bone is available, as an alternative to sinus floor elevation. This avoids invasive grafting techniques and it is believed that healing is quicker with reduced pain. They can be used to support single crowns, bridges or dentures.
- **Zygomatic implants:** these may be used as an alternative to bone augmentation where there is severe resorption of the posterior alveolar crest. They can be used in combination with conventional anterior implants or four zygomatic fixtures can be used in cases of severe resorption. Zygomatic implants (e.g. Nobel Biocare) are between 30 mm and 50 mm long and are placed into the thick bone of the zygomatic buttress through an upper buccal sulcus incision. These can usually be loaded immediately and have success rates nearing 100%.

Complications of implant placement may be immediate such as bleeding, damage to anatomical structures, bone fracture and lack of stability. Early complications include infection and failure of osseointegration. The main late complication is peri-implant disease.

A final word from the expert

The processes of bone resorption and maxillary sinus pneumatization are accelerated in patients with periodontal disease.

A 'restorative-driven' approach should always be utilised, with consideration given to the final desired outcome, thereby working backwards to formulate a plan to achieve this result. Multidisciplinary management, with early involvement of restorative specialists and prosthetists, is essential for the best outcome.

The method of bone augmentation must be selected on an individual basis and the planned result presented and discussed with the patient. Follow-up is necessary to ensure long-term stability and patient satisfaction.

Interpositional grafting is an interesting alternative to traditional techniques of vertical bone augmentation, such as onlay grafting or GBR. It is of major clinical benefit that the soft tissues remain attached to the oral aspect of the bone segment. As a result, the attached mucosa remains on top of the crest where it is needed for the emergence of the implant. This reduces the need for additional soft tissue surgery in comparison with onlay grafts and also reduces the risk of wound dehiscence with graft exposure and potential loss.

References

1. Cawood JI, Howell RA. A classification of the edentulous jaws. *Int J Oral Maxillofac Surg* 1988; 17: 232–5.
2. Lekholm U, Zarb GA, Albrektsson T. Patient selection and preparation. Tissue-integrated prostheses. Chicago: Quintessence Publishing Co. Inc., 1985; 199–209.
3. Sharan A, Madjar D. Maxillary sinus pneumatisation following extractions: a radiographic study. *Int J Oral Maxillofac Implants* 2008; 23(1): 48–56.
4. Schettler D. Sandwich technique with cartilage transplant for raising the alveolar process in the lower jaw. *Fortschr Kiefer Gesichtschir* 1976; 20: 61–3.
5. Bell WH, Buche WA, Kennedy JW 3rd, Ampil JP. Surgical correction of the atrophic alveolar ridge. A preliminary report on a new concept of treatment. *Oral Surg Oral Med Oral Pathol* 1977; 43(4): 485–98.
6. Nyström E, Nilson H, Gunne J, Lundgren S. Reconstruction of the atrophic maxilla with interpositional bone grafting/Le Fort I osteotomy and endosteal implants: an 11–16 year follow-up. *Int J Oral Maxillofac Surg* 2009; 38(1): 1–6.
7. Chiapasco M, Casentini P, Zaniboni M. Bone augmentation procedures in implant dentistry. *Int J Oral Maxillofac Implants* 2009; 24 Suppl: 237–59.
8. Reissmann DR, Dietze B, Vogeler M, et al. Impact of donor site for bone graft harvesting for dental implants on health-related and oral health-related quality of life. *Clin Oral Implants Res* 2013; 24(6): 698–705.

23 Keratocystic odontogenic tumours (KCOT) and orthokeratinized odontogenic cysts (OKOC)

Alan Parbhoo

Ⓒ **Expert commentary** Mike Simpson

Case history

An 82-year-old man was referred by his dentist with a recurrent keratocystic odontogenic tumour (KCOT) in the posterior mandible in the region of the lower left third molar nine years after initial surgical treatment with enucleation. He had been followed up for three years following initial treatment, had no recurrence and good bony infill radiographically and had been discharged. Upon re-referral the patient's main complaint was of a lump on the left side of the jaw and in his throat. On examination there was a small but obvious swelling lateral and inferior to the left angle of the mandible and no lymphadenopathy. Intra-oral examination revealed significant swelling in the ipsilateral lingual and peri-tonsillar region. The patient was partially dentate, wore a lower denture and had no visible teeth in the affected area.

The patient had a multiple medical co-morbidities; chronic obstructive pulmonary disease, ischaemic heart disease with previous myocardial infarction and Hodgkin's lymphoma.

Initial investigation was using plain radiography (orthopantomogram, OPG) which showed a large well-defined, corticated radiolucency extending from region of the first molar into the ramus, extending for the full height of the mandible (Figure 23.1). As the lesion was large and causing pharyngeal swelling a magnetic resonance imaging

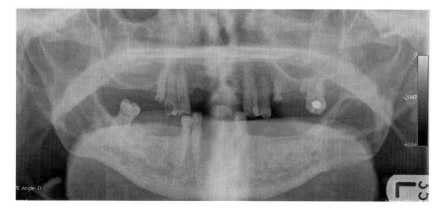

Figure 23.1 Orthopantomogram taken at diagnosis of recurrence showing large corticated radiolucency at the left angle of the mandible.

🐦 **Expert comment**

The first controversy is in the nomenclature. Are we discussing a KCOT or an odontogenic keratocyst (OKC) or an OKOC? We aim to demystify this and explain the differences and its clinical relevance. Please note we have used the term 'keratocyst' in the text to denote cases where the distinction between KCOT/OKOC is not known.

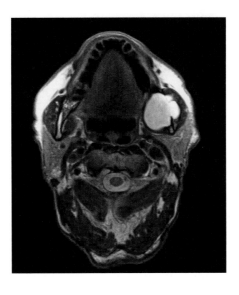

Figure 23.2 T2-weighted magnetic resonance imaging scan in axial section during work-up for treatment of the recurrence. There is perforation of the lingual and buccal cortices of the mandible with extension buccally and lingually causing subtle compression of the oropharynx and displacement of the masseter.

(MRI) scan was performed rather than a computed tomogram (CT) of the mandible. The MRI showed a bilobed cystic lesion measuring 2.9 cm × 2.8 cm with perforation of the buccal and lingual cortices of the mandible with significant extension into the lingual and peri-tonsillar soft tissues as well as sub-masseteric extension. A soft tissue plane was visible around it with displacement of adjacent structures (Figure 23.2). The old histopathology specimen was reviewed and this was confirmed as a parakeratinized cyst (i.e. KCOT) with subepithelial hyalinization (higher risk of recurrence) (Figure 23.3).

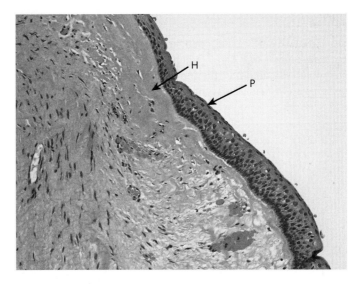

Figure 23.3
Haematoxylin & eosin stain of keratocystic odontogenic tumour removed by enucleation at first presentation showing epithelial parakeratosis (P) and subepithelial hyalinization (H) – both now known to be predictors of high risk of recurrence [1,2]. See colour plate section.

Reproduced courtesy of Dr Jenish Patel, Consultant Cellular Pathologist

A clinical and radiological diagnosis of recurrent KCOT with extensive soft tissue extension was made. This is an unusual presentation of recurrence and potential treatment options were:

- enucleation and packing
- enucleation and primary closure
- wide local resection*
- marsupialization followed by later smaller resection (assuming the size of cyst decreased).*

(* Resection would have required a lip split and mandibulotomy to adequately reach the pharyngeal component.)

The initial treatment plan was to formally excise the recurrence via a trans-oral approach. Enucleation would not have been possible due to the soft tissue extension in multiple directions. An anaesthetic opinion was sought prior to surgery. During the weeks prior to surgery he became systemically unwell with a degree of cardiac failure and an exacerbation of chronic obstructive pulmonary disease (COPD). He subsequently became ASA 3 (American Society of Anaesthesiologists) and risk of extensive surgery under general anaesthesia became high. He also became unable to lie semi-recumbent in a dental chair for any length of time due to his cardiac failure and COPD. The idea of resection was abandoned.

Therefore a relatively conservative approach was taken to marsupialize the cyst only and see what response occurred. This was performed under local anaesthesia and a whiteheads varnish pack placed into the cyst cavity. Antibiotic cover was given pre- and postoperatively for fear of the consequences of surgical site infection that could cause severe airway compromise. After several weeks an impression of the aperture into the cavity was taken with his lower partial denture in situ and his denture was modified with the addition of a loosely fitting bung to prevent the aperture closing (Figure 23.4).

Within two months the soft tissue swelling had resolved completely and there was bony infill into the cyst cavity on OPG. A CT mandible was undertaken seven months following his minor surgery that showed a reduction in the size to 1.6 cm × 1.1 cm. By 19 months post enucleation there was almost complete infill of the cavity. There was partial restoration of the outer cortex of the mandible and resolution of the sub-masseteric extension (Figure 23.5).

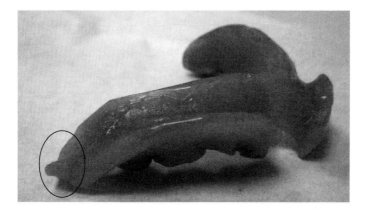

Figure 23.4 Patient's lower partial denture modified with a loose fitting stent (circled) to keep the marsupialized cavity open.

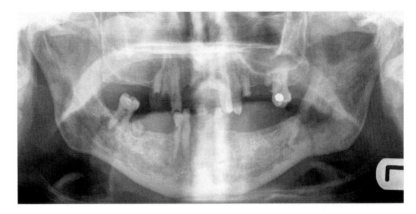

Figure 23.5 Orthopantomogram 19 months after marsupialization showing restoration of much of the cortical bone and good bony infill of the cyst cavity.

⚙ Expert comment

He has been followed up for three years now and OPG shows complete bony infill of the original cavity. He has had no further symptoms or complications of the treatment or disease.

➕ Clinical tip

The parakeratinized variant may be more aggressive due to the increased presence of 'daughter cysts' as budding entities from the sidewall of the main cyst, hence its increased risk of recurrence. This is the variant seen in patients with basal cell naevus syndrome.

★ Learning point Terminology

Keratocysts used to be termed odontogenic keratocyst (OKC). In 2005 they were reclassified as KCOTs that have parakeratinized epithelial lining and a high risk of recurrence. However, this does not include the orthokeratinized variant (OKOC) that has a lower risk of recurrence and can be treated more conservatively. Prior to and after 2005 most authors in the literature fail to distinguish between these two variants and therefore any evidence must be examined with caution.

✔ Evidence base Marsupialization as a definitive treatment for the odontogenic keratocyst [3]

- First case series published; ten patients demonstrating complete resolution of biopsy proven keratocysts after marsupialization alone.
- All lesions resolved to leave a shallow depression that was biopsied to detect residual disease - all biopsies showed normal oral epithelium indicating metaplasia from cyst lining to oral mucosa occurs following marsupialization.
- However: This paper and his subsequent paper in 2005 [4] was partially retracted later [5] following a recurrence in 5 out of 42 patients treated using this method. Pogrel humbly states that marsupialization can result in complete resolution but more aggressive surgery is beneficial in some cases.

Source: data from Pogrel MA and Jordan RCK, Marsupialization as a definitive treatment for the odontogenic keratocyst, *Journal of Oral and Maxillofacial Surgery*, Volume 62, Issue 6, pp.651–655, Copyright © 2004 American Association of Oral and Maxillofacial Surgeons. Published by Elsevier Inc.

✔ Evidence base The case for decompression and marsupialization [4]

- Further to 'Evidence base: Marsupialization as a definitive treatment for the odontogenic keratocyst', Pogrel argued the case for continuing to use this as a viable treatment modality over more aggressive surgery that was becoming favoured due to the high recurrence rate of these lesions regardless of modality used.
- It emphasized existing evidence showing marsupialization reduces the size of large lesions or those in difficult areas that makes subsequent definitive surgery less invasive. There is also a lower risk of damage to vital structures (teeth, inferior dental nerve) and a lower risk of fracture or bony discontinuity following definitive surgery.

Source: data from Pogrel MA and Jordan RCK, Marsupialization as a definitive treatment for the odontogenic keratocyst, *Journal of Oral and Maxillofacial Surgery*, Volume 62, Issue 6, pp.651–655, Copyright © 2004 American Association of Oral and Maxillofacial Surgeons. Published by Elsevier Inc.

> ✓ **Evidence base** Histopathological features that predict the recurrence of odontogenic keratocysts [1]
>
> - Tumours exhibiting subepithelial hyalinization have a greater tendency for recurrence:
> - 46% of recurrent tumours showed hyalinization versus 21% of non-recurrent tumours ($p = 0.006$).
> - Although the title of the paper states OKC, 98% were KCOT.
>
> *Source:* data from Cottom HE et al., Histopathological features that predict the recurrence of odontogenic keratocysts, *Journal of Oral Pathology & Medicine*, Volume 41, Issue 5, pp.408-41, Copyright © 2011 John Wiley & Sons.

Discussion

This case highlights that there are many ways to manage 'the keratocyst' and each senior surgeon has their own opinion as to how they should be managed and even what they should be called. The fact that there are several ways to manage this pathology emphasizes that there is little strong evidence for one modality over another.

The term OKC was described in 1956 but included other keratinizing cysts. The term was reclassified by the World Health Organization (WHO) in 2005 as a KCOT to emphasize its potential for destructive behaviour and recurrence [2]. However, whilst there are some lesions that behave in a more aggressive manner, with the tendency to enlarge or to recur, there are others that do not. Emerging evidence based on histological typing would suggest that there are two distinct subtypes with one having a greater tendency to recur. Knowledge of the histological features of a lesion prior to definitive management appears to be becoming more useful. Compare the management of an oral carcinoma, for example: knowledge of the size, site, differentiation and depth of invasion directly influences the surgical management. With advances in our understanding of the KCOT why should we not apply the same basic principles here?

In general it is thought that the parakeratinized variant (previously named a primordial cyst) has a higher recurrence rate of 25–56% compared to the orthokeratinized variant of 2.2% [6]. The parakeratinized variant may be more aggressive due to the increased presence of 'daughter cysts' as budding entities from the sidewall of the main cyst, hence its increased risk of recurrence. This is the variant seen in patients with basal cell naevus syndrome. The WHO classification of the KCOT only includes the parakeratinized form and does not mention the more benign orthokeratinized variant that we and other authors would consider to be termed an OKOC [7]. This means histological diagnosis is paramount to provide correct management. More recently it has been hypothesized that tumours with subepithelial hyalinization are more likely to recur [4]. With these two characteristics alone we have the ability to treat keratocysts in a more stratified approach based on the risk of recurrence. Subsequent to 2005 the KCOT is now the most common tumour of the jaws [8].

Most of the data in the literature does not distinguish between the two types and that may invalidate any conclusions drawn about treatment modality and recurrence rate. Recurrence can occur up to ten years (up to 41 years has been reported) following initial treatment although the average is within five years [9–11]. Most studies have short follow-up periods, skewing recurrence statistics.

⊘ Evidence base Systematic review of recurrence rate for keratocystic odontogenic tumour in relation to treatment modalities [7]

- There are only 14 papers in the literature up to 2010 investigating recurrence after comparing different treatment modalities of KCOTs.
- Only two of these papers have sufficient follow-up or lack of bias to give reliable data.
- Recurrence rates of 108 cases after 5.3 years have been observed (see Table 23.1).
- Overall recurrence rate of 23% for all modalities but 0% following either enucleation with peripheral ostectomy and Carnoy's solution, or en bloc resection.

Table 23.1 Risk of recurrence stratified by treatment modality for KCOT* [7].

Marsupialization alone	40%
Enucleation alone	26%
Enucleation with Carnoy's solution*	50%*
Enucleation with peripheral ostectomy	18%
Enucleation with peripheral ostectomy and Carnoy's solution	0%
En bloc resection	0%

*Note that the number of patients in each group varied and in some groups the numbers are very small. Hence, although this data is the best available it does have significant limitations.

There were no acceptable studies using cryotherapy.

Reprinted from *International Journal of Oral and Maxillofacial Surgery*, Volume 41, Issue 6, Kaczmarzyk T et al., A systematic review of the recurrence rate for keratocystic odontogenic tumour in relation to treatment modalities, pp.756–767, Copyright © 2012 International Association of Oral and Maxillofacial Surgeons with permission from Elsevier, http://www.sciencedirect.com/science/journal/09015027.

★ Learning point Marsupialization

First described by Partsch as a definitive operation [12]. This was prior to the discovery of antibiotics. The standard prior to Partsch's description was enucleation and primary closure but infection and wound dehiscence was high. Following advent of general anaesthesia, antibiotics and improved surgical techniques, marsupialization tended to be rejected by many as a useful treatment in favour of more aggressive methods. Broadly these can be divided into two groups:

- Conservative: marsupialization, enucleation, curettage.
- Aggressive: peripheral ostectomy (removal of the bone around the cyst cavity with a burr i.e. burr curettage), chemical treatment of the cyst or cavity (Carnoy's solution), physical treatment of the cyst cavity (cryotherapy), en bloc bony resection (marginal or segmental).

⑥ Expert comment Recommendations

At present there is limited strong evidence to support aggressive management of OKOCs. However, it is clear that the KCOT represents a more aggressive disease with a high risk of recurrence. More extensive and aggressive surgery is required to reduce this risk, but for large lesions or those close to vital structures an initial more conservative primary procedure may facilitate a less aggressive definitive procedure.

Knowledge of the histological behaviour prior to making a definitive treatment plan is vitally important, and should be used. Enucleation alone is not sufficient treatment for the KCOT and this raises two questions:

1. Should an initial cyst lining biopsy be performed, even in small lesions, prior to formal removal?
2. Should we demand that all histopathology reports comment on ortho- or parakeratinization and subepithelial hyalinization? We have adopted this in our unit.

If a lesion is shown to be a KCOT after simple enucleation and primary closure, is the surgeon compelled to go back and perform further surgery? This is a difficult question but with a high risk of recurrence presented in the literature each surgeon must make their own choice.

In general we would recommend the following:

1. OKOCs can be treated with conservative surgery.
2. KCOTs should not be treated with conservative surgery.
3. Small KCOTs may be managed with chemical treatment or by peripheral ostectomy. Cryotherapy is probably an acceptable treatment but there is no evidence to support this.
4. Large KCOTs may be better managed by marsupialization followed by chemical treatment or peripheral ostectomy if the patient is able to toilet the cyst cavity to prevent infection. If they are unable to do this then more aggressive surgery is advocated.
5. En bloc resection is not recommended as a primary treatment although it does have the lowest recurrence rate [7]. This operation should be reserved for recurrent cases or where there are multiple KCOTs in a localized area, such as in basal cell naevus syndrome.
6. Beware the KCOT with subepithelial hyalinization, as this appears to have the highest risk of recurrence.

A final word from the expert

As with many aspects of patient care with different pathological entities there will be variations in treatment options chosen based on the histology, size and anatomical location, fitness and patient wishes and expectations.

In dealing with potential KCOT/OKOCs, however, histological diagnosis is of paramount importance for any suspect lesions as the treatment of the two entities is quite different. Furthermore, the biopsy and definitive specimens are best sent to a specialist oral histopathologist with the appropriate experience for comment, rather than a general histopathologist.

For smaller lesions found at operation to be full of keratin squames the use of Carnoy's solution (with ferric chloride) will reduce recurrence rates. It can also be used for larger lesions in difficult anatomical areas where en bloc resection is difficult or one is dealing with a recurrence.

Remember these aspects of using Carnoy's solution: it can be instilled in the cystic 'cavity' to fix the lining and any daughter cysts before removal. Following enucleation/curettage it can be painted onto the residual bony walls to fix any residual cells. Finally, do remember it will be toxic to nerves in close contact for any length of time although permanent numbness is extremely rare (application time <5 minutes).

Overall, remember one can afford to be more conservative in most cases in dealing with these pathological entities. Marsupialization will sometimes cure or at least shrink the lesion to a size requiring less of a surgical resection and therefore less in the way of morbidity.

Once KCOTs have escaped into the soft tissue they can be difficult to deal with and multiple recurrences can take place one after the other. In the case described with the large soft tissue component, surgery would have been difficult with potential spillage of cells and recurrence. Marsupialization worked extremely well with no inflammation or swelling noted by the patient or surgeon, with an excellent outcome, with no distress or morbidity to the patient at any stage.

References

1. Cottom HE, Bshena FI, Speight PM, et al. Histopathological features that predict the recurrence of odontogenic keratocysts. *J Oral Pathol Med* 2012; 41(5): 408–14.
2. Philipsen, HP, Reichart PA, Slootweg PJ, et al. Odontogenic tumours. In: Barnes L, Eveson JW, Reichart P, Sidransky D (eds.) *World Health Organization Classification of Tumours. Pathology & Genetics of Head & Neck Tumours*. Lyon: IARC Press, 2005.
3. Pogrel MA, Jordan RCK. Marsupialization as a definitive treatment for the odontogenic keratocyst. *J Oral Maxillofac Surg* 2004; 62(6): 651–5.
4. Pogrel A. Treatment of keratocysts: the case for decompression and marsupialization. *J Oral Maxillofac Surg* 2005; 63(11): 1667.
5. Pogrel MA. Decompression and marsupialization as definitive treatment for keratocysts: A partial retraction. *J Oral Maxillofac Surg* 2007; 65(2): 362–3.
6. Crowley TE, Kaugars GE, Gunsolley JC. Odontogenic keratocyst: a clinical and histologic comparison of the parakeratin and orthokeratin variants. *J Oral Maxillofac Surg* 1992; 50: 22–6.
7. Kaczmarzyk T, Mojsa I, Stypulkowska J. A systematic review of the recurrence rate for keratocystic odontogenic tumour in relation to treatment modalities. *Int J Oral Maxillofac Surg* 2012; 41(6): 756–67.
8. Gaitán-Cepeda LA, Quezada-Rivera D, Tenorio-Rocha F, et al. Reclassification of odontogenic keratocyst as tumour. Impact on the odontogenic tumours prevalence. *Oral Diseases* 2009; 16(2): 185–7.
9. Gosau M, Draenert FG, Müller S, et al. Two modifications in the treatment of keratocystic odontogenic tumors (KCOT) and the use of Carnoy's solution (CS)—a retrospective study lasting between 2 and 10 years. *Clin Oral Invest* 2010; 14: 27–34.
10. Stoelinga PJW. Excision of the overlying, attached mucosa, in conjunction with cystenucleation and treatment of the bony defect with Carnoy solution. *Oral Maxillofac Surg Clin North Am* 2003; 15: 407–14.
11. Zhao YF, Wei JX, Wang SP. Treatment of odontogenic keratocyst: a follow-up of 255 Chinese patients. *Oral Surg Oral Med Oral Pathol Oral Radiol Endod* 2002; 94: 151–6.
12. Partsch C. Uber kiefercysten. *Deutsche Monatsschr Zahnheil* 1892; 10: 271.

SECTION 9

Paediatric maxillofacial surgery

24 Paediatric temporomandibular joint ankylosis

Kevin McMillan

ⓘ **Expert commentary** Rhodri Williams

Case history

A four-year-old boy was referred to the oral and maxillofacial surgery outpatients department by his general medical practitioner (GMP). The referral letter stated that he had developed severe trismus over the course of the preceding 18 months. This was affecting his ability to eat and as such the child was not progressing along the predicted lines of the growth chart. He was finding it difficult to chew and had resorted to sucking on food. Additionally, his parents had complained that they were struggling to maintain oral hygiene via conventional methods.

The patient was born at term via normal vaginal delivery. There were no complications and he was discharged home the next day. He developed normally for the first 2½ years, meeting all developmental milestones. He was the second child with a healthy sister who was two years older than him.

At age 30 months, he developed a severe right-sided ear infection and was hospitalized for three days. This episode was treated with intravenous antibiotics. He was reviewed in the ear, nose and throat outpatient clinic following his admission. Eight weeks following discharge, he continued to complain of discomfort in the right pre-auricular region. His parents recalled that he preferred a soft diet at the time. There was no known history of trauma to either temporomandibular joint (TMJ).

Over the next year the patient developed an insidious onset of trismus. His parents noted a steady deterioration in his ability to eat. Additionally, his speech became difficult to understand. He was seen on a number of occasions by his GMP and received reassurance that the problem should settle. He attended his dentist for a routine dental check-up and at this point it was noted that the clinical examination was challenging due to his restricted mouth opening.

By the age of four, the situation had deteriorated to such an extent that the boy was only able to drink liquids and has resorted to sucking on pieces of cheese. He was then referred to the oral and maxillofacial surgery department.

On examination, he was noted to be a diminutive child. He weighed 14 kg (9th centile) and was 96 cm tall (5th centile). His speech was difficult to interpret due to poor mouth opening.

He had severe trismus with maximal interincisal opening (MIO) of 2 mm. It was detected that there was almost no movement at the right TMJ. In addition there was a lateral swing of the mandible to the right side on opening. An orthopantomogram revealed a loss of joint space in the right TMJ with some evidence of fusion. He underwent a fine-cut computed tomogram (CT) scan that revealed a complete bony ankylosis of the right TMJ (Figure 24.1).

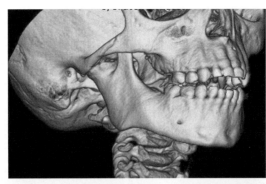

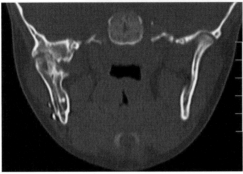 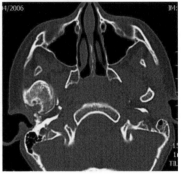

Figure 24.1 Computed tomogram (three-dimensional, coronal and axial formats) demonstrating ankylosis of the right temporomandibular joint. See colour plate section.

Following discussion with the patient's parents, the decision was taken to perform surgery to attempt improvement in the patient's mouth opening. At aged five, the patient underwent a TMJ ankylosis release procedure. This involved a resection of the ankylosed segment, right coronoidectomy and a costochondral graft. Access was obtained via a pre-auricular and retromandibular approach. Post procedure intraoperative mouth opening was noted to be 33 mm.

The patient was discharged at day 2 postoperatively with no complications. Advice regarding intensive postoperative physiotherapy to maintain and improve his mouth opening was given at this juncture. The physiotherapy regime prescribed involved active stretching using a Therabite (Atos Medical, US) appliance on a five times per day basis.

The patient was reviewed four weeks postoperatively and was noted to have a good MIO of 31 mm. He was able to consume a normal diet and complained of little in the way of pain. When questioned regarding his physiotherapy and rehabilitation, the patient's parents stated that they found it difficult to motivate the child to perform all the exercises in the prescribed regime.

The patient was reviewed again six weeks later and his MIO was reduced at 22 mm. His parents stated that they were still struggling to motivate him to continue with his recommended jaw exercises. The importance of the exercises was stressed and further follow-up arranged.

At six months after his initial surgery, the patient had reankylosed his right TMJ. His mouth opening was poor at 3 mm and he was struggling to eat solid foods again. A repeat CT scan revealed reankylosis of the neo joint. Further discussion

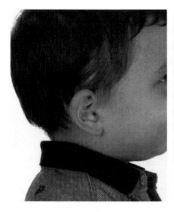 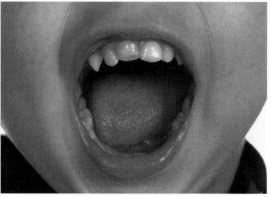

Figure 24.2 (a) Post-operative photographs demonstrating the pre-auricular and retromandibular scars. **(b)** Intra-oral view with mouth opening of 32 mm. See colour plate section.

was engaged with the patient's parents and a decision was taken to re-excise the ankylosed segment. A further procedure was undertaken and excision of the anky-losed segment performed. An interpositional arthroplasty was performed using the right temporalis muscle.

The surgery again proceeded without complication and the patient was dis-charged on day 2 postoperatively. He was given a further intensive rehabilitation programme to undertake. Further to the prior failure of surgery, the patient's parents had renewed motivation to perform the jaw exercises with great discipline.

The patient was followed up for 18 months postoperatively and had excellent function and range of mouth opening (32 mm) (Figure 24.2). His occlusion remained stable.

Discussion

This case illustrates some of the key issues in management of paediatric TMJ ankylosis. TMJ ankylosis is a relatively rare problem encountered by the oral and maxillofacial surgeon. It is also extremely complex and management of young patients increases the challenge faced. This is due to the fact that the growth of the child requires prediction and management involves anticipation of the developing dentition [1].

Ankylosis of the TMJ can manifest with a number of problems including diffi-culty eating and chewing. This may lead to developmental or growth delay as dem-onstrated in this case. Additionally, asymmetrical development of the mandible can lead to malocclusion and facial deformity. This frequently leads to problems with patient self-esteem and bullying is a common complaint in these groups. Restriction of mouth opening may have profound effect upon speech and language development with children unable to develop accurate articulation of specific sounds. Finally, tris-mus provides obstacles to maintenance of oral hygiene that has implications for the developing dentition. Caries is a common consequence in patients with ankylosis.

Ankylosis can be caused by a number of factors. These vary according to the age of the patient and geographic location. In the developed world, the most com-mon cause for ankylosis is trauma to the TMJ. This is most common in fractures

> **⊕ Learning point** Classification of temporomandibular joint ankylosis
>
> Ankylosis can be classified in a number of ways. The disease can be classified according to location (intra- versus extra-articular), type of tissue involved (bone, fibro-osseous, or fibrous tissue), or the extent (complete versus incomplete) [1].

affecting the mandibular condyle. Intra-articular fractures are most commonly associated with development of ankylosis. Young patients and those with comminuted fractures of the condyle are the most likely to develop ankylosis. Patients who have been immobilized in maxillomandibular fixation (MMF) for prolonged periods are thought to be at greater risk as well.

In the developing world, infection is the most common cause of ankylosis. Common causes include severe and prolonged otitis media (as in this case), as well as odontogenic and skin infections. Severe systemic illness is also recognized as a cause of ankylosis.

Other causes of TMJ ankylosis include autoimmune disease, ankylosis following resection of bone tumour/cysts, as well as post radiotherapy changes.

✪ Learning point Causes of TMJ ankylosis

- Trauma
  - particularly intracapsular and subcondylar fractures.
- Infection
  - local (ear, odontogenic, skin)
  - systemic (osteomyelitis from long bones)
- Systemic illness
  - ankylosing spondylitis
  - juvenile rheumatoid arthritis
  - psoriasis
- Radiotherapy
  - parotid, bone and soft tissue tumours, mantle radiotherapy
- Previous surgery to joint

There is no recognized gold standard for the management of TMJ ankylosis in children. A variety of concepts and management strategies have been published in the literature all with varying effect. The essential concept involves release of the ankylosis. This allows free movement of the mandible enabling the child to eat and speak without restriction.

❝ Expert comment

Following release, prevention of reankylosis becomes the goal. This ensures medium-term success of treatment. In the case highlighted here, the patient was young and his parents did not fully appreciate the importance of postoperative rehabilitation. In hindsight, the follow-up intervals of the patient could have been more frequent. In this case the early recognition of the deterioration of mouth opening may have been addressed prior to the irreversible process of reankylosis.

Some authors argue that the most common cause for reankylosis is inadequate excision of the ankylosed segment. Kaban argues that the inaccessible medial segment of the ankylosis can be neglected during excision. This can lead to reossification of the joint and further restriction in mobility regardless of the rehabilitation implemented. It is essential that free movement of the TMJ is easily achievable during the release procedure. If this is not possible during anaesthesia, the patient will not be able to perform an adequate range of motion in the postoperative period.

In reality, success probably revolves around adequate excision of the ankylosed segment and appropriate postoperative rehabilitation.

Other key areas described in the surgical management of ankylosis include the performance of unilateral and bilateral coronoidectomies. In children with ankylosis, the ipsilateral coronoid has a tendency towards hyperplasia. In cases with prolonged trismus, the contralateral coronoid can also become hyperplastic. These changes add further mechanical obstruction to mouth opening. Kaban recommends performing ipsilateral coronoidectomy as a matter of course. He describes the need to remove the entire coronoid along with attachments of temporalis tendon [2]. If this procedure fails to improve mouth opening then a contralateral coronoidectomy should be considered. In this case, a contralateral coronoidectomy was not performed. This reflects the fact that 'on table' range of movement was in the desired range.

Management of the articular disc in the glenoid fossa is a source of debate. Most surgeons will argue that the diseased disc should be excised. Kaban argues that is the disc can be preserved if it remains disease free [2]. Others may argue that excision of the disc should always take place. The use of a temporalis flap to act as a lining is a commonly accepted procedure [3]. The temporalis flap is pedicled on the deep temporal artery from the inferior aspect. Other recognized interpositional materials are listed in 'Clinical tip: Interpositional materials available for arthroplasty'.

Finally, consideration is made relating to the reconstruction of the condyle. Again, this is the source of some debate with some authors suggesting that the costochondral graft should be performed in the first instance [4]. Others suggest that a less aggressive approach may be satisfactory with the use of interpositional arthroplasty using temporalis [3]. The advantage of the costochondral graft is that it has potential to represent a similar anatomical subunit to the resected condyle unit. Additionally, the costochondral graft may offer growth potential thus reducing the impact of mandibular asymmetry with subsequent growth [5]. The disadvantage of the costochondral graft is the involvement of a second operative site and the potential for reankylosis and asymmetric growth [6]. Additionally, many surgeons suggest a short period of MMF following the surgical procedure. As a result, the risk of developing joint stiffness due to delay of active movement is increased.

> **⊕ Clinical tip** Interpositional materials available for arthroplasty
> - Buccal fat pad
> - Temporalis fascia
> - Full thickness skin graft
> - Cartilage
> - Allogenic materials

> **✅ Evidence base** Kaban's protocol for management of temporomandibular joint ankylosis [7]
>
> 1. Aggressive excision of fibrous and/or bony mass.
> 2. Coronoidectomy on affected side.
> 3. Coronoidectomy on opposite side if steps 1 and 2 do not result in MIO of 35 mm or to point of dislocation of opposite side.
> 4. Lining of joint with temporalis fascia or the native disc, if it can be salvaged.
> 5. Reconstruction of resected condyle unit with either distraction osteogenesis or costochondral graft and rigid fixation.
> 6. Early mobilization of jaw; if distraction osteogenesis used to reconstruct resected condyle unit, mobilize on day of surgery. If costochondral graft used, early mobilization with minimal intermaxillary fixation (not more than ten days).
> 7. Aggressive physiotherapy.
>
> Reprinted from *Journal of Oral and Maxillofacial Surgery*, Volume 67, Issue 9, Kaban LB et al., A Protocol for Management of Temporomandibular Joint Ankylosis in Children, pp.1966-1978, Copyright © 2009 American Association of Oral and Maxillofacial Surgeons, with permission from Elsevier, http://www.sciencedirect.com/science/journal/02782391.

The use of distraction osteogenesis (DO) has been described for reconstruction of the excised segment [8]. In this instance the condylar segment is excised as normal but a cortical osteotomy is performed. A mini distractor is placed and active distraction commences after a two to four day latency phase. Distraction proceeds at rate of 1 mm per day until the neo condyle makes contact with the skull base. The advantages of this technique include the lack of donor site morbidity as well as the potential to begin rehabilitation of the joint immediately following surgery. The disadvantages of DO include the risk of infection as well as failure of distraction. Additionally, the proximal 'condyle' lacks a growth centre conferring a risk of developing mandibular asymmetry and malocclusion.

In the immediate postoperative phase, a strict soft diet is recommended. The rehabilitation phase should commence as soon as practically possible. This includes frequent active range exercises as well as manual stretching. These exercises should be performed frequently (four to five times per day) for several minutes at a time. Patients should be seen frequently in the outpatient clinic for follow-up.

If the patient is unable to achieve the immediate postoperative mouth opening at six to eight weeks postoperative period, a manipulation under anaesthesia procedure should be considered. The patient should receive close follow-up for at least one year postoperatively and should be encouraged to maintain aggressive physiotherapy for this period.

A final word from the expert

These patients should be managed in a multidisciplinary setting by a team with experience in treating paediatric TMJ ankylosis. We know that speech therapy and dietetics input are crucial in the early stages of treatment to ensure an optimal outcome. The psychological development is another aspect discussed by Kaban and the involvement of a paediatric psychologist in the multidisciplinary team (MDT) will also prove beneficial. Close liaison with the family dentist (or via a paediatric dentist on the MDT) should be maintained in light of the increased risk of dental disease and the inherent difficulties in providing even simple dental care.

Another key consideration is the difficulty presented to the anaesthetist in view of the limitation in mouth opening. A review by Kundra et al. agrees that the use of video-assisted fibre optic intubation in experienced hands is most effective in managing these challenging airways [9].

From a surgical perspective the aggressive removal of the ankylosis is the first and crucial stage of the process. Inadequate removal will most likely result in re-ankylosis and thus is vital to success. Ultimately it must be borne in mind that a proportion of these patients may require total replacement of the TMJ as adults. As the lifespan of these TMJ prosthesis is not fully understood they will most likely require repeat surgery on the site.

References

1. Perrott DH, Kaban LB. Temporomandibular joint ankylosis in children. *Oral Maxillofacial Clin North Am* 1994; 6: 187.
2. Kaban LB, Perrott DH. A protocol for management of temporomandibular joint ankylosis. *J Oral Maxillofac Surg* 1990; 48: 1145–51.
3. Pogrel MA, Kaban LB. The role of a temporalis fascia and muscle flap in temporomandibular joint surgery. *J Oral Maxillofac Surg* 1990; 48: 14.

4. Lindqvist C, Pihakari A, Tasanen A, et al. Autogenous costochondral grafts in temporomandibular joint arthroplasty: A survey of 66 arthroplasties in 60 patients. *J Maxillofac Surg* 1986; 14: 143.

5. Saeed NR, Kent JN. A retrospective study of the costochondral graft in TMJ reconstruction. *Int J Oral Maxillofac Surg* 2003; 32: 606.

6. Kaban LB, Perrott DH. Discussion: Unpredictable growth pattern of costochondral graft. *Plast Reconstr Surg* 1992; 90: 887.

7. Kaban LB, Bouchard C, Troulis M. A protocol for management of temporomandibular joint ankylosis in children. *J Oral Maxillofac Surg* 2009; 67(9): 1966–78.

8. Dean A, Alamillos F. Mandibular distraction in temporomandibular joint ankylosis. *Plast Reconstr Surg* 1999; 104: 2021.

9. Kundra P, Vasudevan A, Ravishankar M. Video assisted fiberoptic intubation for temporomandibular ankylosis. *Pediatric Anaesthesia* 2006; 16: 458–61.

25 Cleft palate related velopharyngeal incompetence

Christopher Sweet

Expert commentary Simon Van Eeden

Case history

A Caucasian girl was born at 39 + 6 gestation, with bilateral cleft lip and palate (BCLP) deformity. Prior to birth an ante-natal diagnosis of a bilateral cleft lip had been made from a routine 20 week anomaly ultrasound scan.

> **Expert comment**
>
> Ante-natal diagnosis of facial clefts using ultrasound is highly variable. The detection rate for cleft lips is significantly higher than cleft palates and varies according to the skill of the sonographer, the gestational age at scan, the sonographic examination protocol and the severity of the defect. Once a diagnosis has been made the cleft team should be informed of the diagnosis within 24 hours. An appropriately trained member of the cleft team should in turn contact the family within 24 hours of being informed of a diagnosis.

There was no family history of clefting and the mother was fit and well and not taking any regular medication. She was a non-smoker who did not drink alcohol. Following the ante-natal diagnosis the family received counselling from the cleft nurse specialist (CNS). This is to support the family through the diagnosis and also to prepare the family for the possible difficulties with feeding. The birth was uncomplicated and the family and baby were immediately supported by the CNS on notification of the birth. Specialist feeding with soft 'squeezy' bottles and special teats was commenced and the baby gained weight appropriately. The cleft lip and palate were subsequently repaired according to the unit's protocol in three stages. At the first operation at three months the bilateral lip was repaired with a unilateral vomerine flap to close the hard palate on one side. This was followed by a contralateral vomerine flap to close the remaining cleft of the hard palate six weeks later. At nine months repair of the soft palate was carried out using a radical intra-velar veloplasty technique as described by Sommerlad [1]. Her postoperative recovery was uncomplicated.

> **Evidence base** Sommerlad's intra-velar veloplasty [1]
>
> - 442 primary palate repairs.
> - Between 1978 and 1992, with follow-up of 10 years.
> - Technique involves minimal hard palate dissection.
> - Author always uses operating microscope.
> - In 80% palate repair was carried out through incisions at the margins of the cleft and no lateral incisions (Langenbeck flaps).
> - Secondary velopharyngeal surgery decreased from 10.2% to 4.9% to 4.6% in five-year period over 15 years.
> - Radical muscle dissection is suggested to improve speech and reduce velopharyngeal incompetence.
>
> *Source:* data from Sommerlad BC. A technique for cleft palate repair, Plastic and Reconstructive Surgery, Volume 112, Issue 6, pp.1542-1548, Copyright ©2003 American Society of Plastic Surgeons.

At the age of three years, the patient underwent a formal perceptual speech and language assessment by a specialist cleft speech and language therapist (SLT). The GOS.SP.ASS speech profile for children with cleft palate and or velopharyngeal dysfunction was used to assess articulation, resonance, nasal airway emission and voice. The results of this assessment showed features of velopharyngeal incompetence (VPI) (i.e. hypernasal tone and nasal emission) and cleft speech characteristics (i.e. errors of articulation as a result of VPI and/or history of cleft palate) [2].

The patient subsequently underwent lateral videofluoroscopy (VF) for dynamic assessment of her velopharyngeal function. This showed a short soft palate (velum) with muscles inserted into the middle to posterior part of the velum and incomplete closure of the nasopharyngeal port (Figure 25.1).

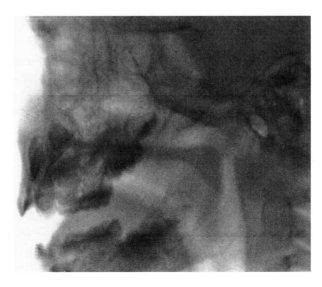

Figure 25.1 An image from a lateral videofluoroscopy illustrating velopharyngeal incompetence. Note the gap between the velum and posterior pharyngeal wall. This was seen consistently during speech on the dynamic images.

Based on these findings a decision to carry out a palatal re-repair with a Z-plasty was made to reposition the velar muscles more posteriorly within the velum and to lengthen the palate. The child's postoperative recovery was uncomplicated and a postoperative perceptual speech assessment was carried out after six months. This assessment showed a marked improvement in the quality of her speech. A repeat lateral videofluoroscopy demonstrated an increase in length of the velum with good movement and closure of the velopharyngeal port.

Discussion

The aims of primary cleft palate repair are closure of the cleft without any fistulae and for normal speech development. A competent and dynamically functional velopharyngeal sphincter is essential for normal eating, breathing and speech production. The ability to close this sphincter, separating the oral cavity from the nasal cavity is called velopharyngeal competence. This complex process requires a functioning velum of sufficient length. In cleft palate deformity the velum is shorter than in non-cleft patients and the muscles of the soft palate are abnormally orientated. The levator veli palatini, the main palatal elevator, inserts into the margins of the cleft. The palatopharyngeus inserts into the margin of the cleft and the posterior aspect of the hard palate medially. The tensor veli palatini inserts into the lateral aspect of the posterior margin of the hard palate. This abnormal orientation, if not corrected, may lead to poor function and subsequent VPI. Releasing the abnormally orientated muscles to reconstitute the palatal muscle slings and repositioning them more posteriorly within the velum can decrease the incidence of VPI. Primary palate repair can, however, be achieved by using a number of different surgical techniques, many of which do not specifically dissect out and reposition the palatal muscles. These different techniques have variable success with a wide range of VPI rates. There are additional confounding factors that contribute to the wide range of reported VPI including the population treated, the cleft type, the presence or absence of syndromes and the skill of the surgeon.

In normal speech the palatal muscles and the pharyngeal constrictor muscles work together to produce velopharyngeal closure. In health the velum normally moves superiorly and posteriorly to meet the posterior pharyngeal wall, which can move in a diffuse pattern or a well-defined ridge can sometimes be identified (Passavant's ridge) (Figure 25.2). In addition to velar movement, velopharyngeal closure is achieved with contributions from the lateral and posterior pharyngeal walls.

> ⭐ **Learning point**
> **Velocardiofacial syndrome**
>
> Pharyngoplasties in patients with VCFS should be undertaken with extreme care as this syndrome leads to aberrant and often medial displacement of the carotid arteries that could be encountered on raising pharyngeal flaps.

> ⭐ **Learning point** Velopharyngeal incompetence
>
> The inability to close the velopharyngeal sphincter is termed VPI. The clinical presentation of VPI includes nasal air escape and hypernasality. Air resonates abnormally within the nose and nasopharynx leading to a hypernasal tone. Air can also frequently be heard to hiss, rustle, or snort from the nose on certain consonant sounds. This is known as nasal turbulence or emission. In an attempt to prevent this nasal escape patients may also be seen to grimace. In the English language, complete closure of the velopharyngeal sphincter is required for the normal production of all but the nasal consonants, 'm', 'n' and 'ng'.
>
> Speech articulation errors can develop secondary to VPI and result in suboptimal speech and poor intelligibility of speech.

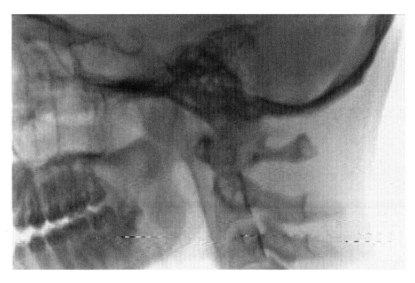

Figure 25.2 An image from a lateral videofluoroscopy illustrating Passavant's ridge.

Patients who are suspected of having VPI should undergo formal perceptual speech assessment by an experienced cleft SLT and in the UK the GOS.SP.ASS protocol is used to do this. This is a comprehensive and standardized screening tool that is validated and used nationally [2]. It is used to describe the features of speech commonly associated with cleft palate and/or VPI. This is a subjective assessment of the speech pattern and helps with diagnosis and treatment planning. Speech therapy is used to correct articulation errors. Errors of resonance are, however, typically related to structural problems that cannot be corrected with speech therapy and usually need a surgical solution.

VPI diagnosed on perceptual speech assessment should then be further investigated using objective assessment methods such as VF, nasendoscopy and nasometry. These special investigations are used to evaluate the movement of the soft palate and pharynx during real-time speech and require good patient cooperation. VF allows visualization of the dynamic function of the velopharyngeal port. The lateral view is the most commonly used view and is usually adequate for preoperative evaluation of velar function. It allows visualization and evaluation of the length, extensibility, velocity, timing and lift of the velum and its relationship to the pharyngeal wall. It can also be useful in determining the position of the insertion of the levator veli palatini muscles into the velum. VF can also be used to rate velopharyngeal closure. This is the fraction of the diameter of the port that is occluded during attempted closure. It is expressed on a scale of 0 to 1 in increments of 0.1 [10]. Lateral VF forms the cornerstone for 'physiological' management of VPI.

It is well recognized that the closure mechanism is complex. In VPI the velum may be too short or narrow to achieve closure of the velopharyngeal port and abnormal positioning of the musculature in the velum may prevent the 'levator knee' from raising the velum in a useful manner.

> **✪ Learning point** Nasometry
>
> This technique can also be used to objectively assess VPI. This measures nasalance, which is the degree of velopharyngeal opening in voiced speech. The system computes the ratio of the amplitude of the acoustic energy at the nares to amplitude of the acoustic energy at the mouth and is expressed as a percentage. Nasometry is not universally used in clinical practice currently in the UK but is used in clinical trials.

> **✪ Learning point** Nasoendoscopy
>
> Nasoendoscopy enables direct visualization of the velum, posterior pharyngeal wall and the closure pattern during speech. A number of closure patterns have been described within the literature (coronal, sagittal, circular and Passavant's ridge pattern) [11].
>
> In the coronal pattern the velum moves to meet a passive posterior pharyngeal wall with a small amount of movement of the lateral pharyngeal walls to complete the port closure. In the sagittal pattern the majority of the movement arises in the pharyngeal walls. The velum moves a small amount to abut with the constricted lateral walls. In the circular pattern there is equal contribution from the velum and lateral pharyngeal walls and in the Passavant's closure pattern there is also a distinct movement of the posterior pharyngeal wall in the form of a ridge. Nasoendoscopy is the investigation of choice for those surgeons favouring an 'obstructive' approach to the management of VPI.

Correction of VPI is usually surgical, although non-surgical options such as prosthetic palatal lifts and speech bulbs can be used. These are, however, often poorly tolerated.

The surgical management of VPI is, however, a controversial issue with no universally agreed treatment and considerable variation between units. Surgical management can be broadly divided into 'obstructive' and 'non-obstructive/physiological' techniques and there is evidence in favour of both approaches. The obstructive approach will permanently close the pharyngeal gap by joining the velum to the pharynx. The non-obstructive approach aims to optimize palatal function and length by operating on the velum and/or reduce the gap size by augmenting the posterior pharyngeal wall while maintaining the nasopharyngeal opening during periods of inactivity (i.e. when not talking or swallowing). The 'obstructive approach' is more popular in North America and the 'physiological approach' is favoured in the UK.

Physiological intervention may follow an algorithm (Figure 25.3) and is usually based on perceptual speech assessment and lateral videofluoroscopy.

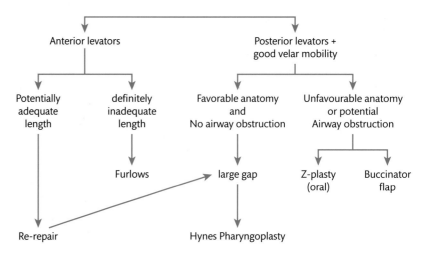

Figure 25.3 Velopharyngeal incompetence physiological treatment algorithm.

For patients with potentially adequate palatal length and anteriorly positioned levators, palatal re-repair is the first procedure of choice. This operation aims to dissect the levator veli palatini muscles from the nasal mucosa and posteriorly reposition them within the velum thereby utilizing the full length of the velum. By dissecting and repositioning the levator muscles more posteriorly it is also hoped that the 'levator sling' within the velum is able to work more effectively to achieve closure with the posterior pharyngeal wall, thereby creating velopharyngeal competence. There are a number of well-recognized techniques for palate re-repair. Sommerlad's 'radical' intra-velar velaplasty technique is commonly used in the UK for both primary repair and palate re-repair surgery. In those cases where the velum is short a Z-plasty of the oral mucosa can be carried out at the same time as the re-repair to increase velar length. Palatal re-repair has been shown to be beneficial but does not correct VPI in all cases [11].

In cases of re-repair that have resulted in posterior muscles but there is still a gap between the velum and the posterior pharyngeal wall, or if the muscles are already posteriorly positioned within the velum, the velopharyngeal gap can be closed by either lengthening the palate further or by augmenting the posterior pharyngeal wall [12]. The decision to choose lengthening over augmentation is usually based on either the anatomy of the pharynx or the potential for airway obstruction. Unfavourable anatomy will include a high angle of velar lift necessitating augmentation high up on the posterior pharyngeal wall or large adenoids in the direction of velar lift. In cases where there is a previous airway obstruction (e.g. sleep apnoea or unfavourable anatomy) then lengthening can be achieved by using an oral Z-plasty with or without a nasal Z-plasty or by utilizing interpositional buccal flaps [13]. Buccal flaps are usually carried out for larger gaps (>5 mm) and Z-plasty for smaller gaps (<5 mm). If, however, there is favourable anatomy and no airway contra-indications then posterior pharyngeal augmentation in the form of a Hynes pharyngoplasty or Coleman fat augmentation will be the procedures of choice. The Hynes pharyngoplasty is a transpositional flap technique transposing a flap containing mucosa and salpingopharyngeus from a vertical position to a horizontal position by suturing the flaps into a horizontal incision made in the posterior pharyngeal wall at a level determined by the angle of velar lift on lateral videofluoroscopy. This, when healed, results in a bulge thereby lessening the anteroposterior distance the velum has to travel to effect velopharyngeal closure. Coleman fat augmentation with deposition of fat into the submucosal tissues may be used for small gaps or in cases of stress velopharyngeal incompetence.

An alternative technique, to lengthen the velum is the Furlow's double opposing Z-plasty [14]. This technique allows realignment of the levator muscles and formation of a muscular sling while also increasing the length of the soft palate. The two Z-plasty flaps are raised with the posteriorly based flap being dissected from the nasal mucosa layer. This flap therefore consists of oral mucosa and musculature. The oral mucosa is dissected free from the underlying musculature and nasal layer in the anteriorly based flap.

These flaps are subsequently transposed and sutured in their new position. Palatal lengthening and muscle repositioning is achieved at the expense of width and it has the advantage of not dissecting the muscle free on both nasal and oral sides, which may preserve greater vascularity to the muscles of the palate. This technique may, however, lead to an asymmetrical repair but can produce good results in cases where there is a small VP gap but is less successful for larger gaps.

❝ Expert comment

Management of non-cleft VPI where there is an element of neuromuscular dysfunction, which may manifest as dysarthria and/or as delayed timing on lateral videofluoroscopy, is difficult to treat with complete success by following a physiological approach. The physiological approach relies on normal baseline neuromuscular function.

This technique is popular amongst cleft surgeons in North America. Modifications incorporating lateral relieving incisions have been described to achieve closure of wider clefts [15].

A final word from the expert

Obstructive techniques, which join the palate to the pharynx permanently, aim to reduce the nasopharyngeal port size and thereby reduce air escape into the nasal cavity. Midline pharyngeal flaps create a central obstruction leaving two open lateral ports, which are then reliant on lateral pharyngeal sidewall movement for closure. The midline pharyngeal flap can be either inferiorly or superiorly pedicled. Alternatively a sphincter pharyngoplasty can be used to reduce the total cross sectional area of the port by inserting flaps taken from the posterior fauces of the pharynx (mucosa and palatopharyngeus) and inserting them into either an inferiorly pedicled or superiorly pedicled posterior pharyngeal flap.

The selection of either a midline pharyngoplasty or a sphincter pharyngoplasty is based on limited evidence in the literature to suggest that preoperative closure pattern of the velopharyngeal port on nasoendoscopy can influence the outcome of pharyngeal flap pharyngoplasty [16]. Some clinicians therefore argue for selected procedures depending upon the preoperative assessment of the closure pattern [17]. If poor lateral wall movement is identified with central closure they may opt for a sphincter type procedure, whereas in those patients with central defects a midline pharyngeal flap procedure may be carried out. The disadvantage of 'obstructive' techniques is permanent narrowing of the nasopharyngeal airway resulting in snoring, hyponasality and, in some cases, sleep apnoea. Death due to airway obstruction in the immediate postoperative period has also been described.

References

1. Sommerlad BC. A technique for cleft palate repair. Plast Reconstr Surg 2003; 112: 1542–48.
2. Sell D, Harding A, Grunwell P. GOS.SP,ASS'98: an assessment for speech disorders associated with cleft palate and/or velopharyngeal dysfunction (revised). Int J Lang Commun Disorder 1999; 34(1): 17–33.
3. Weatherley-White RC, Sakura, Brenner LD, et al. Submucous cleft palate. Its incidence, natural history and indications for treatment. Plast Reconstr Surg 1972; 49(3): 297–304.
4. Garcia Velasco M, Ysunza A, Hernanadez X, Marquez C. Diagnosis and treatment of submucous cleft palate: a review of 108 cases. Cleft Palate J 1988; 25(2): 171–3.
5. Kaplan EN. The occult submucous cleft palate. Cleft palate J 1975; 12: 356–68.
6. Lewin ML, Croft CB, Shprintzen RJ. Velopharyngeal insufficiency due to hypoplasia of the muscularic uvulae and occult submucous cleft palate. Plast Reconstr Surg 1980; 65(5): 585–91.
7. Boorman JG, Varma S, Ogilvie CM. Velopharyngeal incompetence and chromosome 22q11 deletion. Lancet 2001; 357(9258): 774.
8. Saunders NC, Hartley BEJ, Sell D, Sommerlad B. Velopharyngeal insufficiency following adenoidectomy. Clin Otolaryngol Allied Sci 2004; 29(6): 686–8.
9. D'Antonio LL, Snyder LS, Samadani S. Tonsillectomy in children with or at risk for velopharyngeal insufficiency: effects on speech. Otolaryngol Head Neck Surg 1996; 115(4): 319–23.

10. Golding-Kushner KJ, Argamaso RV, Cotton RT, et al. Standardization for the reporting of nasopharyngoscopy and multiview videofluoroscopy: A report from an international working group. Cleft Palate J 1973; 27: 337–L 47; discussion 347–8.

11. Sommerlad BC, Henley M, Birch M, et al. cleft palate re-repair: a clinical and radiological study of 32 consecutive cases. Br J Plast Surg 1994; 47; 406–10.

12. Skolnick ML, McCall GN, Barnes M. The sphincteric mechanism of the velopharyngeal closure. Cleft Palate J 1973; 10: 286–305.

13. Hill C, Hayden C, Riaz M, Leonard AG. Buccinators sandwich pushback: a new technique for treatment of secondary velopharyngeal incompetence.*Cleft Palate Craniofac J* 2004; 41(3); 230–7.

14. Furlow LT. Cleft palate repair by double opposing Z plasty. Plast Reconstr Surg 1986; 778: 724–38.

15. LaRossa D, Hunenko-Jackson O, Kirschner RE, et al. The children's hospital of Philidelphia modification of the Furlow double opposing z plasty: Long term speech and growth results. Clin Plast Surg 2004; 31: 243–9.

16. Armour A, Fischbach S, Klaiman P, Fisher DM. Does velopharyngeal closure pattern affect the success of pharyngeal flap pharyngoplasty? Plast Reconstr Surg 2005; 115: 45–52; discussion 53.

17. Fisher DM, Sommerlad BC. Cleft lip, cleft palate and velopharyngeal insufficiency. Plast Reconstr Surg 2011; 128(4): 342e–60e.

26 Paediatric maxillofacial trauma

Atheer Ujam and Suraj Thomas

ⓘ Expert commentary Simon Holmes

Case history: Paediatric orbital floor fractures: observation versus intervention

A six-year-old boy presented to his local Emergency Department (ED) late in the evening complaining of vomiting and left-sided facial pain. Earlier in the day he was running in his school playground and had collided with another student. The father who attended with him stated that the teachers reported a few seconds loss of consciousness and had called the ambulance. On further questioning he also complained of a headache and blurred vision. The patient reported that he still had severe pain around the left eye and that he had not stopped vomiting since the injury. It was six hours since the injury and the young boy although fully conscious, was clearly in severe distress.

His past medical history was unremarkable and he has had no previous operations. He has no known drug allergies.

He was examined in the paediatric ED following a computed tomography (CT) scan already performed to exclude a significant head injury. The patient was supine and reluctant to engage in the examination that revealed he was clammy and in obvious discomfort. The left eye appeared normal with no subconjunctival haemorrhage as did the right eye. He had normal visual acuity in both eyes when tested separately. There was no enophthalmos. Furthermore, examination of his teeth, soft tissues and face was entirely normal. There was no sign of a fractured zygoma on either side.

On closer inspection of his eyes, it became obvious that his left eye was moving less than his right eye.

This was confirmed by the finding of severe restriction of left eye movements and in particular upward gaze on testing each eye. The patient became more distressed and nauseated on attempting upward gaze motion.

His blood pressure was within normal limits, he was apyrexial but was tachycardic at 130 beats per minute. He was subsequently given intravenous analgesia and anti-emetics but despite this he was still nauseated. See Learning point: Important management considerations in paediatric orbital fractures', which highlights important management considerations.

The CT scans are reviewed and are shown in Figure 26.1 and Figure 26.2.

He underwent emergency surgery at 2 am, six hours after presenting to the maxillofacial unit. The orbit was accessed via a transconjuctival incision. The intraoperative findings were of muscle and fat herniation with entrapment through a trapdoor fracture that was released (Figure 26.3). A small sheet of PDS®

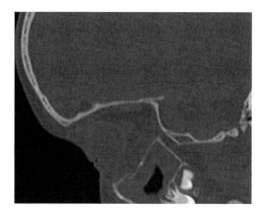

Figure 26.1 Left orbital floor sagittal view.

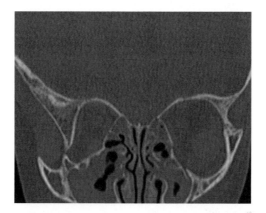

Figure 26.2 Coronal view.

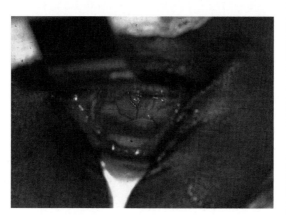

Figure 26.3 Image of orbital floor through a transconjunctival approach. Fat herniation into the fracture can be clearly identified and must be released. See colour plate section.

○ **Clinical tip**

Young patients presenting with restricted eye movement with no significant orbital floor fracture on CT scan require urgent exploration.

Early intervention is associated with better postoperative outcomes and less persistent diplopia and therefore avoids corrective surgery to the extra-ocular muscles.

❝ **Expert comment**

Orbital floor and medial wall fractures are extremely common injuries of the craniofacial skeleton, and the management is well described and understood. However, across the whole population there are still areas where there is conflict of thought. The timing around paediatric orbital injuries is a classic example of this.

(polydioxanone, Ethicon, US) was applied to the orbital floor to prevent further herniation.

Postoperatively the patient had a full range of eye movements and no diplopia. He was discharged home the next day.

⭐ **Learning point** Important management considerations in paediatric orbital fractures.

- History:
  - mechanism of injury
  - vomiting
  - loss of consciousness
  - diplopia.
- Clinical examination:
  - Advanced Trauma Life Support (ATLS)
  - diplopia
  - visual acuity
  - restricted eye movements
  - 'white eye'
  - vomiting
  - restless, unwell patient
  - any age up to late teens.
- Investigations:
  - urgent CT scan including coronal views.
- Operative considerations:
  - significant medical history
  - nil by mouth
  - consent from patient / parent
  - suitably trained paediatric anaesthetist
  - surgeon availability.

The clinical examination at seven days following the repair elicited a full range of eye movements, no enophthalmos and no diplopia. He was referred to orthoptics for formal visual assessments.

💬 **Expert comment**

Considering the orbit as a whole, there is a fundamental design flaw that predisposes to the floor and medial wall fracturing in preference to the lateral wall and roof. This is also true in the paediatric age group; however, this is modified by a number of factors. Firstly the bone quality in the paediatric age group is different to that of the adult. The bone is much more elastic and can yield according to force and recoil back into place causing a so-called trapdoor fracture.

Secondly, children tend to not get involved in high-energy mechanisms of injury, and if subjected to such mechanisms then the orbital fracture is usually part of a wider fracture pattern including middle and upper third facial bone fractured configurations.

💬 **Expert comment**

CT scanning is mandatory in these patients, firstly to diagnose and secondly to quantify the size of the defect. In addition, it is important to exclude other facial injuries and to ensure that the orbit is not part of the wider fracture pattern.

⭐ **Learning point**

Applied anatomy:

- Height of orbital margin 40 mm.
- Width of orbital margin 35 mm.
- Depth of orbit 40–50 mm.
- Volume of orbit 30 cm³.

Key anatomical structures:

- Whitnall's tubercle – a small elevation on the lateral orbital rim approximately 11 mm beneath the frontozygomatic suture. The tubercle has attachments to the following important structures:
  - check ligament of the lateral rectus muscle
  - the lateral palpebral ligament
  - the suspensory ligament of Lockwood
  - the levator palpebrae superioris muscle.

Discussion

The orbit is a quadrilateral pyramidal shaped structure that consists of seven conjoined bones (Figure 26.4).

If a transconjunctival approach is taken, this may be supplemented with a lateral cantholysis and lid swing to aid access. Understanding this anatomy is key to achieving a blood free dissection. The ligaments around the eye are shown in Figure 26.5.

The mechanism of orbital floor fractures remains controversial but two theories are commonly accepted and well described:

1. Buckling mechanism: this theory suggests that force is transmitted through the orbital rim and in a posterior direction through the orbital floor causing a fracture.

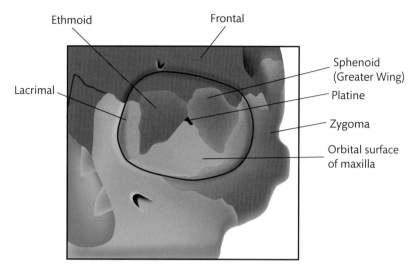

Figure 26.4 Left orbit demonstrating the seven conjoined bones.

Images provided by and reproduced with kind permission from Mr Chris Bridle.

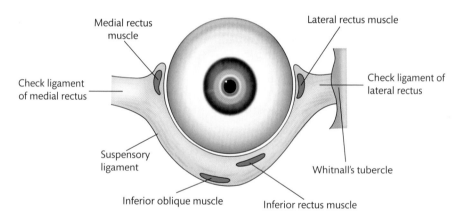

Figure 26.5 The ligaments around the left eye. The suspensory ligament runs from medial to lateral check ligament and prevents downwards displacement of the globe.

Images provided by and reproduced with kind permission from Mr Chris Bridle.

2. Hydraulic: this theory suggests that direct force is transmitted to the orbital floor as a result of increased intra-orbital pressure. Commonly, direct blunt injury to the globe may result in an orbital floor fracture.

> ✪ **Learning point**
>
> Trap door fractures are due to immature orbital floor bones with high elasticity that become minimally displaced, hinged and spring back into its original position following the injury. This leads to entrapment of periorbital tissue and in particular the inferior rectus muscle with risk of severe muscle ischemia.
>
> (continued)

> ➕ **Clinical tip** Paediatric orbital floor fractures evidence
>
> • Are caused by low velocity but high force crush injuries.
> • In the very young – orbital roof fractures are more common.
> • Above the age of 7, orbital floor fractures are more common.
> • More common in males then females (ratio M:F = 4:1).

There are two common presentations of paediatric trap door fractures:

1. **White-eye** presentation: history of trauma with restricted eye movements and usually a negative CT scan. Clinical examination is otherwise unremarkable (see Figure 26.6).
2. **Oculocardiac reflex** presentation: vomiting with bradycardia and syncope. Nausea and vomiting has a positive predictive value of 75 % for a trap door fracture.

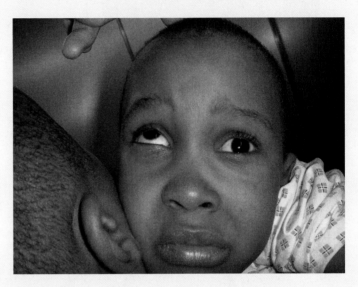

Figure 26.6 White-eye blow-out fracture. The image demonstrates a patient who on initial examination appeared to have no visual disturbance. However, on assessment of ocular movements, restriction of the left eye excursion on upward gaze was clearly apparent.

Images provided by and reproduced with kind permission from Mr Leo Cheng.

Paediatric patients presenting with a history of trauma to the orbital region with key signs of restricted eye movement, diplopia, enophthalmos, nausea and vomiting, severe pain, proptosis and reduced visual acuity should undergo imaging of the orbits. Fine-cut high-resolution CT scan with coronal and sagittal views will allow excellent assessment of the orbital floor and soft tissues. There is evidence to suggest that trap door fractures with muscle entrapment are less easily identified in paediatric cases compared to the adult population, but nevertheless CT remains the gold standard imaging modality. Plain x-ray facial views are often non-diagnostic and should be avoided.

If clinical assessment results in a high suspicion of inferior rectus entrapment and trap door fracture then surgery even in the presence of a negative CT scan may be indicated.

A final word from the expert

In the case of a paediatric orbital floor injury there are number of important points to consider: firstly recognition and secondly optimum management in terms of timing and surgical approach. It is important to understand that whilst the dimensions of the orbit are established surprisingly early on at around six years of age, the maxim that children do not behave as young adults is very true with respect to orbital trauma [1]. There are concerns over interfering with growth, but a number of authors have highlighted the risk of delayed management to development of short, medium and long-term complications.

Because the bone could be described as very elastic in this age group, fractures involving small linear patterns with subsequent entrapment of orbital soft tissues are well known and described. The phenomena of the white-eye blow-out is universally accepted as an established injury and a common trap for the unwary. The question is therefore how do we spot this fracture and as importantly, how do we educate accident and emergency colleagues to flag these injuries to us as specialists?

In reality linear fractures not involving herniation and entrapment of orbital tissues are probably under-diagnosed and of little subsequent consequence. Should the soft tissues around the globe become trapped then there will likely be limitation of eye movement and subsequent diplopia. In addition, pain on movement is a very common finding [2]. Around two-thirds of patients experience this as a symptom.

Often in these injuries the soft tissue swelling is minimal, and unless full movements of the eye tested, then the injury is often missed.

Fractures of the medial orbital wall are much rarer but can behave in exactly the same way as that of the floor, except that the failure of movement is in a medial lateral direction [3].

One of the most significant presenting features of the white-eyed blow-out fracture, is persistent nausea and vomiting. In younger children this may be ascribed to emotional disturbance, or even as a sign of impending head injury deterioration [4]. This is such a significant physical sign that in a recent study of orbital trauma in the primary care setting, presence of vomiting was given a positive predictive value of 83.3% [5].

The physical manifestation of entrapment may also be manifest by the presence of the ocular- cardiac reflex. This physical sign is elicited by traction of the eye muscles causing a bradycardia [4]. This reflex is given the eponymous name of Aschner-Dagnini reflex [6].

There is widespread opinion that patients require immediate surgery. The timing, however, is not widely agreed within the literature. Various timings have been suggested, from two weeks [7] right down to immediate surgery [8], with other authors running in between [2].

Management of these include surgery is well established and mirrors that of the adult population. The paediatric lower eyelid is usually quite distensible and therefore transconjunctival access without the need to perform cantholysis is perfectly possible. The choice of implant material is subject to individual surgeon preference, but we have found PDS membrane to be very reliable for this indication.

In our experience, with a very heterogeneous referral stream we have seen paediatric patients present both early and late and whilst we recognize the need for prompt surgery within the scientific literature, we have not found long-standing diplopia to be an issue for the majority of patients. What however it is critical is that these children are managed within a multidisciplinary team which includes a strabismus surgeon and dedicated orthoptist.

Case history: Paediatric condyle fractures

An 11-year-old boy was taken to the Regional Trauma Centre by air ambulance after a pushbike accident. He reported that he was thrown head first over the handle bars of his bicycle after applying the brakes heavily whilst cycling down a steep slope and that his head had impacted with a stationary lorry. There was no loss of consciousness. He was examined initially by ED staff using the standard ATLS assessment and on secondary survey he was noted to have multiple injuries as listed below:

- Subluxation of the 1st and 2nd cervical spine (C-Spine), as shown in a CT and magnetic resonance imaging (MRI) scan.
- Left tibial shaft undisplaced comminuted fracture.
- Salter-Harris type III left distal radius fracture.
- Bilateral mandibular condylar fractures and mandibular midline symphyseal fracture (as evident on CT scan).

There were no intracranial injuries on CT imaging of his head. After initial resuscitation and stabilization with a C-spine collar he was transferred to the nearest paediatric neurosurgical centre for management of his C-spine injury.

At the children's hospital he underwent manipulation of his C-spine under general anaesthesia and was placed on a hard collar. Post-operative CT and MRI revealed satisfactory alignment of the C-spine. He was transferred back to the Regional Trauma Centre three days later for management of his maxillofacial and orthopaedic injuries. The instructions from the paediatric neurosurgical team were that the patient must maintain strict in-line cervical stabilization during the surgical management of his mandibular fractures.

Following further clinical examination by the maxillofacial team, his specific head and neck injuries appeared to be limited to his mandible. Closer inspection demonstrated a mobile anterior segment fracture and shortening of vertical height of the ramus causing an anterior open bite (AOB).

⊕ **Clinical tip** Assessment

A thorough clinical examination of the paediatric patient with facial injuries is essential to avoid missing potential fractures. Importantly, an ATLS approach to management will identify patients with serious injuries such as to the head and C-spine.

- Head and neck – inspection:
  - asymmetry
  - swelling
  - haematoma
  - skin laceration or defect
  - facial nerve
  - mouth opening.

- Head and neck – palpation:
  - tenderness
  - fracture line / step
  - crepitation
  - trigeminal nerve
  - special attention to posterior ramus of mandible and temporomandibular joint (TMJ)

- Intra-oral assessment:
  - occlusion
  - AOB / lateral open bite   (continued)

○ premature contact
○ sliding
○ deviation of mouth opening.

● Ear assessment:
○ haematoma
○ lacerations
○ obstruction of the external auditory meatus
○ otoscopy - look for haemotympanum
○ consider ear, nose and throat referral.

CT scans demonstrated bilateral mandibular condyle fractures and a displaced symphyseal fracture (Figure 26.7 and 26.8)

It was decided that an open reduction and internal fixation (ORIF) of the mandibular symphyseal fracture should be performed and that conservative management of the bilateral condylar fractures was most appropriate.

This decision in part was influenced by the consultations with the paediatric neurosurgeons who felt mobilization of his jaws should be kept to a minimum to avoid further injury to his C-spine. ORIF of his anterior mandibular fracture was organized in conjunction with the orthopaedic surgeons who performed closed reduction and stabilization of his limb injuries during the same general anaesthesia. ORIF of the mandibular symphyseal fracture proceeded smoothly with the assistance of anaesthetists and operation department practitioners maintaining in-line stabilization of the patient's C-spine. Anatomical reduction of the symphyseal fracture was achieved.

Postoperatively the patient made a rapid recovery from his orthopaedic injuries. His mandibular symphyseal fracture also healed uneventfully. Clinical assessment showed that he had shortening of posterior ramus height resulting in an AOB. The overjet was recorded as 15 mm.

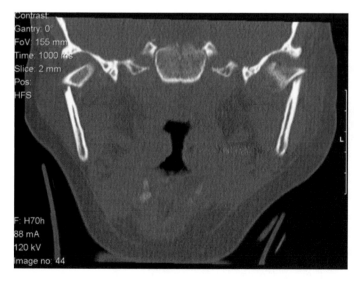

Figure 26.7 Coronal view of bilateral condyle fractures.

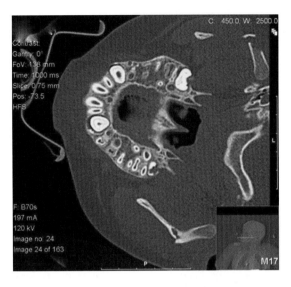

Figure 26.8 Computed tomogram axial view.

> ⭐ **Learning point**
>
> It is important to understand both the anatomy and embryology of the TMJ in order to appreciate potential complications of paediatric condyle fractures.
>
> Key learning points are:
>
> - The condyle is 15–20 mm long and 8–12 mm thick.
> - The condyle rotates and undertakes translatory movements.
> - The condyle is covered by fibrous tissue mostly of type 1 collagen.
>
> Embryological development:
>
> - The condyle is formed from secondary growth cartilage during the 12th week of development.
> - This cartilage becomes bone through endochondral ossification.
> - By the 20th week of development only a thin layer of cartilage remains in the condylar head that persists until the second decade of life, providing a mechanism for growth of the mandible [9].

Following discharge from hospital the patient was referred to a joint clinic for orthodontic specialist input. An orthodontic appliance with twin anterior sliding block (Figure 26.9) was provided to correct the AOB.

> 💬 **Expert comment**
>
> In the paediatric age group adaptive changes around dentoalveolar growth are expected and tend to work in favour of compensatory mechanisms to close dental malocclusions. In addition orthodontic treatment is commonly carried out in this age group, and improvement in the occlusion could be achieved as part of a conventional dental treatment plan.

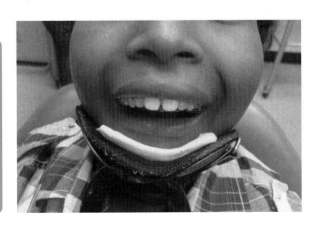

Figure 26.9 Photograph of patient demonstrating anterior open bite, with twin block appliance in situ.

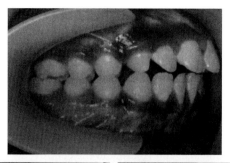

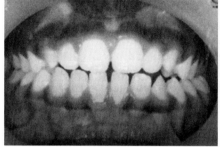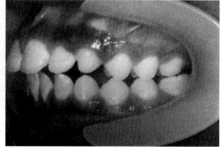

Figure 26.10 Patient at 18 months post trauma following orthodontic management.

Eight weeks post injury he was noted to have no significant improvement in his occlusal relationship due to the chinstrap on his cervical collar, which prevented the anterior sliding movement of his mandible. CT scans eight weeks after injury showed bony healing and remodelling of the condylar heads. The cervical collar was discontinued at this time in discussion with the treating neurosurgical team.

He was followed up and treated by our orthodontic colleagues for over 18 months. Cephalometric analyses were performed in a 16-month interval. The maxilla to mandible plane angle improved from 50° to 39° in this period. His AOB was completely closed and he had a stable occlusion with an acceptable overjet of 4 mm (Figure 26.10). No further orthodontic or surgical treatment is planned for him at this stage.

Discussion

This case demonstrates the potential difficulties in managing paediatric mandibular fractures. Children with maxillofacial injuries and concurrent polytrauma will require input from other surgical specialties and experienced anaesthetists confident in paediatric airway emergencies. Furthermore, suitable post-surgery recovery and paediatric intensive care must be available and taken into consideration prior to surgical intervention. Transfer to a dedicated children's hospital or trauma centre may be necessary.

As this case report has also demonstrated, a detailed examination of the patient followed by CT scan of the mandible is crucial in obtaining both a diagnosis of condyle fracture but importantly the anatomy of the fracture pattern.

There are a huge number of publications on the management and outcomes of mandible condyle fractures in children. In children condylar fractures can account for up to 72% of all mandibular fractures [10]. The evidence from a mixture of case reports, prospective and retrospective studies supports conservative management of condyle fractures in children [11,12]. Outcomes appear to be very satisfactory when a non-surgical approach is adopted. It appears that normal function, occlusion and facial symmetry can be achieved with non-surgical management.

The age group at which the outcome of conservative approach becomes less satisfactory is unclear. However, at about the age of 12 years, there is decreased remodelling capacity and therefore the risk of a resulting abnormally shaped condylar head or shortened ramus heights may lead to persistent malocclusion [12]. ORIF may be required with increasing age, contributing to the controversy of the topic.

Radiological studies of conservatively managed fractures demonstrate that the majority of cases will show incomplete condyle remodelling but that symptoms of TMJ dysfunction, although fairly prevalent, were mild [13].

In conclusion, the overwhelming evidence and clinical opinion is that paediatric condyle fractures of the mandible in children and early adolescents should be managed by a non-surgical strategy that includes the input from orthodontic specialists were a malocclusion is diagnosed. In children, early mobilization and soft diet is recommended.

A final word from the expert

Within the field of craniofacial trauma, there is no other subject that lends itself to a more full and frank discussion than whether or not a fractured mandibular condyle should be treated open or closed. There has been a growing revolution in the management of this fracture pattern over the last 20 years and there is little doubt the current opinion is fast coalescing towards more aggressive management. This has largely been due to increasing surgical confidence towards the open surgical approach and also improvement in osteosynthesis techniques. There are now fixed and firm guidelines (as much as that could be between surgeons) towards which fractures should be treated. Most clinicians now would strongly consider 30° of angulation and 5 mm of shortening as an indication for open surgery. We have come a long way since Zide and Kent first tried to produce hard and fast indications for open intervention. In the academic discord there has been one theme in the management of fractures of the mandibular condyle that has been almost sacrosanct. The 11th surgical commandment could be 'thou shalt not operate on the paediatric mandibular condyle'.

It is important to discuss why this is the case. The intellectual framework around reduction and fixation of adult fractures is to firstly restore posterior facial height and secondly to avoid the need for intermaxillary fixation and therefore restore early mobilization to function.

The significance of the posterior facial height is that in a percentage of cases prompt restoration of this dimension will achieve a better and more predictable dental occlusion than by closed reduction. This is very much the experience of the author.

As I have already commented, in the paediatric age group compensatory mechanisms can result in closure of dental malocclusions.

The question must therefore be asked should all paediatric condylar fractures be managed conservatively? In truth in medicine and surgery: never say never, never say always. We have managed a malunion of a mandibular condylar neck using a functional appliance and in addition we have fixed a number of very displaced low condylar neck fractures. The trend, however, is to be conservative.

Within the practice of paediatric trauma, it is obvious that longer-term follow-up must also be observed because of the fear of growth disturbance of the mandible. In theory growth could be enhanced by increased blood flow, or reduced by damage the growth plate, or somewhere in between. This lack of agreement seen in the literature does not support anything other than an observational approach.

It is also said that children are more likely to develop ankylosis of the mandible due to a putative feeling that uncontrolled bone growth is more common in children. We have not observed this phenomenon in our practice.

The truth is that there are very few centres within the world that have an established series of these fractures with cogent long-term follow-up. This is certainly required, but will need a national study.

References

1. Oppenheimer AJ, Monson LA, Buchman SR. Pediatric orbital fractures. *Craniomaxillofac Trauma Reconstr* 2013; 6(1): 9–20.
2. Egbert JE, May K, Kersten RC, Kulwin DR. Pediatric orbital floor fracture. *Ophthalmology* 2000; 107(10): 1875–9.
3. McCulley TJ, Yip CC, Kersten RC, Kulwin DR. Medial rectus muscle incarceration in pediatric medial orbital wall trapdoor fractures. *Eur J Ophthalmol* 2004; 14(4): 330–3.
4. Cobb A, Murthy R, Manisali M, et al. Oculovagal reflex in paediatric orbital floor fractures mimicking head injury. *Emerg Med J* 2009; 26(5): 351–3.
5. Cohen SM, Garrett CG. Pediatric orbital floor fractures: nausea/vomiting as signs of entrapment. *Otolaryngol Head Neck Surg* 2003; 129: 43–7.
6. Cobb AR, Jeelani NO, Ayliffe PR. Orbital fractures in children. *Br J Oral Maxillofac Surg* 2013; 51(1): 41–6.
7. Burnstine MA. Clinical recommendations for repair of isolated orbital floor fractures. *Ophthalmology* 2002; 109(7): 1207–10.
8. de Man K, Wijngaarde R, Hes J, de Jong PT. Influence of age on the management of blow-out fractures of the orbital floor. *Int J Oral Maxillofac Surg* 1991; 20(6): 330–6.
9. Ten Cate AR (ed). *Oral Histology: Development, Structure and Function*, 4th edition. St Louis: Mosby; 1994.
10. Thorén H1, Iizuka T, Hallikainen D, Lindqvist C. Different patterns of mandibular fractures in children. An analysis of 220 fractures in 157 patients. *J Craniomaxillofac Surg* 1992; 20(7): 292–6.
11. Bruckmoser E, Undt G.Management and outcome of condylar fractures in children and adolescents: a review of the literature. *Oral Surg Oral Med Oral Pathol Oral Radiol* 2012; 114(5 Suppl): S86–S106
12. Chrcanovic BR. Open versus closed reduction: mandibular condylar fractures in children. *Oral Maxillofac Surg* 2012; 16(3): 245–55.
13. Thorén H1, Hallikainen D, Iizuka T, Lindqvist C. Condylar process fractures in children: a follow-up study of fractures with total dislocation of the condyle from the glenoid fossa. *J Oral Maxillofac Surg* 2001; 59(7): 768–73; discussion 773–4.

INDEX

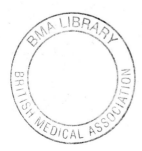